Yellow Fever Years

REGENSBURG STUDIES IN BRITISH
AND AMERICAN LANGUAGES AND CULTURES

Edited by
Prof. Dr. Udo J. Hebel, Prof. Dr. Edgar W. Schneider
and Prof. Dr. Anne-Julia Zwierlein

VOLUME 52

PETER LANG
EDITION

Ingrid Gessner

Yellow Fever Years

An Epidemiology of Nineteenth-Century American Literature and Culture

PETER LANG
EDITION

Bibliographic Information published by the Deutsche Nationalbibliothek
The Deutsche Nationalbibliothek lists this publication in the Deutsche Nationalbibliografie; detailed bibliographic data is available in the internet at http://dnb.d-nb.de.

Cover image:
"Patients in Yellow Fever Hospital, Havana, Cuba ca. 1899."
Library of Congress, LC-USZ62-101537.

Library of Congress Cataloging-in-Publication Data
Names: Gessner, Ingrid, 1972- author.
Title: Yellow Fever years : an epidemiology of nineteenth-century American literature and culture / Ingrid Gessner.
Description: Frankfurt am Main ; New York : Peter Lang, 2016. | Series: Regensburg studies in British and American languages and cultures ; 52 | Includes bibliographical references.
Identifiers: LCCN 2016004641 | ISBN 9783631674123
Subjects: LCSH: American literature--19th century--History and criticism. | Literature and medicine--United States--History--19th century. | Diseases and literature--United States--History--19th century. | Yellow fever in literature. | Epidemics in literature. | Yellow fever--United States--History--19th century.
Classification: LCC PS217.M44 G47 2016 | DDC 810.9/356--dc23 LC record available at https://lccn.loc.gov/2016004641

ISSN 1615-925X
ISBN 978-3-631-67412-3 (Print)
ISBN 978-3-653-06755-2 (E-PDF)
ISBN 978-3-631-69719-1 (EPUB)
ISBN 978-3-631-69720-7 (MOBI)
DOI 10.3726/978-3-653-06755-2

Peter Lang Edition is an Imprint of Peter Lang GmbH.

Peter Lang – Frankfurt am Main · Bern · Bruxelles · New York · Oxford · Warszawa · Wien

This publication has been peer reviewed.

www.peterlang.com

For Markus, Ida and Jonah

Table of Contents

Acknowledgements

The beginning of my first academic probings into the combination of matters medical, historical, and literary can be dated to the fall of 2005. However, my ideas, it seems, had to be stimulated, like a dormant virus if you will. My play with metaphors ends here since the 'virus' which had been planted was positively stimulating and not at all destructive. My general interest and original questions were further influenced by the works on literature, medicine, and biomedical discourses by Carmen Birkle in Marburg and Rüdiger Kunow in Potsdam.[1] Their work has been instrumental in the development of my project. It is an honor that both of them have seen the project evolve over the years and have continuously offered their generous advice.

I am greatly indebted to Udo Hebel, whose continuous support and belief in this project, paired with generous professional and knowledgeable advice, made this book possible. I am also most grateful to Volker Depkat and Christoph Meinel for serving as mentors and for expertly supervising the Habilitation process. I thank Volker Depkat for his pertinent and continuous questioning of the arguments I presented at various research colloquia. Christoph Meinel saw this study emerge from a very early stage, and I thank him for his thoughtful questions and comments. The project has received substantial financial support from the State Government of Bavaria in the form of a Habilitation scholarship, which allowed me to advance the project in the year 2011–2012.

This book would not have come into being but for the wise guidance and inspiration of my teachers at the University of Mainz, Winfried Herget and Alfred Hornung. I have significantly profited from, as well as enjoyed fruitful discussions and conversations about, literature, visual and memory culture, medical history, and American Studies with Erika Doss, Shelley Fisher Fishkin, Karsten Fitz, Gesa Mackenthun, Miles Orvell, Gregory Tomso, and Werner Sollors. Marc Priewe's comments have greatly helped in advancing my thinking in terms of health and illness. Conversations with scholars also working in the fields of literature, culture, and medicine were invaluable in terms of exchanging ideas and sources as well as providing encouragement: I wish to thank Antje Dallmann, Marcel Hartwig, and Andrea Zittlau. Some arguments presented in this book

---

1 In October 2005 I heard Professor Kunow's talk "In Sickness and in Health" at Mita Banerjee's conference entitled *Virtually American?* Carmen Birkle presented at the EAAS biennial conference in Oslo in May 2008.

have been tested at conferences and invited lectures. On these occasions, and when preparing presentations for publication as articles in collections of essays, I have received instrumental feedback from Heike Paul, Christopher J. Lukasik, and again, Rüdiger Kunow and Carmen Birkle. I wish to thank the anonymous readers of Peter Lang Press for their reading of my manuscript and for nominating it for the Young Scholars Award 2015. It is through them that the book came 'home' to Regensburg and appears in the Regensburg Studies in British and American Languages and Cultures series, generously edited by Udo Hebel, Edgar W. Schneider, and Anne-Julia Zwierlein.

In between revising manuscripts, teaching, and speaking at many stimulating conferences, I have attended the most important 'firsts' in anyone's life, notably the first day of school of our daughter Ida and of our son Jonah, as well as Ida's First Holy Communion. Writing a book on yellow fever discourses and raising kids at the same time has been both a challenging experience and one full of joy and happiness. I studied the biomedical threat and presence of yellow fever in the nineteenth century while nursing ailing backs, and fighting real bouts of scarlet fever in the twenty-first. In this sense, while nursing a book to life, I also self-schooled myself as a nurse. However, most of the time, no one is sick and you just live in the moment, which is something you re-learn by having kids, and you simply enjoy what is happening in front of your eyes.

I want to thank those that helped and steadfastly accompanied me in academic and non-academic ways on parental, medical, and academic paths. My current and former colleagues in American Studies at Regensburg offered critical feedback when I presented several parts of my book to them as it was taking shape. I would like to thank Susanne Leikam and Nassim Balestrini for their helpful suggestions and their friendship. I thank Katharina Fackler for sharing my academic curiosity in regard to a forgotten author, Mary Faith Floyd, as well as for her continuous friendship and support. I am indebted to the questions and succinct comments of Birgit Bauridl, Katharina Boehm, Anna Farkas, Alexandra Herzog, Klara-Stephanie Szlezák, Claudia Trotzke, Florian Weinzierl, and Doris Wess. I also thank my students over the years who shared my various academic interests and whose questions helped me to clarify many of my arguments.

A book like this is not possible without the help and guidance of knowledgeable librarians. With this work I am greatly indebted to the incredible and ever so kind Christopher Dagleish at Regensburg's university library. He taught me to tap into resources I had only dreamt existed: There are no words to describe what you made possible. And a book like this would also not be possible without the incredible friends I am blessed to have. For their kindness, inspiration and unrelenting support I thank Birgit Däwes, Veronika Hofstätter, Juliane Schwarz-Bierschenk, and Amy Gebauer.

I thank my incredibly calm and knowledgeable father-in-law, Dr. med. Klaus Gloede, with whom I not only discussed such medical problems as the (im)possibility of in utero yellow fever infection, but who also took a keen interest in my pursuing a university career. I also thank my belligerent and uncompromising, but equally sensitive mother-in-law, Christiane Gloede, who taught me to believe in and fight for what is important (to me). My brother Ansgar and his wife Susann Park-Gessner always offered support at very critical times. I thank the strong women in my family, my aunt and godmother Elisabeth Gerster and my grandmother Meta Gerster. Many thanks go to my kind and thoughtful father, Ingwald Gessner, with whom I share a love for writing, and who supported me in all the ways parents do, by not asking questions when there were none to be answered and by asking questions and encouraging me when I needed support. I am also thinking of my mother, Ursula Gessner, who always knew I would do this—although she did not live to see it. I thank you all. My husband Markus Gloede not only discussed many of the novels with me, read my drafts, and made thought-to-be lost documents magically re-appear on my computer screen, he also gave me strength during the most trying times. Without him this book would not have been written. The most important acknowledgement thus goes to those with whom I share every single precious day in life, in sickness and in health: Ida, Jonah and Markus, this book is dedicated to you.

March 2016

Preface

As a child I received vaccinations against a wealth of diseases that have threatened mankind for most of its history. I am one of the last of my larger generation to bear the smallpox-immunization marks on my upper left arm. My slightly younger brother was already spared the procedure as smallpox was certified as eradicated by 1980.

However, my teenage years were not free of disease threats and affected by the discovery of and growing concern with HIV/AIDS. The disease was covered prominently in the media and has inspired federal educational campaigns until this day. In its Safe Sex campaigns of the 1980s, the German Ministry of Health flooded schools with flyers and educational material, and it pioneered the demonstration of correct condom use in the classrooms. I remember the first time the disease hit (close to) home, when our next-door neighbor, "who had gotten *it* in San Francisco" (the word went), died of HIV/AIDS in the late 1980s. And I remember the day when a friend who was late for school that day broke the silence of our algebra classroom on the morning of November 25, 1991 to announce: "Freddy Mercury is dead." In the 1990s, with outbreak suppressant medication available, Western societies in particular seemingly learned to live with the disease and have accepted it as a negligible risk of modern life. This is the biggest problem related to HIV/AIDS today: it is no longer perceived as an immediate threat. Other diseases took over its prominent place in the 1990s.

While HIV/AIDS was the disease of the 1980s, 'Mad Cow' or Creutzfeld-Jakob disease took over in the late 1990s. The threat of the disease seems to have lingered from the late 1990s until the 2000s. The 2000s were marked by a perceived flow of epidemic diseases beginning with SARS (Severe Acute Respiratory Syndrome), which nearly became a pandemic with initial infections in the southern Chinese province of Guangdong in November 2002, and an outbreak in Hong Kong only four months later which spread worldwide in early 2003. Within weeks, global air-travel brought SARS to 29 countries across five continents and infected over 8,000 people, of whom 774 died ("WHO: Summary of Probable SARS Cases"). In late May 2003, *FIFA*, world soccer's governing body, decided to move the *Women's World Cup* tournament (September 23 to October 11, 2003) from China to the United States because of *SARS*.

The panic surrounding avian influenza, 'bird flu' or H5N1, which had been spreading throughout Asia since 2003 and reached Europe and the Middle East with the first cases in 2005, is a particularly interesting case. H5N1 literally prospered in the shadow of SARS and is an example of the incongruence between perceived threat and actual infections (320 by 2007), while bird flu's case fatality rate of over 60 percent is admittedly high (WHO Sept. 10, 2007; http://www.wikibirdflu.org/). The litany of health threats continues with the 2009 H1N1 swine flu pandemic and the 2011 epidemic of the Hemolytic-uremic Syndrome (HUS) caused by a strain of E. coli bacteria EHEC, a foodborne illness.

In 2010, a special surveillance was established for several mosquito-transmitted diseases, such as the West Nile virus (WNV), dengue virus (DENV), and the chikungunya virus (CHIKV), in the Veneto Region of northeastern Italy. These arthropod-borne viral diseases have spread in the Western Hemisphere, with dengue in the 1990s, West Nile virus since the 2000s and the chikungunya virus more recently (2010s).

Between March 2014 and early 2016 the Ebola epidemic in the West African states of Liberia, Guinea, and Sierra Leone killed more than 11,300 people. The fear of Ebola—fueled by the extensive media coverage—spread faster than the actual virus. The United States immediately reacted with measures of biocontainment, screening and surveillance. Immigration officers began questioning airplane passengers and screened them for fever at U.S. airports, while specialized biocontainment units were set up to isolate patients. One year later, in May 2015, the first Zika virus infections were confirmed in Brazil. This illness, which—like yellow and dengue fever—is transmitted by the bite of an infected Aedes aegypti mosquito, is usually mild with symptoms lasting from several days to a week. Many times those infected do not even realize that they are carriers of the virus, which has been related to the Guillain-Barré syndrome and to pregnant women giving birth to babies with birth defects and to poor pregnancy outcomes. Like yellow fever in the United States until the early twentieth century, the Zika virus poses a risk that is seemingly indeterminable in its spread over time. As a disease that is not gender-neutral because it affects men and women differently and could potentially be transmitted sexually, it represents a socio-cultural time-bomb.

Oftentimes, a seemingly incongruous assessment of a health risk and media-induced panics over certain diseases generate and feed into a "culture of fear"—to use Barry Glassner's term. In the 2000s the escalation from limited outbreaks to global media attention and panics seems to have happened in ever shorter periods of time. For example, cholera received major press attention in October 2010 due to an outbreak on Haiti. Some media sources connected the epidemic to Nepali peacekeepers that had been stationed there on an UN mandate. The presumption led to riots as Haitians believed the UN to have lied about the true origin of the outbreak (a UN resolution on November 12, 2010 had denied the

Nepali contingents' responsibility for the outbreak). This news item, apart from exemplifying the spiral of anxiety, panic, and public mistrust in the face of a national health crisis, reminds us of the crucial role that Haiti plays metaphorically (with respect to the 1793 Philadelphia Yellow Fever epidemic and Charles Brockden Brown's fictionalization of it in his gothic novel *Arthur Mervyn*) yet also politically to this day in race and disease relations of the U.S. and the Caribbean.

Entering the names of epidemics that have induced global health threats in the 2000s into the search field of my browser, the following alphabet-soup laced headline caught my eye: "Swine Flu Lessons from SARS, Mad Cow & Bird Flu of Past (GILD, BCRX, NVAX, GNBT, VICL, AVII, CRXL, RHHBY, GSK, SFD, EWW, MXF)" ("Swine Flu Lessons"). These abbreviations are not codes of the respective diseases but the stock ticker symbols of pharmaceutical companies that were expected to prosper during the swine flu season: most notable among them are Roche (RHHBY), the maker of Tamiflu and GlaxoSmithKline (GSK), the maker of Relenza (the two approved drug treatments of—not vaccines against—swine flu). Most of the other abbreviations represent tier-two and tier-three stocks, i.e. makers of drugs that block key enzymes in viral diseases.

Of course this headline is not needed to establish a connection between economy and health, but it emphasizes it. Health and its opposite, disease, are inherently linked to economic questions. If a cultural historian were to name the key concerns of the early twenty-first century, the economic/financial crisis, the ever growing cost of health care and attempts at its reform would be among them. For example, the 2010 health care overhaul law that is President Obama's signature legislation, continued to be challenged in court until the Supreme Court ruled to uphold it in 2012 (Liptak). Until then, public polls showed more people to be against the law than in favor of it. The ruling actually bolstered public support in the aftermath. Another eminent concern of the twenty-first century—from a health, science, and medical perspective—is the state of preparedness in light of the sporadic but consistent threats of pandemics.

Recent Hollywood outbreak narratives pick up on people's anxieties as well as the enjoyment to be found in fear. Over ten years after *Outbreak* (1995), movies such as *I am Legend* (2007), *The Invasion* (2007), and *Contagion* (2011) show the continued popularity of the genre. In *I am Legend* (2007) a plague kills most of mankind; the film portrays a sole immune survivor's quest for a cure. The African American virologist Robert Neville (played by Will Smith) is stranded in New York and tries to create a remedy while defending himself against human mutants. The fictional representation of these post-apocalyptic disease phenomena has a long Hollywood tradition that relies on large casts and multiple storylines.

The narrative translation of epidemic diseases onto the big screen usually works by pitting the protagonist against a mob of infected. For example, both *The Invasion* (2007) with Nicole Kidman and *Contagion* (2011) with Kate Winslet feature female protagonists who try to avert and cope with the medical disaster that has created a zombie-like crowd of infected whose collective experience is the effect of a loss of individuality. While Kidman as a heroic mother is fighting against a mass of people who are not able to feel ("you won't feel a thing"), medical scientist Winslet attempts to control what is referred to as MEV-1, a bird-flu like disease, but eventually also succumbs to the disease. Steven Soderbergh's *Contagion* is the more ambitious project in content and visual representation: by presenting individual frames of the protagonist's suffering, and thus condensing one disease biography, it seeks to individualize the disease and also shed light on a national phenomenon. In the exceedingly popular television series *The Walking Dead* the infected are not even disguised as zombies, they are zombies. Zombieism is presented as a communicable disease: when human beings are bitten, they not only die from the inflicted wounds, but they also 'turn' and rise again from the dead. When at the end of the first season, a group of survivors reaches the headquarters of the Center for Disease Control in Atlanta, it does not provide the shelter and protection they seek at all, but the building explodes in front of their eyes. This does not only signal the breakdown of institutional power and state control, but the viewer learns that the zombie pathogen has been transmitted to the entire population, so that everyone still living will also inevitably 'turn,' even without being bitten. Birgit Däwes has rightfully pointed out *The Walking Dead*'s questionable reactionary celebration of "masculinity, xenophobia, patriotic heroism, and [...] Social Darwinist implications (22–23).

Dan Brown's international bestseller *Inferno* (2013) taps into the same popular fascination with killer viruses and builds on the constant threat of unstoppable pandemics. Protagonist Robert Langdon fights along with the WHO against the release of a genetically engineered virus which is hidden in a dissoluble container in Istanbul. Only after solving a sequence of riddles connected to Dante's *Divine Comedy* is Langdon able to locate the hiding place. Too late, it seems, since the virus that stimulates gene mutation resulting in infertility has spread across the city and will ultimately conquer the world. What was designed to regulate overpopulation by the novel's antagonist is released, thus demonstrating the uncontrollability and continuing risk of diseases. The popular fascination is, however, not limited to the fictional form. The popularity of scientific books like Christopher Wills' *Yellow Fever, Black Goddess: The Coevolution of People and Plagues* (1996) and John Booss and Marilyn J. August's *To Catch a Virus* (2013) shows that "our interest in epidemics is not going to wane in the near future" (Schell 824). Countering public assumptions of epidemic revenge made popular in the mid-1990s in such novels as Richard Preston's *The Hot Zone* (1994) and Laurie Garrett's pseudo-scientific *The Coming Plague* (1994), Wills, a geneticist, locates disease as a central part of human history (Schell 824). He introduces a general audience to the germ theory of history by forging a bridge between the great epidemic outbreaks from bubonic plague, cholera, typhoid, malaria, and syphilis to HIV/AIDS. The gripping title of the book—in contrast to its original British title *Plagues: Their Origins, History, and Future*—and the illustration of a yellow fever-transmitting Aedes aegypti mosquito on the book's cover seems like a marketing trick, given the mere three pages in which he discusses the disease (Wills 33, 161, 163).

This nexus of disease and panic is certainly nothing new; maybe the connection was not always as instantaneously created and distributed globally by news feeds or tweets, but it is not new. How were issues of health and disease negotiated and put into place in earlier times? As an Americanist my first inclination is, of course, to look at American history and culture. And this is where I begin, by looking at the history of North America and the United States in connection with epidemic disease, yellow fever and its cultural negotiation.

1 Representing Yellow Fever: Contagion, Crisis, and Control

1.1 Approaches to Reading Yellow Fever Texts

This study on the representation of yellow fever focuses on American foundational literature from the end of the eighteenth century until the late nineteenth and early twentieth century (with the exception of aesthetic representations of yellow fever that date just beyond this frame). With its diachronic focus, the book is situated before and within Cynthia Davis' investigation (1845–1915) into the influence of medicine in American literature in light of the emerging germ theory. Since there is no linear development in the trajectory from post-revolutionary to post-Civil War novel writing, it comes as no surprise that this also holds true for yellow fever texts. Especially after the Civil War, diseases seemed not to fit into narratives that were "to heal the nation's wounds by highlighting the brave deeds of its northern and southern heroes" (Bell 116).[2] Furthermore, with the emergence and growing acceptance of the Pasteurian germ theory (Louis Pasteur gave his famous lecture at the Sorbonne on April 7, 1864) and other microbiological findings (e.g. Robert Koch's bacteriological discoveries) and medical innovations since the 1860s and 1870s, a new era of medical history and understanding of medicine sets in that is also reflected in fictional texts of the era. The end of the nineteenth century in particular witnessed a biomedical and technological revolution with discoveries and major innovations that helped cure diseases and treat previously deadly conditions. Pasteur and Koch had convincingly demonstrated the association of a specific disease with a specific microorganism, and for many American physicians in the late 1870s and 1880s it seemed only a matter of time until the connection of yellow fever with a still unknown organism could be proven.

---

2 For the purpose of the study I will deal with the category of nation in the sense of Benedict Anderson's "imagined communities" and not necessarily in terms of a juridical entity. I am aware of the "problematic associations of nationalism with evolving state practices that were often quite repressive" such as endorsing "slavery and the removal of other nations claiming territorial boundaries." Although the ideology of a white nation was "expanded during the nineteenth century to include members of other races and nations, […] the earliest expressions of nationalism in American fiction refer most often to a nation composed of male citizens" (Samuels, *Reading the Novel* 20–21n1; see Berlant; Castronovo, *Fathering the Nation*; Robert S. Levine; Nelson).

Yellow Fever Years explores the ideological, socio-political, and cultural productivity of yellow fever epidemics in the formative nineteenth century of U.S. American history and culture. Reading yellow fever texts as representations of crisis phenomena and experiences of crisis, the following questions seem pertinent: How is the disease aestheticized and explained as meaningful; how is the textual representation, in Jane Tompkins's words, "doing cultural work"? Which cultural and medical 'knowledges' are articulated in the writings? Do these narratives also undermine or subvert hegemonic structures and practices, which are otherwise strengthened through the general panic and fear caused by epidemic diseases?[3] For example, is expert medical knowledge undermined or transformed? Especially with regard to visual representations in particular, scenes of disease and death require us to ask what kind of ethics emerges. Which forms of control are suggested through the narratives in times of perceived danger to minimize health risks, contain yellow fever and its outbreak, and to regulate human action?[4] For example, both Cindy Patton and Priscilla Wald have shown in their respective works that "pathogens reify nationalist impulses" which they originally appear to undermine through their 'transnational' behavior of unimpeded border crossing (Silva 9; Patton; Wald, *Contagious*; Wald, "Imagined Immunities"). The reification takes place through laws and legal power and the social performance of control, such as quarantines, and mandatory vaccinations that are enacted in order to protect national health.

The social and political importance of yellow fever (or rather the threat or risk yellow fever posed), I argue, is reflected in the cultural productivity (texts and writing produced, promoted and read) throughout the nineteenth century. Following Pierre Bourdieu, one could speak of a "cultural field" of yellow fever that is defined by certain agents, most prominently physicians and politicians, from which visual and textual accounts (and all other manifestations of the yellow fever field) derive their meaning and function. The fictional texts are symbolic practices that operate in the specific field of disease memory. Yellow fever serves as a metaphor for crises and engages with the many -isms (expansionism, sectionalism, racism, feminism, and abolitionism) of the nineteenth century, while

---

3 With a nod to Stephen Greenblatt I am proposing a subversion-containment dialectic of narrative cultures of fear here (Greenblatt, *Shakespearean Negotiations* 21–65).

4 Winfried Fluck points out that the novel, which recomends itself as a means of control, contributes to the opposite in the long run, contributing to an imaginary justified struggle for independence: "Der Roman, der sich als effektives Mittel sozialer Kontrolle empfiehlt, trägt somit langfristig gesehen, gerade umgekehrt zur Formierung eines imaginär begründeten Unabhängigkeitsstrebens bei" (*Das kulturelle Imaginäre* 36).

never losing its factuality as a very real health risk.[5] An analysis of the use of pathos as a device to appeal to an audience's emotions, which are often based on the underlying values of readers, will shed light on the nexus of health and anxieties about it. In the language of affect theory, pathos may be used to appeal to fear in order to sway the audience in the desired direction.

The focus is on yellow fever and its representation in nineteenth-century U.S.-American writing and the ways in which these literary and cultural representations operated as a means of justifying and critiquing prominent concerns of the period. I should make clear from the outset that this study is not another medical history of yellow fever. I approach the disease as a literary and historical scholar interested in the productivity and cultural meanings of published writing on it. The fictional and visual texts describe diseases as events that reflect wider cultural categories of nation, race, and gender.[6] While it is my hope that the argument presented in the following pages might be of interest to the history of science, medicine and medical history, *Yellow Fever Years* is situated in the field of cultural (primarily visual and literary) studies. In contrast with earlier studies on yellow fever and writing (e.g. by scholars such as Joann P. Krieg) which have based their analyses on the by now well-known corpus of disease literature of the nineteenth century, I will expand this corpus with novels, short fiction, and poetry that specifically 'treat' yellow fever, but have not been regarded together in earlier studies. The retrieval of such a wide variety of yellow fever texts as well as access to their existence has become possible through the increased availability of a growing body of digitized and scanned writings of the period in research libraries that allows for full text searches.

I propose a critical investigation of these texts, some of which might never be reprinted or see the light of a critical scholarly edition due to their lack of aesthetic value (e.g. Wesley Bradshaw's writing) or outrageous moral content (e.g. *The Mysteries of New Orleans*), yet offer a view into nineteenth-century United States culture which could not previously be pursued, also with regard to questions of readership. Or, as Shirley Samuels argues:

> The possibility that critical study might profitably venture into the realm of the aesthetically and morally outrageous as well as making continued excursions in the world of the

5 Regarding feminism and abolitionism I follow Karen Sánchez-Eppler who has successfully argued that "the social and political goals of both feminism and abolition depend upon an act of representation, the inscription of black and female bodies into the discourses of personhood" (93).

6 On the nexus of disease and gender see Zwierlein and Heid.

> acknowledged classic has been a steady development in American Studies as well as cultural studies during the past decades. The results are still contested. (*Reading the Novel* 157)

The critical discourse here returns to Jane Tompkins' seminal question "But is it any good?" that addresses the dichotomy between works celebrated for their aesthetic quality and works that are examined "through the lens of the historical circumstances of their production" (Samuels, *Reading the Novel* 157). It is my belief that the circumstances and contexts producing these texts are informed by social and medical discourses, political discourses, and identity discourses—to name but the most important ones.

I follow Tompkins in selecting the works discussed not for their supposed literary value but for the cultural work they do with regard to constructing knowledge about disease in relation to issues of nation, gender, and race. Whether the texts have achieved the status of canonical works or works that have only been rediscovered in the past 25 years in a critical or scholarly context or that have lent themselves particularly for this book on yellow fever and heretofore lay buried in the archives for their lack of literary value and misguided moral stipulations under today's critical understanding or for mere lack of knowledge about them is noteworthy, yet of secondary importance behind an assessment of their reflexivity of nineteenth-century United States culture. Moreover, a simple binary between reading nineteenth-century fiction as a subversive act or a complacent endorsement of separate spheres ideology is no longer tenable (cf. Samuels, *Reading the Novel* 153).

Tracing the representation of yellow fever in historical, fictional, and visual texts, *Yellow Fever Years* takes up developments in American Studies, Hemispheric and Atlantic studies, and the transnational turn in American Studies (Fishkin; Hornung), to explore an interdisciplinary field that is continually listed among the key topics for the American Studies Association's (ASA) annual conventions: "the political dimensions of disease (mental and physical), disasters, and epidemics; politics of the body" (ASA Website 2009). The 2011 Call for Papers explicitly stresses an interest in discourses of the "literary and visual arts" and "health and medicine" from an interdisciplinary perspective. American studies practitioners in Germany and Europe in particular have strengthened the field with their research at the interface of literature, culture, and medicine in recent years.[7]

---

7 See in particular the work of Carmen Birkle, Rüdiger Kunow, Marc Priewe, Astrid Haas, and Antje Dallmann. The 2012 biennial conference of the *European Association for American Studies* focused on research regarding "The Health of the Nation." The proceedings were published with the same title. In German studies the field of research

Textual analyses show how the different texts approach the specific depiction of yellow fever. Additionally, on different and more complex layers, Stephen Greenblatt's New Historicist approach is employed to situate the texts within the cultural framework and within specific crises (e.g. the future of racial relations) and issues (nation, gender, and race) of nineteenth-century United States. For Greenblatt literary works "are not neutral relay stations in the circulation of cultural material," but rather "[s]omething happens to objects, beliefs, and practices when they are represented, reimagined, and performed in literary texts, something often unpredictable and disturbing" ("Culture" 230–31). Literary texts are thus carefully constructed "variations upon received themes" (Greenblatt, "Culture" 229) that feature the culturally specific encoded meanings and messages of a society and its identity with the creators of texts serving as skilled masters and interpreters of these codes and of cultural interaction (Greenblatt, "Culture" 230). Cultural productions and as such, works of literature, function as agents in the interaction of circulating identity constructs and role models of a given time (Greenblatt, *Shakespearean Negotiations* 12). They are places of negotiation and are read as "interested interpretations of the real" (Howard and O'Connor 3). This pertains to pictures as well: they present "only possibilities of meaning, yielding specific semantic outcomes through its placement within particular discourse systems" (Reynolds 6), which need to be deciphered.

I take into account the generic forms, themes, and structural techniques of what I subsume under the label 'yellow fever texts' and situate them in their specific U.S. cultural contexts. The texts are approached in a combination of surveys and more detailed analyses with the overarching aim to unveil fictional strategies to represent crises and control disease. In order to do this, the study relies on a paradigm of 'culture' dependent on the revisionary ideas (the questioning of the essentialism of history) about the relation of literature to history (developed since the 1980s): cultural anthropology and New Cultural History, the New Historicism, postmodernism and history. It relates to the fields of cultural studies, cultural and literary history and the medical humanities. The groundbreaking text in the latter field is Michel Foucault's *Birth of the Clinic*, which critically explores discourses of sickness and healing and the new practice of medicine since the late eighteenth century. The institutionalization of medicine with the medical clinic and teaching hospital is essential in the development and distribution of medical knowledge.

---

is lead by Bettina von Jagow and Florian Steger, editors of the *Jahrbuch Literatur und Medizin*, published annually by Winter Verlag Heidelberg since 2007 (see also Jagow and Steger, *Was treibt die Literatur zur Medizin?*).

Foucault describes the changed perception of physicians as representing scientific enlightenment after they have put medieval medical superstition and ignorance behind them. They are seen as experts who will win the war against disease, and the decisive new element of control is the clinical physical examination. Foucault characterizes modern medicine by a changed "relation between the visible and invisible" because "gaze and language [disclosed] what had previously been below and beyond their domain" (xii). What Foucault terms the 'medical or clinical gaze' can be described as the physician's detached pose and his scientific power that enables him to see the hidden truths beyond the appearance of sickness and connected symptoms to understand the fundamental reality of disease: "The observing gaze refrains from intervening: it is silent and gestureless. Observation leaves things as they are; there is nothing hidden to it in what is given," writes Foucault (107). It is also the supreme example of surveillance. The method of visually framing the body as a set of structures—an 'anatomical atlas'—to be studied, leads to "a 'biologization' or 'medicalization' of socio-political discourses" (Haas 23). The decisive question is, whether and in how far the yellow fever texts under discussion circumvent or subvert the observing gaze.

One of the central issues for the study of literature and medicine is the acknowledgement of the constructedness of disease. A disease is not discovered but created through its representation in medical-scientific discourse as well as in the culture at large (Theriot 3). *Yellow Fever Years* is based on an understanding that epidemic diseases are created and experienced within social, political, cultural, and economic contexts (cf. Wald, Tomes, and Lynch 618). Consequently, it is only by identifying the contexts involved in the representation of a particular disease, i.e. yellow fever in this study, that that we may understand the relationship between cultural production and epidemic experiences. The focus remains on 'literary' texts that will be read within a cultural-historical framework and an understanding of literature as 'symbolic action.'

1.2 Yellow Fever Fiction as Symbolic Action

I read literary texts as symbolic action, going back to Kenneth Burke's interest in a sociological criticism of literature by identifying the historical context and inherent criticism of a literary text through analyzing its symbolic action. Frederic Jameson has formulated Burke's idea into a method of cultural and textual analysis that assumes fiction to be a strategic response to historical situations and conditions. Fluck calls this "[t]he text's constant [...] attempt to restructure and renegotiate the materials of a culture ("Literature as Symbolic Action" 367). Language and fiction comment and (re)define the non-fictional. In *Valences of the Dialectic*

(2009) Jameson defends the proposition that 'everything is narrative,' the production and consumption of which he understands as a socially symbolic act (*Political Unconscious*). While Jameson is interested in rereading Burke's work as a model for contemporary ideological analysis ("Symbolic Inference"; "Ideology and Symbolic Action"), Fluck stresses the concept's applicability for understanding the uses and functions of literary texts, including pre-modernist and non-experimental texts ("Literature as Symbolic Action" 370). Referring to Burke, Cynthia Davis also considers form as "a strategy for confronting or encompassing [a literary or historical] situation" (Burke qtd. in C. J. Davis 4). With regard to the negotiation of yellow fever, the fictional and visual representations of and cultural responses to the disease since the eighteenth century shape the (changing) responses to it. The negotiation may lead to different results, which the analysis of the examined texts and pictures will show. Conventional images, e.g. of suffering women and children, which the cultural storehouse of disease accommodates, are symbolically employed as sites of crisis in different ways: While they may be confirmed or confronted with counter-images and interpretations, they are also approached critically in the texts. Where applicable, analyses will trace intertextual and interpictorial relationships between textual images and pictures with special attention to the "functionality of the semantic surplus produced by the participation in and, particularly significant, possible transformation and resignification of conventions, repertoires and traditions" (Hebel, "'American' Pictures" 414).

But why primarily novels? Due to their specific representational options as fictions they provide space for experimental constructions of reality which mirror and problematize cultural tensions particularly well. In this respect, Emory Elliott has astutely observed that "literature teaches us about dimensions of society and of ourselves in ways that often penetrate more deeply into our consciousness and our lives than other vehicles of knowledge" ("Diversity in the United States" 3). Winfried Fluck speaks of literature as a testing-ground ("Literature as Symbolic Action" 365, 370, 371). He continues:

> In its freedom to arrange, to construct and to correct reality according to our own norms and interests, fiction permits us tentatively to reformulate, complement, or oppose the social and cultural constructions of reality, and it is exactly in this tentative, playful nature that one unique value of literature as a symbolic strategy can be found. (Fluck, "Literature as Symbolic Action" 365)

Fictional texts thus contribute to and shape social reality (Tompkins 141); they present, as Jane Tompkins has pointed out for the nineteenth century, "an affective alternative that not only gave political actions their emotional significance, but beyond that, intimately linked individual bodies to the national body" (Tompkins 4).

Literary texts, i.e. 'fiction,' should, of course, also not be understood as the opposite, but rather the complement of 'reality' (Iser 73). Edward Said has expressed it similarly: "Therefore novels are aesthetic objects that fill gaps in an incomplete world, they satisfy a human urge to add to reality" (48). Sentimental fictions also often include biographical or autobiographical reportage besides the fictional elaboration of the stories they tell and thus rightfully make claims to a "realistic" representation of actual experience.

Frederic Jameson has similarly argued for the melodramatic narrative as "a socially symbolic act, as the ideological—but formal and immanent—response to a historical dilemma." In this way melodrama becomes an instrument to manage social tensions and conflicts (*Political Unconscious* 139, 171). Melodramatic narratives were not only read by those who suffered with the victims/victimized, but also by those who enjoyed the suffering in a masochistic way (Herget). In this sense, an alleged classic like Charles Brockden Brown's *Arthur Mervyn* will be read alongside Wesley Bradshaw's popular sentimental novellas or children's literature (such as A. Tracy's *Dear Little Marchioness*). While canonical works might be discussed on a more cursory level, close and detailed readings are provided for many texts that are less well known or have been buried in the archives for years. In the texts discussed in *Yellow Fever Years* the treatment of yellow fever ranges from a referential mentioning, to plot device, to full-fledged literary portrayal, as in *Arthur Mervyn*. Analyses of these yellow fever texts will help us to better grasp how disease is both constituted and experienced within social, political, cultural, economic and representational contexts.

Literature serves as a major vehicle for shaping responses to disease. Narratives on disease experiences and events of epidemic disease fever offer generic 'templates' on how to deal with and potentially control diseases. As a major form for the dissemination of knowledge pre-twentieth century they acquire a particular importance. It seems that different diseases suit different forms of literature and different types of representation. For example, the fine line between abhorrent and tragic is often determined by the fashionability of disease (Lawlor). Regarding fashionability, diseases retain a cultural and social function, for example the paradoxically attractive fragility of the consumptive body celebrated in nineteenth-century literature (from Little Eva in Harriet Beecher Stowe's *Uncle Tom's Cabin* (1852) to Alexandre Dumas' Marguerite Gautier in *La Dame aux camélias* [engl. *The Lady of the Camellias*], 1848). Susan Sontag describes the metaphorical discourse of romance regarding the disease: "The tubercular look had to be considered attractive once it came to be considered a mark of distinction, of breeding. [...] [It] symbolized an appealing vulnerability, a superior sensitivity" (*Illness as Metaphor* 27–28).

Yellow fever was certainly not a fashionable disease with regard to its gruesome range of symptoms. It was generally feared but was equally adapted into the social and cultural nexus of literary representation. A large number of novels about yellow fever epidemics exists that offer differing interpretations of the respective crises. They will be analysed with regard to the interaction of their thematic and formal strategies which provides the scaffolding against which cultural claims and constructs are tested (cf. Fluck, "Literature as Symbolic Action" 371). The literary texts are grouped under thematic rubrics (nation, race, gender) and with regard to yellow fever's impact on the novels' protagonists. With regard to structural aspects, yellow fever epidemics mark a conflict or crisis; they are also, in Fluck's terms, "characterized by [...] negotiation and 'eventfulness'" ("Literature as Symbolic Action" 367). For the protagonists, for example, they often trigger a process of initiation. They find themselves in borderline situations as a result of an epidemic and have to reveal their 'true' characters. At the same time, disease outbreaks are decisive times for the whole nation. In this way, yellow fever describes both an individual experience (initiation, chance, trauma) and an American experience (test for the nation).

Based on these insights *Yellow Fever Years* explores how (literary) narratives—complemented by non-fictional accounts—symbolically negotiate the disease experience and how it is ideologically functionalized. Sacvan Bercovitch has formulated an anthropologically grounded definition of ideology as "cultural symbology" which means "the system of symbolic meanings that encompasses text and context alike" and "a network of complex reciprocities between social construction and textual creation" (Bercovitch xvii, xviii; Hebel, "New Historicism" 336). I do not mean to reduce aesthetic expression merely to ideology, but want to point to the interdependency of aesthetic form and ideological context (cf. C. J. Davis 3). In *Criticism and Ideology* Terry Eagleton maintains, that "[t]he text does not merely 'take' ideological conflicts in order to 'resolve' them aesthetically, for the character of those conflicts is itself overdetermined by the textual modes in which they are produced" (88). In his readings Jameson is equally interested as much in the choices of form and theme as in the unconscious framework that determines these choices. Going beyond a formerly purely aesthetic assessment, he is interested in recovering literary practices and norms, the historical framework, with the aim of developing a systematic typology of the constraints imposed on the artist and the creative project.

Yellow Fever Years is a contribution to the study of nineteenth-century American literature and culture and visual studies. It takes the idea of symbolic action and its implications to engage in a cultural reading of fictional and also non-fictional texts and examines a previously untapped body of discourses under the focus of a socio-political and bio-medical lens. Based on an inclusive understanding of texts, historical accounts and popular and pulp fiction are similarly of interest, as are canonized works of literature and illustrations, and make for the survey character of the book. They follow and mix the forms of epistolary,[8] gothic, sensational, sentimental, and historical novel, as well as naturalist and realist fiction toward the end of the nineteenth century. I have grouped this mixture of canonical and hitherto widely disregarded novels under new rubrics.

1.3 Conceptualizing Yellow Fever Representations: Nation, Gender, and Race

The conceptualization of the book follows the diachronic orientation of the project. To ensure the comprehensive character of each of the larger chapters brief theoretical considerations introduce the thematic complexes of nation, visuality, gender, and race at the beginning of the respective sections. While providing an overview of my line of argument in the following I ask readers to turn to the specific chapters where concepts and insights are evaluated more fully. In order to explain the character of the disease until the early 1900s yellow fever epidemics are explored in the latter part of chapter 1 in their historical dimension and etiology, the study of causality. Chapter 1 also provides an overview of the research literature and of the textual and visual material.

The preamble of the Constitution stipulates the formation of 'a more perfect Union,' and the larger project of the United States in the nineteenth century can roughly be surmised by the construction of that union. The building of a nation based on republican ideals was at the center of the early Republic, which was not without setbacks and political and social crises that helped to sharpen the contours. Chapter 2 treats the 1793 yellow fever epidemic in Philadelphia as a case in point. Representations of the epidemic served to disclose the early republic's problems and to project the nation's future. The probably best known yellow fever narrative of the period is Charles Brockden Brown's gothic novel *Arthur*

8 With reference, for example to Charles Brockden Brown's *Edgar Huntly* (1799) Shirley Samuels has pointed to the mobile quality of letters and the epistolary form as a device. The private space of home was occupied by letters and letter writing, and novels were carried around in pockets just like letters (Samuels, *Reading the Novel* 13).

Mervyn, or, Memoirs of the Year 1793 (1799/1800). The fever-stricken Philadelphia serves Brown as a laboratory for his considerations and predictions about the future of the nation. Matthew Carey's *Short Account of the Malignant Fever, Lately Prevalent in Philadelphia* (1793) and Richard Allen and Absalom Jones's *Narrative of the Proceedings of the Black People during the Late Awful Calamity in Philadelphia in the Year 1793* (1794) will be considered as sources and blueprints for the spaces functionalized in the fictional text. Carey's *Short Account* is a racialized pamphlet that chronicles the epidemic. In their *Narrative* Allen and Jones base their main criticism on the fact that Carey had actually fled the infected city and published his account upon his return, suggesting that Carey lacked any first-hand experience. The continuously felt need of mastering (medical) crises as part of the national project is furthermore exemplified in the recurrent fictional representations of the Philadelphia yellow fever epidemic, thus also manifesting the epidemic's cultural status in the storehouse of memory.

Indebted to cultural memory studies, chapter 3 analyzes visual practices and patterns of yellow fever pictures from the perspective of affect studies. Establishing an iconography of calamity in American visual culture from colonial times and stressing the role of popular print culture by tracing the rise of nineteenth-century illustrated newspapers, this section covers examples from the yellow fever field from the early nineteenth until the early twentieth century (cf. *Iconographies of the Calamitous*; Gessner and Leikam 533–37). An aesthetics of the 'destructive sublime,' famously applied by Miles Orvell to the mediation of the terror attacks of 9/11, is applied to the analysis of the yellow fever pictures. Readers familiarize themselves, if not empathize, with the experiences of yellow fever represented in the newspapers of the time. I term this process the touristic or distant gaze. The illustrations and the military photographs of yellow fever victims convey—*at a distance*—other people's pain. The disease and its particular symptoms remain largely unrepresentable in the photographic medium, which unfolds its power through its suggestiveness. The political nature and affective potential of the visual representations presented in "Displaying Disease" recurs to issues of nation(-building), gender, and race.

Gendered accounts of the yellow fever experience are scrutinized in chapter 4. Taking into account that the social and political development of the nineteenth century was mirrored in writing both by and for women, this chapter looks at works of the postbellum and post-Reconstruction period, including one set in New Orleans during the Gilded Age. Besides fictionalizing yellow fever crises, Wesley Bradshaw's two sentimental novellas, the novels by Mary Faith Floyd and Mollie E. M. Davis, and Elizabeth Stuart Phelps's short story all focus on the figure of a medical practitioner (nurse or physician) who symbolically acts to resolve the crisis situation. In the narratives these roles are taken up by both men and women, leaving room to suggest the transformative potential of facing medical crises for both genders.

Chapter 5 focuses on the increasingly hybrid makeup of American society and the connected issue of racism throughout the nineteenth century. The growing diversity and difficulty of ethnic and racial relationships is reflected in the imagined and real spaces of yellow fever and slavery. Beginning with the sea as such an imagined space, the presence of yellow fever and race as part of an oceanic paradigm (cf. Boelhower; Esty) and within—what Paul Gilroy has termed—the Black Atlantic will be examined. Another such space is created with the cultural imagination of New Orleans as the Crescent City, the *Big Easy*, the City That Care Forgot, and—especially in the context of this book—the capital of race, sin and yellow fever. African American as well as Irish American, German American, and Creole experiences with the disease are represented in quite a few texts focusing on New Orleans. Last, but not least, texts by African American writers that politically explore the connection of yellow fever and race are analyzed. Beginning with the *Narrative* by Absalom Jones and Richard Allen these writings by William Wells Brown, Frances Harper, and Ida B. Wells furthermore shed light on community building efforts as a means to control the disease.

The sixth chapter presents four major conclusions emerging from my analysis of nation, gender, and race in connection with visual and textual yellow fever representations. It also points toward further fields of research such as an even broader hemispheric and circum-Atlantic approach which would connect voices, images, and texts from the Caribbean, North, Central and South America with West African ones. The continuous relevance of nineteenth-century yellow fever texts and their transformation as part of a storehouse of cultural disease memory is equally exemplified. An extensive bibliography of primary yellow fever sources also testifies to the disease's unceasing cultural significance.

1.4 Etiology and History of Yellow Fever

The history of North America and the United States has always been accompanied by the presence of diseases: from smallpox in the colonial period to swine flu today. Scientists agree that many acute viruses, such as smallpox, measles, yellow fever, chickenpox, and influenza were introduced infections. Some bacteria (anthrax, whooping cough, and typhus) and some parasites (malaria and schistosomes) were equally imported (cf. Ramenofsky, Wilbur, and Stone 242, 243).

Debates about the pre-contact status of long-lived infectious agents, such as tuberculosis and syphilis, are still not fully resolved.[9]

Both bacteria and viruses are incredibly mobile, and their mobility links what is otherwise kept apart by means of social or ideological constructions (people and nations). Diseases, as Rüdiger Kunow has argued, are inherently transgressive phenomena ("In Sickness and in Health" 24). This holds equally true for concepts related to disease, such as (im)migration, infection, and transmission, or more precisely the fear or risk of transmission and spread of panic accompanying the outbreak of epidemic diseases. Besides a transgressive quality, epidemic diseases also display a 'transnational' quality, as they are capable of traveling from host to host across national borders (sometimes with the help of a non-human carrier). The invisible transgression of (national) borders also feeds into a culture of fear and evokes panic. The concept of contagion in its figurative and literal usage may link the history of epidemics and panic.[10] As Martin Pernick points out, "[r]eferences to contagious fear were not necessarily or wholly metaphorical" (861) since fear was seen as a direct cause of disease. It is also reflected in yellow fever narratives, in which fear and "senselessness with terror" (Souvestre, *Isle of the Dead* 51) induce yellow fever. In this line of argument panic could be defined as an "epidemic of fear" and also as the agent that intensifies the speed and extent by which epidemics spread (Pernick, "Contagion" 861). In 1798 the British military surgeon Robert Jackson commented on yellow fever as inducing an 'epidemic of fear' or—in his words—a "contagion of fear": "Though the contagion of

9 In a 2008 genetic study scientist Kristin N. Harper (Emory U) and colleagues have found what they say is the strongest evidence yet linking the first European explorers of the New World to the origin of sexually transmitted syphilis (Wilford). In an online media gossip and popular culture news source, the same story reads "Study: Indians Gave You Syphilis" (Pareene) which, of course, gives the story a whole new—or very old (in the framing of Native Americans)—twist.

10 Although *contagious* has been replaced in medical dictionaries by *communicable*, in the sense of 'capable of being transmitted' the concept of contagion remains important with respect to speculations about the cause of diseases. Contagion is entangled with politics and ethics: the assumption "that another person is the source of disease makes the links between contagion and personal blame [...] especially close and visible. When 'other people' have been seen as the source, contagion has been used to blame outsiders and outcasts, especially immigrants and minorities. However, when the emphasis has been placed on 'close contact,' contagion has also blamed intimate intracommunal communications, especially sexual and family contacts" (Pernick, "Contagion" 862). Pernick also cautions researchers not to reduce contagionist medicine to politics or morality alone, but also to see it in its relations and the dependencies of its specific time and place.

yellow fever may prove to be a fiction, the contagion of fear has so impressed the minds of men, that things are seen through a false medium, and common sense cannot obtain a hearing" (*Outline of the History and Cure of Fever* 223).

With regard to the twentieth century, yet equally applicable to earlier times, medical historian Allan M. Brandt has pointed out that "the way any society comes to understand patterns of health and disease and their causes reveals basic cultural norms and expectations" (71). In terms of North America and the United States, a double helix of health (and emphasis on the purity of the body) and fear (or anxiety about losing health) seems to have been ingrained in society and culture from colonial times. In a 2012 *Atlantic* article, Maura Kelly argues that anxiety might well be considered a "peculiarly American phenomenon."[11] Significantly, "[a]nxieties about border crossings pervade the early novel" as Shirley Samuels points out and refers to "the boundary of the ocean, of the nation, of the alien territory" (*Reading the Novel* 15) and—one could add—to health and disease. This culture of fear (to once again borrow Barry Glassner's contemporary term) has been fed through various real and perceived threats from smallpox-infected blankets, through 'undetected' immigrant carriers of disease such as Typhoid Mary, to the post-9/11 anthrax scare. Throughout the nineteenth century, when waves of mass immigration fostered an ethnic and cultural diversification of society, U.S.-America anxiously sought to define itself against threats to the national body. In their collection of essays Stefan Brandt and Astrid Fellner point out that the body as a trope became popular during in the post-revolutionary era of emerging nationalism; infections and purity became key terms in describing the body politic and the nation (3–4). Notions of health crises were figuratively linked to the period's experience of a highly complex layering of several social and political conditions such as slavery, immigration, urbanization, and expansion. The crisis experiences were often woven into discourses of progress and nation-building since the construction, confirmation, and assurance of a national identity seemed imperative for the social and political advancement of American nationhood during this period. At least "since the middle of the 19th century, crisis has become a catchword in cultural rhetoric" and, as Rüdiger Kunow furthermore points out, "narrative has always been concerned with the human experience of change, and as Aristotle already pointed out, the most basic human stories have always dealt with, if not focused on *peripeteia*, the movement of reversal of crisis" ("Rhetoric of Crisis" 474, 478). The field of medicine

11 Kelly's dictum was taken up in a special issue of the American studies journal *aspeers* on *American Anxieties*.

also found itself in a profound state of flux in the nineteenth century, and many new discoveries forced physicians to change and adapt old presumptions to fit current findings.

While we know and describe disease by "the severity of its symptoms and their effect on our body's systems [...], we categorize it by the extent to which its symptoms are shared" and then designate it an "outbreak, epidemic, or pandemic" (Koch 1). In other words, it is a matter of degree, which epithet is applied. While Samuel Johnson in his *Dictionary of the English Language* (1755) defines an epidemic as a disease that "falls at once upon great numbers of people, as a plague" (S. Johnson 243), epidemiologists Fox, Hall, and Elveback simply describe an epidemic as a deviation from the normal, as an incidence of a disease (16). According to Astrid Haas,

> [m]odern medicine defines an epidemic as a highly infectious disease that affects many individuals at a time and is not restricted or peculiar to a specific locality. However, the classical medical understanding of epidemics and its religious/moral interpretive framework continue to thrive in popular notions of such diseases: to this day, societal and media discourses commonly attribute an inexplicable origin to serious epidemics and modes of transmission appear to be either unknown or difficult to control, which raises fears of a potential exposure of large segments of a population to the disease in question. (21)

When the term 'outbreak' is used in this study in connection with disease in the nineteenth century, I follow Robert DeSalle and Marla Jo Brickman's definition of "a suddenly occurring and explosively rapid increase of an infectious disease in a population" (113).[12]

The analogy of medical knowledge-making (i.e. categorization) and cultural knowledge-production is striking. Narratives are crucial both for medical diagnosis and for literary representations of disease that spread medical knowledge. In cultural terms, not only the extent of symptoms *shared* in order to make a prediction about or identify a specific disease, but also the extent of disease discourses and narratives *shared* are relevant to an assessment of healthy or diseased body politic. With regard to disease narrative, Carmen Birkle points out that they "are always also studies of societies or individuals under extreme pressures, in which memory is often lost, denied, ignored, or simply in crisis and in need of recovery" ("Saving the Circum-Atlantic World" 60). I also follow Priscilla Wald, Nancy Tomes, and Lisa Lynch, who have pointed out that "[a]ppropriate emotional, economic, and medical responses to disease depend upon our recognizing the processes that

---

12 DeSalle's collection of essays accompanied the American Museum of Natural History's exhibit *Epidemic!* shown in Washington, D.C. in 1999 and San Diego in 2001.

produce the experience of and responses to it." In order to explore the "multifaceted relationships between culture and transmissible disease" (618), I will focus on the disease that has caused the most fatal epidemic outbreaks and consequently posed a constant threat throughout the nineteenth century, yellow fever.

By the end of the eighteenth century, smallpox, the disease of the colonial period, no longer posed an epidemic threat due to the wide acceptance of inoculation and vaccination (at least in urban areas).[13] Between 1793 and 1905 the most severe epidemic outbreaks of diseases in the U.S. accompanied by panics were due to yellow fever and cholera. Regarding yellow fever, historian Andrew McIlwaine Bell points out that "no other disease produced more public panic throughout the nineteenth century" (6). Cholera first appeared in North America as well as in Europe in 1826–1837. During the 1832 cholera epidemic three thousand people died in New York (July-August) and over four thousand people in New Orleans (October).

At the end of the eighteenth century the threat that smallpox had caused was replaced by yellow fever as the most feared epidemic disease. From July to November 1793 between four and five thousand Philadelphia residents, or about 10 percent of the city's population, died from yellow fever. Many more left the city for a temporary home in the country. Among them were the infected Alexander Hamilton and his wife, and Matthew Carey, who published his *Short Account of the Malignant Fever* soon after his return in November 1793. Carey estimated that 17,000 fled the city (77). Benjamin Rush, a physician and signatory to the Declaration of Independence, stayed in the city. He became highly regarded by issuing guidelines for avoiding infection and helping set up a fever hospital for victims. However Rush, who believed in the immunity of people of African descent, also had to stand corrected on this issue, thus complicating his role as benefactor. Charles Brockden Brown's gothic novel *Arthur Mervyn* (1799/1800) probably provides one of the most thorough literary portrayals of the 1793 Philadelphia epidemic. It will be read together with several other texts in chapter 2 which provide a spotlight on the epidemic that was so decisive for the still young nation.

Philadelphia, then the capital of the United States, experienced repeated outbreaks of yellow fever between 1793 and 1805, and then again in the 1820s. Concurrent epidemics actually affected the nation's three major cities in the early years of the republic. Medical historian John Duffy asserts that the period from 1793 to 1806 "deserves to be known as the yellow fever era" (Duffy, *Sanitarians* 38). New York, which had turned away Philadelphia refugees in 1793, was

13 George Washington had promoted an inoculation policy for the American army in 1777 (cf. Dine 414, 419).

hit in 1795 and again in the summer of 1798. The 1798 epidemic under whose direct influence Charles Brockden Brown penned his novel in New York also affected Boston and again Philadelphia and left more than 5,000 dead. Two years later, Baltimore was hit and lost over 1,000 of its residents. The combination of the very high mortality in the early epidemics with the political (most of those politically in charge fleeing the city), social (e.g. the hospital system and organization of burials), and economic (the halt on trade) impact of the disease, affected the nascent United States that found itself in a period of consolidation and nation-building. In particular the lack of organization of hospitals, physicians and nurses as well as undertakers led to catastrophic conditions (cf. esp. Carey, *Short Account*; see also Allen and Jones).

After 1820 yellow fever outbreaks were increasingly confined to the southern and south-eastern United States. By the 1840s yellow fever had retreated from northern port cities to the South, where its frequency and malignancy seemed to rise concurrently with almost yearly epidemics in southern maritime cities. The disease took more than 40,000 lives in New Orleans from 1817–1905. The 1853 yellow fever epidemic alone claimed the lives of eight to nine thousand people, or 9 percent of the population, and needs to be counted among the deadliest in American history. More than 2,000 died of yellow fever in Norfolk, Virginia between June and October 1855. The outbreak could be traced to the arrival of a ship from the West Indies, which furthered a contagionist view of the disease (see G. D. Armstrong).

Yellow fever was also often referred to as 'strangers' disease' in the nineteenth-century United States. This corresponds to contemporary descriptions as well as to modern studies that point toward a greater vulnerability of new residents and temporary visitors from northern states, interior southern states, and Europe (Patterson 861). Furthermore, the fatality rate of men was higher than that of women, "adults were more likely to contract fatal cases than children. Poor people seemed to be singled out in some epidemics [...] partly because they lived near the docks, where [...] infected ships would bring the disease first, and partly because many of the poor were immunologically naïve newcomers" (Patterson 860).

By the 1870s yellow fever also reached cities further inland that were increasingly connected through a growing and commercially active system of rail transportation.[14] A "new anxiety about regional disparities" between North and South could be detected in the writings of medical southerners, Margaret Humphreys

14 Up until 1905 yellow fever epidemics in the South "renewed historical public health concerns over the hygienic dangers of rail transportation" (J. Brown, "Purity and Danger" 106).

observes (*Yellow Fever* 46). The fact that yellow fever was curtailing the Southern economy and social growth influenced the Northern view of the South as backward especially in the Reconstruction era in the 1870s. Several outbreaks of yellow fever during the decade culminated in the devastating 1878 epidemic during which, by one estimate, twenty thousand people or 10 percent of the population died in the lower Mississippi Valley (Patterson 857–58; "Major U.S. Epidemics").[15] From New Orleans the epidemic had spread up the Mississippi Valley to Memphis, where half of the city's population of 47,000 fled the city. More than 5,000, or 10 percent of the original population, died of yellow fever. With mortality rates of 9–10 percent during these major epidemics a certain congruence of perceived and actual threat can be asserted. However, not every yellow fever epidemic was equally devastating, yet the perceived threat remained. Military physician John R. Pierce and his co-author Jim Writer speculate in their 2005 history that the horror a nineteenth-century yellow fever epidemic was able to induce was due to its relative rarity and arbitrariness (2).

It was not until 1881 that a Cuban physician, Carlos Juan Finlay, suggested that mosquitos might actually be the culprits in the transmission of the disease.[16] And even after Finlay's proposal in 1881 scientists struggled to reconcile the geographical and the bacteriological-contagionist perspective of yellow fever. The establishment of a military-medical complex and necessity eventually paved the way for a groundbreaking confirmation. The Spanish-American War was accompanied by a yellow fever outbreak on Cuba in the summer of 1898. Yellow fever and other diseases killed more than five times as many American soldiers as enemy bullets (Gessner, "Heroines of Health"). The disease's direct impact on military power and performance resulted in the establishment of a U.S. Army Yellow Fever Board chaired by Major Walter Reed. Together with Acting Assistant Surgeons James Carroll, Aristides Agramonte, and Jesse Lazear, Reed was able to prove Finlay's hypothesis that yellow fever was transmitted through the female *Aedes aegypti* mosquito (fig. 1). Yellow fever was the first of many viral diseases shown to be arthropod-borne.

---

15 Although the death toll in Memphis alone was over 5,000, President Rutherford B. Hayes called pleas for help 'greatly exaggerated.' The federal response was unusually slow (Roach).

16 As early as 1848, Josiah Clark Nott published papers in which he proposed some connection between insects and disease. Writing at a time when the term 'insect' was loosely used, and before the germ theory of disease had taken hold, Nott made no clear distinction between insects as pathogens and as vectors of pathogens (see also Humphreys, *Yellow Fever* 20) and thus cannot be credited as the originator of the mosquito theory.

Fig. 1. Dedication of the Camp Lazear National Monument, 3 Dec. 1952. Philip S. Hench Walter Reed Yellow Fever Collection 1800-ca. 1998, University of Virginia Claude Moore Health Sciences Library.

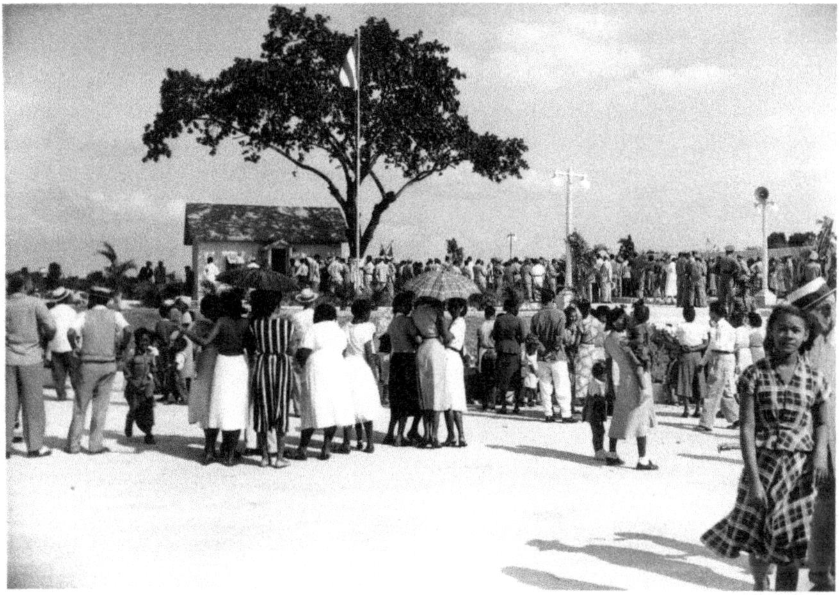

Until 1900, the authors of medical treatises and the authors of historical accounts, novels, short stories, poems, articles and dramas had to rely on presumption and speculation when it came to the origin, the best prevention method and the transmission of yellow fever. Only when the arthropod vector in the transmission was confirmed was a scientifically reliable prevention possible, namely by suppressing the mosquito population. Today we know that yellow fever is an acute viral disease transmitted to humans by the bite of the female *Aedes aegypti* mosquito, unspreadable through human contact and noncontagious (Patterson 855). The finding eventually led to the eradication of the disease in North America, and the 1905 New Orleans epidemic with more than 900 dead was the last in the United States. Yellow fever's viral nature was established in 1927 and a vaccine developed in 1937. Today yellow fever remains endemic in South America and in West and Central Africa, which still suffer from occasional serious outbreaks (Barnett 850).[17]

One source of anxiety about yellow fever and also a reason for its late eighteenth and nineteenth-century construction as an American disease may have been the fact that it was never experienced in its epidemic form in continental Europe, with the exception of local epidemics in Gibraltar and the coasts of Spain and Portugal (Coleman).[18] The disease was not indigenous to America, and—with the benefit of hindsight—can be called an 'imperial' disease since vector and virus originated in Africa and entered the New World through the slave trade (Patterson 856); yellow fever probably first occurred in Spanish Florida in 1649–1650 (Swagerty and Dobyns 279, qtd. in Patterson 855). Epidemiologist Robert S. Desowitz describes a "concatenation of conditions" around the mid-seventeenth century that "led to near simultaneous outbreaks of a previously unknown disease in Havana, Barbados, Guadeloupe, St. Christopher, and Mexico's Yucatan peninsula (99). We know that those conditions included the importation of African slaves to work plantations, and presumably the accidental inclusion of the *Aedes aegypti* mosquito in the holds of ships whose sailors and cargos of slaves carried the flavivirus that causes yellow fever. Once in the New World the virus prospered, as did its mosquito carrier, in European settlements across the tropical and subtropical latitudes" (Koch 73–74). The National Library of Medicine lists an even earlier date for the introduction of yellow fever to North American, namely 1616. In that year an estimated 45,000 people, two-thirds of the Wampanoag, died of yellow fever. According to the source, European traders carried yellow fever to the area between Provincetown, Massachusetts and Narragansett Bay, Rhode Island, where the Wampanoag resided ("Yellow Fever Kills Two-Thirds of the Wampanoag"). It is historically confirmed that in 1693 Boston and other towns were infected when ships from the West Indies brought it to then British North America (Krieg 49; Pierce and Writer 15). The disease

---

17 The mosquito species *Aedes aegypti*, the vector of yellow fever, is also primarily responsible for transmitting dengue fever. On June 20, 2013 a medical company made a first release of engineered *Aedes aegypti* mosquitoes to control the dengue mosquito in the town of Jacobina in the State of Bahia, Brazil ("Moscamed Launches Urban Scale Project Using Oxitec GM Mosquitoes in Battle Against Dengue").

18 Historian William Coleman examines the occurrence of yellow fever cases in Gibraltar (1828), and the European port cities of Saint Nazaire (1861), and Swansea (1865). The few major yellow fever outbreaks in nineteenth-century Europe were confined to Spain and Portugal: Cádiz, 1800; Barcelona, 1819–21; Gibraltar, 1828; Lisbon, 1857 (see Coleman 18).

struck irregularly. Sometimes communities were afflicted yearly by epidemics in the summer and early fall, then yellow fever completely disappeared and did not come back for decades. Yellow fever's symptoms include high temperatures, chills, body aches, nausea and vomiting; more severe cases brought jaundice, internal hemorrhage and thus bleeding from nose and mouth, stool stained dark with blood, and copious black vomit. In the nineteenth century yellow fever had a case-fatality that fluctuated between 15 and 50 percent and higher; these very high mortality rates may indicate that milder cases were not recognized as yellow fever (Pierce and Writer 246). Survivors of yellow fever gain lifetime immunity (Patterson 855). The horrifying symptoms together with the high case-fatality rate created panic and fear incomparable to other diseases. Not surprisingly, several yellow fever narratives such as Charles Brockden Brown's gothic novel *Arthur Mervyn* that detail the 1793 Philadelphia yellow fever epidemic testify to the cultural significance of the disease threat.[19] Even more than the relative risk of infection, the panics stirred by outbreaks of epidemic diseases in the late eighteenth and nineteenth century may be connected to anxieties stirred by an imperial expansion and the crossing of previous boundaries and extension of trade routes between Europe, Africa, the Carribbean and the United States (cf. Harrison, *Medicine* 266). When yellow fever, primarily perceived as a tropical disease, appeared in the Mediterranean (in Cadiz in 1800) and caused a major epidemic in Philadelphia in 1793, it raised the "grim spectre of contagious pestilence spreading out [...] to infect more 'civilized' lands" (Harrison, *Medicine* 208; cf. Harrison, *Contagion* 63). Yellow fever was linked to imperialism, colonial expansion, commerce and the slave trade.

1.5 Making Yellow Fever American: Medical Discourses and Atlantic Conversations

The task of our immune system is to protect the body against infection by microbes (bacteria, fungi, parasites, viruses) and tumor cells. To ensure this it constantly discriminates between 'self' and 'foreign.' The system is specific and it is 'remembering.' Once overcome, viruses leave their 'scripts' in the body, making it

---

19 The first German translation of Charles Brockden Brown's yellow fever tale was published in 1859 as *Arthur Mervyn oder die Pest in Philadelphia: Denkwürdigkeiten aus dem Jahre 1793*. The plague as a general stand-in for a devastating disease is featured in the title instead of the mere reference to the year 1793 (as in the English original) that would conjure up the yellow fever outbreak for a contemporary U.S.-American audience, since the disease was not as widely recognized in Germany.

immune against attacks by the same kind of intruder. Viral diseases do not only leave scriptural traces in the body, they are also investigated through writing, both medical and cultural: "symptoms are identified, listed, and then somehow projected in the search for clues to its origin and possible prevention" (Koch 4). By studying this textual production regarding diseases over the centuries, one may formulate a chronology of diseases (and their investigation): the plague is the disease of the seventeenth century, yellow fever of the eighteenth and nineteenth century, and cholera of the nineteenth century (yet only as a particular British colonial threat) (Koch 4).[20] In contrast with their British colleagues, nineteenth-century Caribbean and North American physicians remained focused on an investigation of yellow fever that continued to pose a particular threat to the United States. Molly Caldwell Crosby juxtaposes the late eighteenth-century European with an American understanding of yellow fever when she titles her 2006 book "The American Plague [...] that shaped *our* history" (emphasis mine) and created panic and fear incomparable to other diseases.[21] Not surprisingly, yellow fever narratives testify to the cultural significance of the disease (threat) as well as to the America-specificity of yellow fever. The clear distinction of yellow fever and cholera further exemplifies what might be termed 'disease exceptionalism.' As Charles Rosenberg, the major medical historian on cholera, argues, "America did all in its collective power to distance itself from [cholera] by assuming the attitude that, since the disease was of foreign origin (unlike yellow fever, which was unknown outside the Western Hemisphere), it reflected nothing of the American experience, and that its victims were limited to those whose way of life invited such disaster" (qtd. in Krieg 71).

Yellow fever has a long and notorious history in the United States; it has also been called "West-India and American yellow fever" (Rush, "Facts" 156). My contention is that yellow fever was constructed as a specifically American disease and used to exemplify the particular and specific American condition(s), struggles and crises of the nineteenth century: the slave trade, connected with sea travel and foreign trade, and immigration. The many names given to the disease illustrate the association with these issues: "Bronze John, dock fever, stranger's fever, yellow jacket, Barbados distemper, and Palatine fever" (Brooks 155). In

20 Cholera ravaged in several European cities in the period and affected large and quickly growing industrial cities, such as Vienna and Berlin in 1831, London in 1832, and Munich in 1836 (see Evans).

21 Crosby writes: "Yellow fever became the most dreaded disease in North America for two hundred years. It did not kill in numbers as high [...] as cholera or smallpox, and it was not contagious; yet it created panic and fear few other diseases, ancient and contemporary, can elicit" (11).

order to accomplish an interpretative sovereignty American physicians had to emancipate themselves from their colleagues especially in Great Britain (and also France). British colonial expansion afforded new challenges and opportunities regarding diseases. Colonial British surgeons and physicians pursuing tropical medical practice had made important contributions to British medicine.[22] Great emphasis was placed on firsthand experience and on seeing for oneself. As an example historian Mark Harrison cites military practitioner George Pinckard, who dissected a soldier in Stabroek, Guiana (later Georgetown, British Guiana) who had died of yellow fever:

> From experience, and examination of the diseased appearances, I may hope for more accurate elucidation, and perhaps be enabled to arrive at some general maxim, which, in vain, I have looked for in the discordant opinions of the ingenious men who have devoted their pens to this great—this interesting, and most important subject. (Pinckard 2: 324)

This strategy of claiming firsthand experience and knowledge over replicated findings was later taken up by U.S. American physicians who argued for their superiority of interpretation due to their direct exposure to the disease. Colonial practitioners in the Caribbean and North America sought to establish the primacy of experience and direct observation over what they regarded as the merely speculative hypotheses of their Europe-based colleagues.

An important factor in promoting the new genre of medical literature were the imperial wars of the eighteenth century, combined with the increasing economic value attached to the lives of soldiers and sailors (Harrison, *Medicine* 27). Furthermore, fear that the devastation yellow fever had caused in North America could spread to Great Britain led to greater efforts in improving its treatment and prevention. It had claimed the lives of thousands of British and French soldiers on St. Domingue in the 1790s.

> The ravages which this fatal Disease have [sic] made, during the present war, in our fleets and armies, are beyond all precedent. [...] It has offered the severest obstacles to military operations [...]: the chief victims of its fury being the young, the robust, and those free from other diseases; by which means a campaign in the West Indies is now considered as little better than a forlorn hope. (Trotter 322)

---

22 For example, James Makittrick, based his Edinburgh MD thesis of 1764 on his own post-mortem dissections conducted in the West Indies (6–7). Although there was a substantial minority that regarded yellow fever to be contagious due to its mostly epidemic appearance, most physicians at the time, including Makittrick, attributed it to a putrefying quality of the atmosphere (23–26). The theory of putrefication combined with a humid climate as culprit of the disease was also maintained by army medical practitioner William Lempriere who was practicing in Jamaica in the 1790s (2–4).

Equally, literally called to arms by frequent and devastating outbreaks on their own soil since the 1790s (Philadelphia, New York), the U.S. American medical profession used yellow fever outbreaks as objects of study. Besides speculation about its origin, treatment and prevention the disease was used to promote interpretational sovereignty and reject 'old world' understandings of disease in such 'American' publications as the newly founded *Medical Repository*. Edited by Samuel Latham Mitchill, a professor of chemistry and a senator from New York, it was the first scientific journal in the United States (Mott, *1741–1850* 149). Among the writers were Benjamin Rush and Charles Caldwell, a former student of Rush's, both of whom corresponded and collaborated with Noah Webster.[23] The *Medical Repository* was first published in 1797 as "a venue for many medical and natural historical topics; the editors made the disease [yellow fever] a primary subject" (Arner 453).[24] The special attention given to epidemics is a recurrent theme in the twenty-three volumes of the journal (Mott, *1741–1850* 149). Noah Webster, in his *Brief History of Epidemic and Pestilential Diseases*, "fashioned his History as a domestic source by an American about American environs and most applicable to interpretations of what he and others thought to be an American disease" (Arner 455; esp. Webster, *Brief History* 26–27). Most of those who wrote about yellow fever from personal experience in this period argued that it was not contagious. American scientists who believed in the non-contagionist nature of the disease not only presented yellow fever as something that originated in America but also claimed it as their domain of research, invoking 'American intellectual independence.' Charles Caldwell wrote: "As well might the parliament of Great Britain, in their present ignorance of our circumstances as a nation, attempt to legislate for all our emergencies, as her faculty to decide for us with regard to the nature, prevention, or cure of *our* epidemics" (Caldwell, *A Reply to Dr. Haygarth's*

23 For Benjamin Rush smallpox inoculation since 1769 played a large role in establishing his practice (Dine 419).

24 Arner cites a 1799 oration by Charles Caldwell (*A Semi-Annual Oration, on the Origin of Pestilential Diseases*), in which he identifies the cause of a late Philadelphia outbreak as of local origin, thus countering the college's assertion of importation (qtd. in Arner 454). Arner continues: "When many American non-contagionists fought against contagionism, they gave a political inflection to their arguments. A domestic disease became associated with the domain of the American interpreter—one who witnessed first-hand not only the disease, but also the local natural environs of which it was a product. Advocating their views involved promoting themselves as the most credible arbiters in the disputes" against British medical writers, such as Colin Chisholm and John Haygarth (455). In Chisholm's view yellow fever's origin lay in a specific agent of contagion with definite symptoms and pathological signs.

Letter 10–11; qtd. in Arner 457; emphasis mine).[25] Benjamin Rush and the editors of the *Medical Repository* thus worked towards defining yellow fever as an American disease. Their medical discourses and the initiation of Atlantic conversations on yellow fever represent a transnational network, which will be further investigated in the chapter on the Philadelphia yellow fever epidemic of 1793 (ch. 2.2).

On both sides of the Atlantic, controversies about the contagiousness of the disease also entailed the heavily debated question whether measures such as quarantine were necessary and advisable. In this sense the contagiousness of yellow fever was a political issue because it was inseparable from the question of quarantine, which did not fit the general climate of reform in a post-revolutionary era and was deemed repressive and inhumane. The fierce debates over the contagiousness of yellow fever in the 1790s and early 1800s can be traced to two publications in 1794 that reached two different conclusions: firstly, Benjamin Rush's *An Account of the Bilious Remitting Fever* based on the 1793 Philadelphia epidemic that had followed the arrival of French refugees from the slave revolt on St. Domingue, and secondly, Colin Chisholm's *Essay on the Malignant Pestilential Fever introduced into the West Indian Islands from Boullam*, which he based on the 1793 yellow fever epidemic he witnessed as a military surgeon stationed in Grenada. While not ruling out the role of contagion altogether, Rush argued for a miasmatic cause of the epidemic and pointed to mouldering coffee beans left on the city's wharves as the culprit. In contrast, Chisholm believed in an importationist cause and cited the fact that it conferred immunity on those who had survived it. He argued that the immunity of some places put yellow fever in the same category as smallpox, a disease which was generally regarded as contagious at the time. Chisholm believed—in hindsight probably correctly—that the specific epidemic had been imported from Bulam, Guinea, on the west coast of Africa.[26] Quarantine measures seemed a wise precaution to Chisholm, whereas Rush rejected the policy as not only medically unjustified but as curtailing liberty and free trade (Haakonssen

25 It needs to be noted that the West Indies complicates the picture of American identity politics. Arner writes that "Americans contended not only with metropolitan relations, but also networks linking them to the Caribbean—a peripheral setting that presented another set of epistemological, as well as cultural and political relations to the new nation" (459).

26 His view was later backed by Gilbert Blane, an important figure in British naval medical reform, who speculated that the disease was imported into the Caribbean on board slave ships from West Africa (285). William Pym, a military surgeon who had been in medical charge during a yellow fever epidemic on Martinique, insisted—with Chisholm—that it be called 'Bulam fever' for its supposed origin (Pym).

214–16; Harrison, *Medicine* 261–62; Harrison, *Contagion* 55). Rush insisted on a more enlightened reaction, namely improving the drainage of marshy ground. Such improvements had also worked in Northern and Western Europe to curtail the plague there (Rush, "Facts").

In the 1810s no consensus on the question of contagiousness was reached in medical-military circles, and the controversy arose anew with yellow fever outbreaks in the United States (Mobile and New Orleans 1819, Savannah 1820) and on the coast of Spain in the 1820s (Barcelona 1821). French physician Étienne Pariset (a contagionist) entered the stage of yellow fever discourse in 1820 when he published his *Observations sur la fièvre jaune, faites à Cadiz, en 1819*. Pariset's book includes colored illustrations by Charles Philibert, Comte de Lasteyrie du Saillant (fig. 2). They are perhaps the first illustrations showing the early and late stages of yellow fever in color. Plate 2 (of four) emphasizes the patient's red face, bloodshot eyes and purple lips. Plate 4 shows the same young man in the final stages of yellow fever, bleeding, with black vomit. Jaundice is not noticeable in either plate. A staunch contagionist, Pariset points to the coincidence of the yellow fever appearances in the Caribbean, North America, and the Mediterranean. Consequently, he also saw France at risk and argued for a systematic quarantine to be effected (Mazet and Pariset i–ii, 96–97, 106–08, 123–24, 126–28).

Fig. 2. Plate 2 and Plate 4. Étienne Pariset and André Mazet, Observations sur la fièvre jaune, faites à Cadiz, en 1819. *Paris: Audot, Libraire, 1820. Illustration by Charles Philibert, Comte de Lasteyrie du Saillant. Wellcome Library, London.*

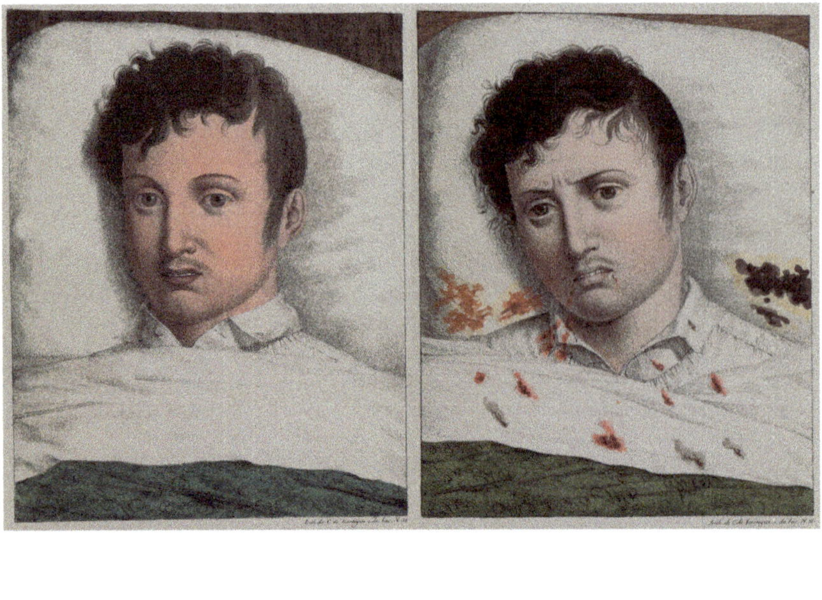

However, by the mid-1840s the sentiment had again changed toward a more trade-oriented paradigm, and although quarantine was not abolished in Great Britain it was much more leniently applied (see Harrison, "Disease, Diplomacy and International Commerce"; Harrison, *Contagion* 100). The strictness of quarantine remained a topic in the mid-nineteenth century American South, whose port cities remained most affected by yellow fever. The rigidity of quarantines varied with the level of public anxiety about the epidemic, and it significantly burdened Southern commerce and, in turn, commercial growth of the South, as historian Margaret Humphreys points out (*Yellow Fever* 8). Beginning in the 1840s and through the 1870s a belief in the germ theory of yellow fever, and thus in the transportability by some—yet unknown—agent, took hold among Southern physicians.[27] In the 1880s a scientifically based technological apparatus was first installed in Louisiana that enabled the large-scale disinfection of ships, trains and their cargo with gases (Humphreys, *Yellow Fever* 14).

Finally, it should be asserted that the need to control yellow fever was the main stimulus for the creation and development of public health institutions, most prominently the U.S. Public Health Service, in the nineteenth century (Humphreys, *Yellow Fever* 1).[28] Marine Hospital Service surgeon general John Woodworth reported to Congress on January 29, 1879, shortly after the worst yellow fever epidemic in U.S. history had declined: "Yellow fever should be dealt with as an enemy which imperils life and cripples commerce and industry. To no other great nation of the earth is yellow fever so calamitous as to the United States of America" (n.pag.). We are, in fact, dealing with an example of U.S. disease exceptionalism here. As a consequence, "yellow fever was the disease that inspired the most permanent public health reform in America" (Humphreys, "Appendix II" 192). On March 3, 1879, the National Board of Health (NBH) was created through an Act of Congress (Pierce and Writer 74). Humphreys cites a federal public health official, who—in 1897—still states that "it is only yellow fever whose shadow ever crosses our path, and is always a source of dread, a constant source of expense, and at once a danger to our people and an onerous

27 Southern physicians Benjamin B. Strobel (1840), John W. Monette (1842) and Wesley M. Carpenter (1844) supported the transmissablity of yellow fever (Humphreys, *Yellow Fever* 21, 27). A belief in the transportability doctrine was independently voiced by European authorities and based on several outbreaks in Gibraltar (1828), Saint-Nazaire (1861) and Swansea (1865) (Coleman).

28 The National Board of Health was created in 1879 in response to the biggest epidemiological catastrophe of the nineteenth century, the 1878 yellow fever epidemic that affected the Mississippi River Valley and killed up to 20,000 people.

burden upon commerce" (H.D. Geddings qtd. in "Appendix II" 192). It should also not be underestimated that the 'American' disease was conquered by a U.S. American team of military physicians, which, of course, rendered any quarantine equipment useless. The American discovery is noteworthy as it stands out against the European medical successes, such as Alphonse Laveran's discovery that the cause of malaria is a parasite (1880); Robert Koch's discovery of the causative agents of tuberculosis (1882), cholera (after Filippo Pacini) and anthrax (after Pollender, Rayer and Davaine); and Friedrich Loeffler's discoveries of the causes for diphtheria (1884).

1.6 Perspectivizing Yellow Fever Historiography and Literature

Several medical-historical studies on epidemics and yellow fever exist. John Harvey Powell's *Bring Out the Dead* is probably the earliest and most comprehensive historical study on the 1793 yellow fever epidemic in Philadelphia. The emotional pattern Powell lays bare in his book (first published in 1949) also informs *Yellow Fever Years*. Powell writes that an epidemic "is compounded not of disease alone, but of people's reaction to disease, how they recognize the pestilence, how they fear it or flee from it or fight it, how they are unnerved or gather resolution to conquer it" (26). In Philadelphia people "acquired the habits of living with fear," yet "[t]error and numb dismay overwhelmed people" who gave in to "a coarsening fear" (John Harvey Powell 46, 90). The endurance of Powell's argument is proven by Simon Finger who, in his history of Philadelphia from 1682 to the yellow fever outbreak of 1793, cites the disease as the "central fact of early national Philadelphia, touching every facet of society in the nation's capital (120).

J. Worth Estes and Billy G. Smith present a collection of essays on the public response to the 1793 epidemic with *A Melancholy Scene of Devastation* (1997). The themes tackled in the volume by some of the leading medical historians on yellow fever include the role of the newspapers, the role of the African American community and public health measures as well as the social, demographic and historiographic dimension of the epidemic. Estes and Smith also reprint Martin Pernick's influential 1972 article ("Politics, Parties, and Pestilence"). The timing of the epidemic and its location in the capital city denotes its national significance. With regard to Philadelphia Eve Kornfeld points out that "learning, manufactures, and human improvements of every kind thrive and flourish" (191). To this day countless publications search for meaning in the tragic events. In her appendix to Estes and Smith's volume, Susan E. Klepp points out "that this particular epidemic stands out in the collective memories of Americans" (176). That Klepp's assessment is accurate is a major argument of my first analytical chapter, in which

I trace the significance of the Philadelphia yellow fever epidemic as a case in point for the continued medical, historical and literary attention paid to it (ch. 2).

Andrew McIlwaine Bell's *Mosquito Soldiers* focuses on the environmental and biomedical factors as agents for historical change during the American Civil War. By the time the war broke out "yellow fever was a terrifying and mysterious southern disease that could appear out of thin air at any moment and wipe out an entire unacclimated brigade, division, or crew in a matter of weeks" (Bell 3). The anxiety was grounded in knowledge of the yellow fever epidemics that had ravaged Charleston, Galveston, Mobile, New Orleans, Norfolk, Savannah and other southern cities, particularly in the 1850s. Yet there was no unified central military response from Washington or elsewhere in how to treat yellow fever patients as medical science still disagreed about the etiology of the disease (Bell 34). While the Confederates might have hoped that yellow fever would act in their favor, they had to realize that it could work against their own troops as well. An insidious plan of distributing clothes previously worn by yellow fever patients was cooked up by Kentucky physician Luke Pryor Blackburn with the knowledge of high Confederate government officials. It was most probably carried out in Norfolk and New Bern in 1864. Although the outbreaks in North and South Carolina in fall 1864 cannot sufficiently be linked back to Blackburn's trunks of clothes, Bell concludes his brief analysis of the purportedly biological warfare episode by stating that "[b]y all appearances the Confederate government was willing to wage biological warfare, even at the risk of killing its own citizens, in order to secure southern independence" (109). Blackburn's plot was later turned into a novel by Dion Haco as *Dr. Blackburn: The Yellow Fever Fiend* (1866).

Medical-historical studies with a regional focus are able to analyze epidemics and the changes they induce in a limited space. Results may be applied to the larger experience. Jo Ann Carrigan's *The Saffron Scourge* on the history of yellow fever in Louisiana between 1796 and 1905 sheds light on the many outbreaks New Orleans suffered in the course of the nineteenth century (see also Carrigan, "Yellow Fever"). The largest city of the nineteenth-century South served as the principal port of entry for yellow fever, which arrived via ship from the Caribbean and Central America (Carrigan, *Saffron Scourge* 1). Carrigan takes the title of her study from the common epithet for yellow fever in the nineteenth century: the "scourge of the South" (Carrigan, *Saffron Scourge* 2). In a brief excursus Carrigan also looks at the cultural production the yellow fever epidemics stimulated. Her most elaborate example is *Doctor Dispachemquic: A Story of the Great Southern Plague of 1878* (1879), a satire with the typical elements of the genre (Dugan). The highly ironic narrative satirizes the attitudes and activities of so-called physicians and members of the benevolent associations. The telling names of the three protagonists already reveal the gist and attitudes of the story's main characters: the physicians Dr. Dispachemquic, Dr. Kwarentenus, and Dr. Kancurum. The first, a recent medical graduate from a distant state, i.e. the North, is employed by one of the benevolent associations and freely tests his scientific theories without any great regard for his patients, many of whom die. Dr. Kwarentenus promotes quarantine measures as a means of control and is otherwise Dispachemquic's friend, colleague, and mirror image. Dr. Kancurum, on the other hand, has studied yellow fever for years and is skillful in treating his patients. He argues for a training school for nurses and thus highlights the mostly inadequate medical education of the time and the conflicts resulting from competing medical systems. He furthermore criticizes the practice of some associations in hiring inexperienced nurses who are solely interested in the money or conceited members of female societies who merely visited the sick to bring them flowers. Carrigan interprets the satire as an argument for a solidified education and commitment of those entering the medical profession as physicians and as nurses (*Saffron Scourge* 357).

Besides Carrigan, several other historians have written regional histories of yellow fever. John Duffy's *Sword of Pestilence* also focuses on New Orleans by detailing the devastating 1853 epidemic, and Deanne Stephens Nuwer's *Plague Among the Magnolias* looks at the 1878 yellow fever epidemic in Mississippi. The 1878 epidemic is also the focus of Thomas H. Baker's article and Khaled J. Bloom's study. Shorter essays on the 1878 Memphis epidemic, the Virginia epidemic of 1855 and the South Carolina epidemic of 1877 have appeared in medical journals with a local history interest (Wright, "1878 Yellow Fever Epidemic"; Lewis and Lewis; Newsom). John H. Ellis's *Yellow Fever & Public Health in the New South* is like a companion piece to Margaret Humphreys' similar study with the same geographical focus on the U.S. South. While Ellis assesses the public health movement's early development from 1878 to 1888 by focusing on yellow fever experiences and reactions in urban southern centers (New Orleans, Memphis and Atlanta), Humphreys' book more broadly analyzes the ways in which yellow fever engaged the American South, its commercial and scientific communities, and its federal authorities which eventually formed public health boards in the late nineteenth century. Her research spans the time from the 1840s until the beginning of the twentieth century and presents a historiography of yellow fever and public health.

Mariola Espinosa's *Epidemic Invasions* (2009) is located at the nexus of disease and empire studies. With her focus on yellow fever in Cuba between 1878 and 1930, Espinosa shows that the disease, which had been endemic on the island probably since the seventeenth century when slave ships from Africa brought it there (2), had a decidedly different impact on Cuba than on the United States. Cubans did not suffer greatly from yellow fever, as most gained immunity through mild childhood infections, whereas the United States encountered it as a severe threat to commercial and military expansion into the Caribbean. The public health component and control of the disease was thus of much greater interest to the U.S. than to Cuba.

William Coleman's *Yellow Fever in the North* (1987) reveals the little known fact that yellow fever also reached continental Europe and Britain through trans-Atlantic commerce in the nineteenth century. By recounting three epidemics of yellow fever in Gibraltar (1828), Saint-Nazaire (1861), and Swansea (1865) his main aim is to shed light on the development of epidemiological methods such as case-tracing which had acquired a certain methodological autonomy by the 1860s.

The following three studies are crucial for my argument, not necessarily because of the historical narratives they tell but because they exemplify the continued applicability and functionality of yellow fever as a metaphor for diverse crises. John R. Pierce and Jim Writer's *Yellow Jack* (2005), Molly Caldwell Crosby's *The American Plague* (2006), and James L. Dickerson's *Yellow Fever: A Deadly Disease Poised to Kill Again* (2006) can be counted among the more popular historical studies. All three books were published in the mid-2000s, a time of social and military insecurity that could be easily applied to general fears about health. John R. Pierce and Jim Writer present American yellow fever history with a focus on Reed's discovery and end with a view on yellow fever today. Molly Caldwell Crosby's *The American Plague* is a journalistic account that picks up the yellow fever storyline with the 1878 epidemic in the Mississippi Valley, tells the medical detective story of Walter S. Reed and his team on Cuba and ends in the present-day United States with the discovery of the Asian tiger mosquito in Memphis and a visit to the Elmwood cemetery in Memphis, where many victims of the 1878 epidemic lie buried (Crosby 235–39). Crosby's book is remarkable for its rhetorical Americanization of the disease and reference to a storehouse of memory regarding yellow fever with her descriptions of memorial markers at Elmwood and elsewhere. Dickerson provides the most ambitious historical account by beginning with the 1793 Philadelphia epidemic and ending with three chapters that cash in on the culture of fear of the mid-2000s: "Weapons of Mass Destruction," "Global Warming Casts Ominous Shadow," and "The Disease That Won't Go Away" (Dickerson 187–252).

With *Epidemic Disease and Human Understanding: A Historical Analysis of Scientific and Other Writings* (2006), Charles De Paolo presents a survey of responses to epidemic disease spanning a period of over 2,500 years, from epidemic evidence in the first Book of Samuel (composed between 630–540 BCE) to the history of Ebola from 1976 into the twenty-first century. In his chapter on the Havana yellow fever epidemic of 1899–1900 he relies on memoirs (Moran) and letters of the involved parties and—like others before him—tells a fascinating 'detective story' with Major Walter Reed and his colleagues solving and thus successfully closing a long open case. The "other writings" De Paolo bases his yellow fever chapter on are limited to two renditions from the 1920s and 1930s: Firstly, Paul de Kruif's *Microbe Hunters* (1926) presents a version of the Reed story. Secondly, de Kruif turned his narrative into a play together with screenwriter Sidney Coe Howard. Their collaboration, entitled *Yellow Jack: A History*, heavily dramatizes the events. The play premiered on Broadway in 1934 with James Stewart in one of the leading roles. *Yellow Jack* was also turned into a major Hollywood movie in 1938, directed by George B. Seitz and starring Robert Montgomery, Virginia Bruce, and Charles Coburn (Seitz). As with the memoirs De Paolo analyzes, his focus with the plays and the movie is on representations of yellow fever that are produced after the discovery of transmission and thus after contemporary representations of yellow fever that have an imaginative quality regarding the disease. The fictitious and factitious accounts De Paolo engages with are more representative of the time of their production (late 1920s until late 1930s United States and the time of the Great Depression) than of the immediate cultural representation and imagination of the disease in the late eighteenth and nineteenth century I am interested in.

Robert S. Desowitz asks "Who Gave Pinta to the *Santa Maria*?" in his study of tropical diseases, which he defines as "Anglo-American as the heart attack" (11). The book's chronological focus is as broad in focus as that of De Paolo, yet Desowitz focuses almost exclusively on the so-called New World and on colonial interdependencies regarding diseases; his actual discussion of yellow fever from 1885–1900 is rather limited.

In *Disease and the Novel* (1985) Jeffrey Meyers has analyzed fictional writings from 1880 until 1960 from a comparatist's perspective, mostly focusing on tuberculosis. Analyzing works from Leo Tolstoy, Thomas Mann, and Ernest Hemingway, he contends that "[d]isease has always been a great mystery: a visitation, a curse, a judgement" (Meyers 2). Detailed medical and (pseudo)scientific descriptions of diseases and psychological conditions entered the realm of mainly naturalist fiction writing at the end of the nineteenth century together with major advances in scientific medicine (Herzlich and Pierret 29). Similar to Meyers only in the fact that she is not concerned with epidemic occurrences of disease or yellow fever in particular, Cynthia J. Davis in *Bodily and Narrative Forms* (2000) investigates the influence of medicine on American literature (1845–1915) in light of the emerging germ theory. In her literary case studies Davis analyzes narrative structures as sites of bodily representations. What I take from Davis in my study is related to her understanding of form "to indicate that I am addressing not just what a story means but how it works, how it is structured" (C. J. Davis 4).

With *Contagious* (2008), Priscilla Wald has defined what she calls outbreak narrative as a literary form that systemizes “individuals, groups, populations, locales (regional and global), behaviors and lifestyles” (*Contagious* 3). Immunity as well as susceptibility to diseases are used to imagine and bind communities together, and outbreak narratives make these processes visible. Wald’s biomedical framework enables us to discover “imagined immunities” (*Contagious* 29–67) as stabilizing factors and to question and critique the politics of nationhood and nationalistic discourse that enable them. The threat of epidemics actually triggers those nationalist impulses. What Wald has formulated, mainly with regard to the twentieth and twenty-first century, seems equally applicable to the nineteenth and will be tested in *Yellow Fever Years*, although I will not speak of outbreak narratives with reference to the narratives I will be looking at because the formulas seem not to follow as clear a path as charted by Wald.

Despite these numerous medical-historical and partly literary studies on epidemic diseases and yellow fever in particular, so far no scientific study has been concerned with the relationship of historical yellow fever epidemics, their literary representation in a previously inaccessible body of writing, and the political and social conditions from the late eighteenth to the beginning of the twentieth century. Joann P. Krieg’s chapter “The American Plague” in her book *Epidemics in the Modern World* (1992) comes closest to this approach. Her discussion is limited to a single chapter that focuses on the 1790s, while *Yellow Fever Years* takes a broader view beginning in that period, spanning the whole nineteenth century and concluding at the beginning of the twentieth century. This enables me to draw comparative conclusions about the negotiation of the disease at the end of the eighteenth century and the second half of the nineteenth century. I attempt to rectify a dearth of attention given to race in relation with yellow fever in chapter 5 of this study.[29]

The literary history of disease or plague narratives probably dates back to Thucydides’ description of the plague that killed Pericles and many other Athenians during the Peloponnesian War (430 BCE) (Thucydides 97–101). Biblical writing and the *Iliad* have used disease as symbol for divine providence. The tales in Giovanni Boccaccio’s *Decamerone* (1353) are told after the flight from plague-ridden Florence, and Daniel Defoe’s *Journal of the Plague Year* (1722) is a historical novel about the Great Plague of London in 1665. On the North American continent John Winthrop introduced a rhetoric of infection

29 With regard to yellow fever and race Kiple and Kiple; Kiple; and Watts have specifically taken up the issue of black immunity.

as part of his justification narrative by describing the epidemics that decimated the Native American population between 1616 and 1619 as follows: "God hath consumed the natives with a miraculous plague, whereby the greater part of the country is left voide of inhabitants" (Winthrop 120). Winthrop's account is echoed by Edward Johnson, who observed that the epidemics in New England created "roome" for English settlers (17). Edwards also justified their endeavor with the connection between migration and providence. Cristobal Silva comments that

> [e]pidemics certainly facilitated settlement in New England, but as important as these effects were, the seventeenth-century colonial justification narratives that described diseases rendered them legible to English audiences by providing settlers with the language through which to understand and legitimate their migration. (Silva 26)

Especially in the early eighteenth-century, the writings surrounding the Boston smallpox inoculation debate come to mind (Cotton Mather, Zabdiel Boylston, Otho Beall and Richard Shryock) (see Priewe 303–15; Silverman). From the nineteenth century on several American plague narratives appear, beginning with the literary representations of the 1793 yellow fever epidemic in Philadelphia, Charles Brockden Brown's *Arthur Mervyn* (1799/1800). The list might be followed by Edgar Allan Poe's short story "The Masque of the Red Death" (1842), and Herman Melville's *Redburn: His First Voyage* (1849).

The impact the Philadelphia yellow fever epidemic of 1793 had on literary production is particularly striking. Besides Brown, Philip Freneau's "Pestilence: Written during the Prevalence of a Yellow Fever" (1793), John Searson's "Mount Vernon: A Poem…" (1800), and Henry Wadsworth Longfellow's *Evangeline: A Tale of Acadie* (1847) took up and reflected on the devastating event. The poetological discourses are equally tied to the yellow fever epidemics as the political ones that find their expression in, for example, ideology of the purity of the Anglo-Saxon race, or the Alien and Sedition Acts (1798), a legislative package aimed to protect the young nation against spies and unwelcome strangers.

Textual representations of the later nineteenth-century include Wesley Bradshaw's (aka Charles Wesley Alexander) *Angel Agnes* (1873); George Washington Cable's *The Grandissimes* (1879); Elizabeth Stuart Phelps's "Zerviah Hope" (1880), Mollie Davis's novel *The Queen's Garden* (1900), Roland Williamson's short story "Uncle Phil," collected in *The Star Well, and Other Stories* (1916); William Wells Brown in *Clotel; or, The President's Daughter: A Narrative of Slave Life in the United States* (1853) also inserts a brief yellow fever episode. J. F. Simmons's *The Welded Link and Other Poems* (1881) contains several poems that thematically employ the yellow fever epidemic of 1878/1879 in the lower Mississippi

Valley, especially Memphis. A judge in Memphis, J. F. Simmons negotiates the devastating yellow fever epidemic of 1878 as he experienced it in his collection of poetry entitled *The Welded Link and Other Poems* (1881). The longest of the poems, "Evening Meditations," was written during the fall of 1878, at the high point of the epidemic, when yellow fever—as Simmons writes in his preface—"to a certain extent isolated us from the world abroad" (14). Yet Simmons first and foremost claims that northern generosity and kindness toward the South in 1878 accomplished "what arms never could have done. It conquered the Southern people and the Southern heart" (Simmons 14). Simmons expressed a common feeling, that the epidemic and Northern help managed—at least temporarily—to soften the Southern bitterness left after the war and the years of reconstruction (Carrigan, *Saffron Scourge* 357). The poem "The Phantom-Train" refers to a train (Memphis, Grenada, Hernando, Horn Lake, Senatobia, Garner) that was constantly employed during the epidemic in Memphis to convey contributions and nurses to the stricken villages, but it was only allowed to stop at quarantine stations. Yellow fever is equated with the "storms" in "The Storm-Beaten Barque," and "I am Ready" describes the yellow fever alarm in Sardis, 5 September 1878. "A Brave but Sad Martyrdom" is an elegy to Reverend F.M. Howell who died of yellow fever at Somerville, Tennessee on 21 October 1878. American journalist Richard Harding Davis published his comedy/farce *The Dictator* in 1904. Set in an imaginary Central American country, the protagonist Brooke Travers, alias 'Steve' Hill, finds himself replacing the nation's dictator. He accepts life under the constant threat of yellow fever at Porto Banos—a "fever swamp"—which he prefers to being "hanged" (Richard Harding Davis 10, 42). The farcical character of the play becomes more than apparent when Hill initiates a revolution and eventually rescues the heroine Juanita.

Yellow fever is reflected in a variety of forms extending beyond the fictionalized, lyrical, and dramatic accounts mentioned hitherto. Far from creating a totalizing effect of categorization, the variety of cultural production pertaining to yellow fever will be illuminated by example in a chapter on visual representations. In *Disease and Representation* Sander Gilman argues that the iconography of an illness shows how societies perceive and conceptualize disease, how a disease and sick patients are treated by others. He writes,

> The portrait of the sufferer, the portrait of the patient, is therefore the image of disease anthropomorphized. [...] [T]he image of all disease, the very face of the patient, is a continuous one, and through a study of its continuities comes a sense of the interrelationship of all our projected fears of collapse. This continuity, however, reflects changing functions that the image of disease has within an age's or an individual's overall sense of control. In some cases, the fearful is made harmless through being made comic; in some cases it

> looms as a threat, controlled only by being made visible. How we see the diseased, the mad, the polluting is a reflex of our own sense of control and the limits inherent in that sense of control. (Gilman 2–3)

"Displaying Disease: Yellow Fever Visualized," the chronologically most expansive and inclusive chapter (in that it covers the whole of the nineteenth century), sheds light on the vast field of yellow fever production in lithographs and illustrated newspapers, and photography. The act of making visible what needs to be controlled will be a major focus in this chapter.

The newly emerging art and technology of photography in the nineteenth century represents a striking resemblance and connection to the process of a medicalization of society. I am not only thinking in terms of the clinical and photographic gaze that often served medical practitioners with the help of photographers to frame deviant or diseased bodies, but also in terms of medical language as applied to the photographic process. As Tanya Sheehan in her study on the medicine of photography in the nineteenth-century points out, "photographic negatives were often said to contract 'a sort of leprous disease,' to develop 'Yellow Fever,' or to become afflicted with the dreaded 'green fog,' once dubbed 'the measles of photographic childhood'" (Sheehan 119; "The Open Corner" 20). Mass communication via visual media started through the technologies developed in the nineteenth century. With it "[i]conographic representations of health, illness and disease have become more important," Deborah Lupton rightfully observes (75). As a powerful means of communication, especially photographs can be "realizations and instantiations of ideology" (Kress and van Leeuwen 14) that serve political purposes.

While they will not be the sole focus of this book, quite a number of texts with a specific yellow fever-theme have been published in the United States since the 1980s. They speak to the continued efficacy and potential of a collective yellow fever memory in U.S. history. Many of the historical neo-realist novels cater toward young, mostly female readers or fall into the category of fiction for 'young readers.' The commercially most successful novel among them is probably Laurie Halse Anderson's *Fever, 1793* (2000). In the typical coming-of-age narrative set during the 1793 Philadelphia yellow fever epidemic, the sixteen-year-old protagonist Matilda Cook is separated from her sick mother and forced to cope with the crisis. Also set during the Philadelphia epidemic, Paul Fleischman's young readers' novel *Path of the Pale Horse* (1983) merely borrows the idea of a story around a doctor's apprentice from Charles Brockden Brown's *Arthur Mervyn* (1799/1800). In Fleischman's novel the fourteen-year-old Lep is apprenticed to Dr. Peale in fulfillment of the wish of his late father for his son to become a physician. When yellow fever breaks out in Philadelphia Lep helps his master take care of the victims.

Two of Denise Patrick's popular and heavily didactic Cécile novels are set during the devastating 1853 New Orleans yellow fever epidemic. The series is part of the long-time-running American Girls Collection. The series' protagonist, Cécile grows up in an affluent black New Orleans family and witnesses the epidemic hitting home when her older brother falls sick in *Troubles for Cécile* (2011). The sequel, *Cécile's Gift* (2011), is set in the aftermath of the epidemic. Cécile and her white friend Marie-Grace (the title heroine of another interwoven series) become volunteers in an asylum for yellow fever orphans. The asylum plot is continued and sporadically paralleled in another American Girls Collection series centering on Marie-Grace. In Sarah Buckey's *Marie-Grace and the Orphans* (2011) the protagonist disobeys her physician father and stays in the disease-ridden city. He, meanwhile, is swamped with yellow fever cases. Marie-Grace stays in the city and first saves her music teacher and later takes care of an orphaned infant. Also set in New Orleans, Josh Russell in his novel *Yellow Jack* (1999) combines the almost constant threat of yellow fever epidemics in the 1840s with the technological innovation of photography. The protagonist is a French daguerrotypist called Claude Marchand who profits from the epidemic by taking memorial pictures of the dead. A quite stereotypical image of mid-nineteenth-century New Orleans is conjured up with a hero who is racially and sexually entangled in a love triangle plot. Two women vie for Marchand's affections: the wealthy daughter of a prominent New Orleans family and an octoroon who uses voodoo.

Another set of novels focuses on the 1878 epidemic in Memphis and environs during which about twenty thousand people, or 10 percent of the population, died in the lower Mississippi Valley. Anna Myers' *Graveyard Girl* (1995) is the story of three young teenagers in yellow-fever-devastated Memphis. Eli has lost his mother and sister to the disease and his grieving father has fled the city without him. He befriends orphaned Addie and—in a magical realist twist—both are haunted by the ghosts of their loved ones. The title-giving character, angelic Grace tries to help both of them. Referred to as the Graveyard Girl, she tolls the bell for each dead soul in the graveyard. Diana Brown's novel *The Hand of a Woman* (1984) opens in New York City during the Civil War and culminates with the decline of the Memphis epidemic. It chronicles the life of impoverished and partly black Damaris Fanshawe who aspires to become a medical doctor despite the odds. In fact, she moves from nursemaid, to outcast, to nun, to become a physician.

While recurring outbreaks affected the Eastern seaboard of the United States in the nineteenth century, yellow fever posed a constant threat to those venturing to and from the West Indies. At least two recent novels take on the formulas of the seas, recreating the fact that the United States used to be much more dependent on the sea as a means of transportation, with all the inherent dangers this included. Bodie Thoene's *Winds of Promise* (1997), an adventure tale in the true vein of sensation fiction with religious overtones, follows the impulsive steamer pilot Rafer Maddox on his eighteen thousand mile journey from New York around the Horn to California where the Gold Rush is just erupting. The steamer, significantly called the *New World*, is in danger of being pursued and the crew suffers from the perils of yellow fever even before they round the Horn and encounter a corrupt ring of thievery. In *Ransome's Crossing* (2010), the second book in the highly sentimental Ransome trilogy by Kaye Dacus, readers follow the protagonist Charlotte Ransome across the Atlantic to Jamaica, where her secret fiancé awaits her. Disguised as a midshipman as part of her brother William Ransome's crew, she falls sick with yellow fever and her identity is discovered. She is cared for by her brother's young wife Julia and by first officer Ned Cochran. Her illness and his affections only temporarily complicate the marriage plot. Sally Armstrong bases her historical novel *The Nine Lives of Charlotte Taylor* (2007) on the life of her great-great-great-grandmother. Twenty year-old pregnant Charlotte Taylor is stranded in Jamaica after losing her black lover, the family's butler, to yellow fever soon after their arrival from England. Allying herself with a naval commodore, she reaches British North America and finds refuge with the Mi'kmaq tribe, where she gives birth to her child. In a blend of fact and fiction readers follow Charlotte Taylor who marries three times and has nine more children as well as a lifelong relationship with an aboriginal man.

In *A Separate Country* (2009) Robert Hicks fictionalizes the post-Civil War life of ex-Confederate general John Bell Hood and his battle with yellow fever in New Orleans. William Waring even puts the disease into the title of his novel *Yellow Fever: The Slave's Revenge* (1994). Yellow fever epidemics in the late 1800s and early 1900s also function as plot devices in Susan Kohl's *The Ghost of Gracie Mansion* (1999) and in Melissa Forney's *The Astonishing Journey of Teddy Bodain* (2009). In the former, a New York epidemic decides the fate of Esther and Archibald Gracie who move their family from Manhattan to their country home. *The Astonishing Journey of Teddy Bodain* is the story of an eleven-year-old girl who is separated from her parents during the 1792 Florida outbreak.

Set only one year later during the Philadelphia epidemic, John Edgar Wideman's yellow fever fiction certainly does not fall into the category of popular historical or young adult fiction of the novels previously discussed. I am particularly referring to Wideman's short story "Fever" (1989) (cf. Gysin) and his novel *The Cattle Killing* (1996). In *The Cattle Killing*, a novel about the Xhosa cattle killing in South Africa in the 1850s, the Philadelphia yellow fever epidemic of

1793 serves as an archetypal situation of black-white relations that is applicable throughout United States history (Eschborn 18–19). Wideman frames the Philadelphia yellow fever epidemic as "historical metaphor" of African American experiences of oppression. Ulrich Eschborn explains:

> African-American workers rendered Philadelphia a valuable service during the yellow fever epidemic, but, instead of being rewarded, they were later accused of having taken advantage of helpless infected white people. Wideman interprets this constellation as a situation characterizing the black-white relationship in American history: African-Americans wanted to support the nation and become part of it but were rejected and denied the treatment as equals because of racist prejudice on account of their skin color. The historical metaphors in Wideman's texts transcend the narrow limits of their place and time and refer to the whole nation and American history in general. (19)

Despite the services rendered by African Americans during the epidemic, their situation does not improve in the aftermath of the epidemic.

While acknowledging the obvious differences between primarily didactic, popular sensation, and sentimental novels and John Edgar Wideman's critical postcolonialist stance, it needs to be noted that the locations in which many of the yellow fever discourses take place—namely Philadelphia, New Orleans, Memphis, and the Caribbean—are similar, if not identical, in the late twentieth and twenty-first century accounts as well as in those of the nineteenth century. While this might not be surprising as the places most affected and devastated during recurring epidemics also feature most prominently in the contemporary nineteenth-century accounts, it also documents the creation and existence of a collective disease memory, a storehouse of yellow fever experiences, tapped and re-fictionalized by authors of the late twentieth and twenty-first century (cf. Tompkins xvi; see also Fisher 3). Furthermore the connection of race, racial identity and disease, as well as the role of women are themes that remain present in yellow fever fiction from the eighteenth to the twenty-first century. The twenty and twenty-first century texts have the potential to wholly demystify the representation of yellow fever. While mostly presenting historically accurate accounts and introducing characters that do not know about the origin or prevention of the disease, these texts are written after the discovery of the vector of disease transmission and make use of the storehouse of yellow fever memory. They shed as much light on the respective yellow fever experience as on the events surrounding their time of production.

2 Yellow Fever in 1793—A Case in Point: Resolving Crises and Building the Nation

2.1 Introducing Yellow Fever in 1793

The relation of fiction to the building of a nation is often based on Benedict Anderson's "imagined communities." Recently, both Samuel Otter and Carroll Smith-Rosenberg have exemplified the workings of fiction on the formulation of nationalism by analyzing works by Charles Brockden Brown. In *Arthur Mervyn* and *Edgar Huntly* fiction becomes "a carrier zone for the nation" (Samuels, *Reading the Novel* 96). Smith-Rosenberg sees the national project being carried out in the struggle of the lost white man in the wilderness that is depicted in *Edgar Huntly* (*This Violent Empire*). Otter, on the other hand, reads Philadelphia, the nation's capital at the time, as a microcosm of the national project, "a laboratory for testing character and evaluating freedom, in which 'race' is seen as crucial" (66). It was "the first great national American epidemic" (Dine 431). I follow in Otter's footsteps when analyzing *Arthur Mervyn* as a nation-building narrative in this chapter. The Philadelphia yellow fever epidemic—that is so central in Brown's narrative—serves as a case in point on how to control and overcome a crisis and solidify the nation (cf. Gessner, "Contagion, Crisis, and Control"). Mathew Carey's *Short Account of the Malignant Fever, Lately Prevalent in Philadelphia* (1793) and Richard Allen and Absalom Jones's *Narrative of the Proceedings of the Black People during the Late Awful Calamity in Philadelphia in the Year 1793* (1794) can be read in the same vein and will equally be treated in this chapter. The fact that the yellow fever crisis and the need of an interpretation of what the nation should and would look like came together in 1793 in Philadelphia might explain why it remains the epidemic most written about in the city's history (Otter 28).

Between July and November 1793 about four to five thousand Philadelphia residents, approximately ten percent of the capital city's population, died of yellow fever. Many more left the city for a temporary home in the country. Among them were Alexander Hamilton and his wife, and Matthew Carey, who published his *Short Account of the Malignant Fever* shortly after his return to the city in November 1793. Carey estimated that 17,000 fled the city (*Short Account* 77). Altogether Carey published six versions of his *Short Account* between 1793 and 1830. All later editions included meticulous revisions in response to criticism voiced particularly with regard to the role of African Americans during the epidemic. Benjamin Rush, a physician and signatory to the Declaration of Independence, stayed in the city. He became highly regarded after issuing guidelines for avoiding infection and helping to set up a fever hospital for victims. However, Rush, who believed in the innate immunity of people of African descent, also had to stand corrected on this issue, thus complicating his role as benefactor. Rush wrote about his experience in letters and medical essays and—most prominently—in his *Account of the Bilious Remitting Fever*. He later justified his actions during the 1793 and 1797 yellow fever epidemics in his autobiography *Travels through Life*. Alongside these medical and historical accounts, Charles Brockden Brown's gothic novel *Arthur Mervyn, or, Memoirs of the Year 1793* (1799/1800) probably provides one of the most thorough literary portrayals of the Philadelphia epidemic. I will address his and other evocative narratives, letters, and accounts of the epidemic in terms of their spatial dialectic between the rural and the urban, and their significance in a period heavily involved in building the nation against threats from within and without (see also Gessner, "Spatial Dialectics").

In addition to Brown's novel, Matthew Carey's *Short Account* and Richard Allen and Absalom Jones's *Narrative of the Proceedings of the Black People* (1794) will be considered as blueprints setting the stage for the spaces functionalized in the fictional text.[30] Yellow fever provides a dramatic setting for Brown's *Arthur Mervyn* and represents the complex experience of crisis the young nation was facing. It "becomes symbolic of a society out of joint [...] a fitting metaphor for expressing this state of flux and this fear" (61; 63), as Gesa Mackenthun has argued. The "epidemic of fear" (Pernick, "Contagion" 861)—the rumors Arthur Mervyn picks up in rural Pennsylvania—precedes his actual experience of the disease. The ideological and spatial dialectic of city versus country serve as structural device and means to control the epidemic and thus stabilize the nation. Ties between country and city were not completely severed, so that, for example, the contagiousness of fear and actual infection also reached the countryside.

With his narrative of the yellow fever epidemic Brown constructs a representation for a culture of fear, but also offers a way of interpreting and controlling what seems incomprehensible. With his novel he questions existing social power structures, inherent in the practice of slavery, and puts forward an alternative vision for a nation eagerly trying to define itself against threats from within and without.

---

30 The exchange between Carey and Jones and Allen has been recognized for its "development of an early national literature" (Otter 28) in recent scholarship (see Lapsanksy 61–78; Stern 219–23; Gould 157–86; Brooks 151–78).

2.2 Infecting the Nation: Charles Brockden Brown's *Arthur Mervyn, or, Memoirs of the Year 1793* (1799/1800)

The Evils of pestilence by which this city has lately been afflicted will probably form an era in its history.

Charles Brockden Brown, *Arthur Mervyn* (1799/1800)

Brown's *Arthur Mervyn*, a gothic novel in the true vein of social critique, was published in two parts in 1799 and 1800 respectively. Choosing the gothic form in this period served to address unprivileged readers because it "questioned the rules of rationalism that, for those in power, conveniently ordered their interest and their status" (Davidson 335). In what Brown calls a "brief but faithful sketch" his observations provide an "instructive" model of "benevolence" and "virtue" for his readers to copy (3).[31] In *Arthur Mervyn*, yellow fever, which had befallen the city in 1793 after a hiatus of some 30 years, provides a dramatic setting and metaphorically represents the complex experience of crisis and transformation the young nation was facing. Gesa Mackenthun refers to the representation of disease as "symbolic of a society out of joint" and a fitting metaphor for expressing this state of flux and this fear" (61; 63). Samuel Otter similarly points out that Brown has turned "his novel into a metonymy of the epidemic" (29). Yellow fever also has a de-hierarchizing function and provided Brown with an opportunity to present himself as historiographer. Instead of interpreting the epidemic outbreak of yellow fever in Philadelphia through a Puritan lens as God's punishment and a transgression of the perceived purity of the body, as one may have done in the seventeenth century, Brown fictionally explores the epidemic from the perspective of the Enlightenment. His fascination with medical and scientific discoveries already becomes apparent in his preface, where he introduces his rational approach, stating that he "has ventured to methodize his own reflections" upon the "medical and political discussions which are now afloat in the community" (*AM* 3), referring to a wealth of written and oral material, of which his novel is only a part (Waterman, "Arthur Mervyn's" 216). Brown proposes to engage the discussions in a two-fold manner: first, he wants to present a morality tale, and second, he uses the medical knowledge and political discourse available to him at the time in his fictional account in order to offer a means of control in the face of a medical and also socio-political crisis of the 1790s. Especially the latter crisis was played out on the field of the dichotomy between the rural and the urban.

31 In the following, for simplicity's sake, I will use *AM* for *Arthur Mervyn, or, Memoirs of the Year 1793.*

Jeffersonian Republican Democrats argued for a rural lifestyle, while Federalists upheld a general need for cities, which, however, required better protection from outside influences.

In 1793, without concrete medical evidence or knowledge of the Pasteurian germ theory that emerged over half a century later, debates around the origin of the fever were almost instantaneously politicized: a xenophobic contagionist school saw the origin in infected products imported to the city and thus in ship passengers of French and African origin (Pernick, "Politics, Parties, and Pestilence" 568; see also J. H. Powell 16). Beyond the social and economic catastrophe yellow fever created, it "acquired the status of a powerful metaphor [...]. [It] increasingly served a rhetorical purpose within the political debates between Jefferson's Democratic Republicans on the one hand and Alexander Hamilton's Federalists on the other" (Mackenthun 53–54; see also Arner). Federalists in particular used the disease to express anti-Republican ideas and blame the epidemic on French revolutionaries. They declared a need to isolate America from the revolutionary 'contagions' that—in the trans-Atlantic and global reverberations of the French Revolution—had passed from France to the West Indies and were about to spread to the United States. Hamiltonian Federalists argued for the exclusion of French immigrants in order to quench revolutionary sympathies. A growing xenophobia was mainly directed against the refugees who fled to Philadelphia in the wake of the slave uprising on the island of St. Domingue in the summer of 1793. "Epidemic disease," writes historian Mark Harrison, "was synonymous with disorder and the importation of alien maladies was feared for much the same reasons as 'alien' revolutionary ideas" (*Medicine* 264–65). The age-old anxiety over foreign bodies as carriers of disease was translated into a Federalist political imperative of greater security of the United States' national borders.

This policy was heavily opposed by Republicans and many of the city's merchants as they feared a curtailment of their profitable trade with the Caribbean. They sided with a miasmatic, environmentalist school which argued against the fever's transportability and believed in the domestic origin of the disease due to poor urban sanitation and hygiene. The latter theory served a Jeffersonian Democratic Republican rhetoric of separation of city versus country. Already William Penn had warned his wife, "of Citys and towns of concourse beware... a country life and estate I like best for my children" (qtd. in Clarkson 316–17). And Noah Webster also shares the view, when asking: "Why should cities be erected, if they are only to be the tombs of men?" (*Collection of Papers on the Subject of Bilious Fevers* 208). Thomas Jefferson believed that social health required a rural lifestyle and wrote to Benjamin Rush:

> The yellow fever will discourage the growth of great cities in our nation & I view great cities as pestilential to the morals, the health and the liberties of man. True, they nourish some of the elegant arts, but the useful ones can thrive elsewhere, and less perfection in the others, with more health, virtue & freedom, would be my choice (qtd. in White and White 17).

He planned a checkerboard development and wanted to reduce population density by providing trees which in turn would provide country-like fresh air amidst urban settings. Jefferson's plan was mainly prompted by the experience of the Philadelphia epidemics in the 1790s; he promoted his outline as "the best means of preserving the cities of America from the scourge of yellow fever" (qtd. in White and White 28–29).

It should, however, be pointed out that the correlation of contagionists and non-contagionists to a specific partisan affiliation is more complicated than this model of historian Martin Pernick suggests. Physicians of the 'Friendly Club' with whom Brown was associated supported the, at the time, more progressive view of non-contagionism (see also Waterman, "Arthur Mervyn's" 219–20). The physicians of the club were connected to allies in other parts of the country. For example, the New York-based Noah Webster chronicled the disease in his newspaper, the *Commercial Daily Advertiser*, and in his *Brief History of Epidemic and Pestilential Diseases…* (1799), in which he pointed out the threat and the meaning of the disease for the nation (see also Arner 453). Dr. Elihu Hubbard Smith, a physician and poet from New York City and a mentor and close friend of Brown's as well as a member of the 'Friendly Club,' equally adhered to the Republican local-origin theory. When Brown visited his friend in the Pine Street neighborhood in the summer of 1798, both contracted yellow fever, which was sweeping through New York City at that time. While Smith died, Brown survived and, deeply affected by the epidemic, turned his experience also into a tribute to his friend, the novel *Arthur Mervyn*. It was already in print less than one year later (May 1799). Although Smith and another friend of Brown's, Benjamin Rush, were Jeffersonian Democratic Republicans, not all members of the club and Brown's circle shared this affiliation; some were closer to a Federalist stance in political terms. It also needs to be pointed out that the miasma theory supported the idea of a home-grown plague, which in turn contradicted the patriotic image of a young and healthy nation. Rush's main adversary, the physician William Currie, a contagionist, argued for retirement to the country in times of disease:

> It is well known that all who shut themselves up in their houses, retired into the country, and shunned every substance which had been in contact or near to those actually infected, and that everyone who observed these precautions, though daily abroad in the open streets and markets, escaped the disease. (Currie 10)

Given today's knowledge we know that both scientific schools were somewhat correct. Contrary to the widely held medical opinion of the time, the Philadelphia epidemic was most probably introduced through French refugees from Haiti/St. Domingue (Patterson 856), a circumstance which would have confirmed the Federalist hypothesis. In Philadelphia mosquitoes who fed on the sick refugees would spread the disease among locals. Yellow fever is a primarily urban disease because it did not spread easily in rural areas where neither human nor mosquito populations were sufficiently concentrated to induce an epidemic (Carrigan, *Saffron Scourge* 1). In North America it was referred to as 'West-India' or 'American yellow fever' and was also categorized as one of "our epidemics" in the late eighteenth century (Rush, "Facts" 156; Caldwell, *A Reply to Dr. Haygarth's Letter* 16; cf. Arner 458).

Brown's novel includes speculations both that the disease was of domestic miasmatic origin, as Brown's circle, including his friend Benjamin Rush, proposed, and that it was a menace from abroad. The character Vincentio Lodi, for example, brings both money and fever from Guadeloupe. The villain Welbeck meets Lodi, who has contracted "a violent disease [...] in the tropical islands" in chapter 10 (*AM* 72). This is also the first time "Yellow or Malignant Fever" is identified by name (*AM* 72). Mervyn's tale, however, begins with the story of his sad boyhood in rural Pennsylvania. His journeys, as Shirley Samuels contends, also "tend to be rural" (Samuels, *Reading the Novel* 111). And Emory Elliott states that "on first examination the story appears to present the struggle of a virtuous country boy against the corruption of the city" (*Revolutionary Writers* 235). Mervyn is driven out of his family's country home by his father's widow and sets out for Philadelphia in pursuit of education and the wealth he hopes to find in the city.[32] While the stepmother is the main reason for his departure, Louis Kirk McAuley furthermore points out that the father, i.e. the family farm, is not able to support another inhabitant. The inability of Mervyn's father to pay his son for his work on the farm reflects "shifting American values: a revolution towards commercial enterprise and away from agriculture" (McAuley 319–20). En route to Philadelphia, Mervyn encounters wagons traveling from the city—only to learn upon his arrival that yellow fever has struck there. Once in the city, Mervyn falls prey to a swindler, loses his clothing and money, and—in this dire situation—is hired by the apparently wealthy Thomas Welbeck to copy what turns out to be a stolen manuscript.

32 As in many early American novels we find the theme of displacement from home and confinement in what in Arthur Mervyn's case is represented in the maze of the city of Philadelphia.

He thus symbolically exchanges the plough for the pen. Yet, Mervyn's preference for the country and his proposed return remains a leitmotif in the first part of the novel: "I saw that the city was no place for me. [...] [A]nd my ancient occupations rose to my view enhanced by a thousand imaginary charms, I resolved forthwith to strike into the country" (*AM* 36). When young Mervyn finally realizes the criminal activities of his employer, including murder and fraud, he flees the city fearing his own demise.

Mervyn's experience of corrupted morals and yellow fever in the city leads him to develop a theory of an outside origin of the disease, which is later contradicted by the enlightened Quaker and physician Medlicote:

> He combated an opinion I had casually formed respecting the origin of the epidemic, and imputed it not to infected substances imported from East or West, but to a morbid constitution of the atmosphere, owing wholly or in part to filthy streets, airless habitations, and squalid persons. (*AM* 123)

In chapter 8 the atmosphere and unbearable heat already serve to foreshadow the fever scenes and hint at environmental causes of the disease: "The air was remarkably sultry. Lifted sashes and lofty ceilings were insufficient to attemper it. The perturbation of my thoughts affected my body, and the heat which oppressed me was aggravated, by my restlessness, almost into fever" (*AM* 58). The "contagious atmosphere" (*AM* 153) or "an atmosphere so contagious and deadly" (*AM* 133) remains a theme throughout the section of the novel that narrativizes the yellow fever epidemic in the first part of the novel. The effect is enhanced by Brown's hasty writing habit which Mackenthun aptly describes as "feverish" (67).

Although Brown includes contagionist and non-contagionist speculations about the fever's origin, he primarily constructs yellow fever as "a symbol for social crisis" (Grabo 103): yellow fever, along with commercial corruption and the slave trade, is spreading from within. The "spirit of materialism" sweeps Philadelphia "like the contagion of yellow fever" (Davidson 314). In this sense, I follow symbolic-figurative interpretations of the disease that entail consequences for the treatment of the real and the figurative disease(s). The symbolic reading of disease as 'national allegory' (cf. Jameson) and fever as social allegory has been put forward by several critics—Robert Levine, Jane Tompkins, Shirley Samuels, Julia Stern, and Philip Gould—who have linked 'contagion' to "the French Revolution, [...] the Alien and Sedition Acts, the rise of a market economy, patriarchal anxieties, and a breakdown of fellow feeling in the highly partisan Federal era" (Waterman, "Arthur Mervyn's" 219; see also Waterman, *Republic of Intellect* 189–230). Otter adds interpretations of the fever as "irrationality, sympathy, conspiracy, egocentrism, revolution (American, French, Haitan), sexual anxiety, market economy, and rascism" (60). Louis Kirk McAuley furthermore argues for reading yellow fever as a metaphor for the impact of print—that is, a booming partisan publication culture of the 1790s—upon the body politic (311). This would then demonstrate Brown's anxiety—although he and his protagonist Mervyn were participants and beneficiaries of the print culture as well—regarding an uninhibited and contagious print system that followed a technological revolution in America, an early example of yellow journalism (McAuley 335, 340; see also Kley 177). In the novel, the vices of commerce, corruption, and an overheating, i.e. fever, of the financial markets as the result of an unhealthy social environment are equally tied to the disease. The fever, as Bill Christophersen describes it, is the "social toll of America's money ethic" (113). For example, the morally corrupt character Thetford consequently dies together with his whole family. Wallace, in pursuit of financial independence under Thetford's corrupt stewardship, ignores his loved one's plea to leave the infected city, contracts the disease, and dies. And even Mervyn's infected body could be read as a result of his earlier involvement in the character Welbeck's moral corruption. At the infamous Bush Hill hospital of the poor, the attendants are described as only putting their health at risk for the sake of monetary compensation. While Brown conveys a shift towards a post-agrarian society (as represented in the economic demise of Mervyn's father), he still pits the innocent country boy Mervyn against the corrupt city in the first part of his novel. In many instances, such as his problematic and biased description of the Bush Hill hospital attendants, Brown relied on Mathew Carey's problematic and biased account regarding the hospital attendants (see ch. 2.3).[33]

Familiar with Carey's account as well as Jones and Allen's rebuttal of Carey's accusations, Brown was very aware of the racial implications of the disease. In one scene we encounter Arthur Mervyn in front of a mirror recognizing a figure with light yellow-black skin behind him: "One eye, a scar upon his cheek, a tawny skin, a form grotesquely misproportioned" (*AM* 113). Besides a sign for the outbreak of yellow fever, the skin-color and the scar of the reflected figure points to the man's former experience of slavery. Moreover, when Mervyn sees the reflection in the mirror, he also recognizes himself (cf. S. L. Brandt 147). Thus the difference between self and other is blurred. Readers witness an imperial transformation of Mervyn into the racial other. The man reflected in the mirror and the African American figures in Brown's novel are neither named nor do they

---

33 Carey writes: "A profligate, abandoned set of nurses and attendants (hardly any of good character could at that time be procured,) rioted on the provisions and comforts prepared for the sick, who (unless at the hours when the doctors attended) were left almost entirely destitute of every assistance" (*Short Account* 32–33).

speak, but they are all associated with service or mortality: for example, Mervyn witnesses a hearse driven by a black man; a black man carts Thetford's servant to Bush Hill hospital, while a black woman cares for Thetford's wife and child; and a "faithful black" (*AM* 123) remains with Medlicote. The social disease that underlies Brown's novel structurally is the violence associated with the slave trade, which Brown does not attribute as a fault of Africans, who remain largely body- and speechless,[34] but to the merchants who prosper from slavery's benefits and a nation that allows this practice. In Medlicote's words, the fever is not contagious nor can it be attributed "to infected substances imported from east or west, but to a morbid constitution of the atmosphere" (*AM* 123). Medlicote's theory of origin can also be understood as referring to the unhealthy geographic location of the American constitution and nation, or—yet more figuratively—to the American "constitutional defect" (Christophersen 108), the toleration of slavery. The national defect (slavery) is mirrored by a literal constitutional defect Mervyn is sure to harbor in his body; he believes that: "[t]he seeds of an early and lingering death are sown in [his] constitution" (*AM* 104). The threat of black revolution in St. Domingue spreading to the United States as a direct result of the slave trade's aberrations and the overheating of the markets is also broadly associated with a "fever" in the novel. Brown was—like many of his contemporaries—concerned that revolutionary ideas would spread from the Caribbean and threaten the still fragile political system of the United States. While the abolition of slavery would curtail the immediate cause for slave uprisings in the United States, Brown did not include this stance as fervently in the novel as three years later in his nonfiction writing "An Address to the Government" (see also Christophersen 108).

Yellow fever is first introduced in chapter 1 when the fever-stricken Arthur Mervyn is picked up by Dr. Stevens, and it is predominantly represented in the last chapters (15–23) of the novel's first part. Although Dr. Stevens serves as prime narrator of the novel, readers are not given the name of Mervyn's benefactor until chapter 4 of the second part of the novel. Returning to his house in the evening Stevens quite literally stumbles over a sick man, and immediately infers "that [Mervyn's] disease was pestilential [which] did not deter [him] from approaching and examining him more closely" (*AM* 5). Stevens diagnoses Mervyn on the basis of observation and takes the fever-stricken stranger into his home, thus acting benevolently and without profit in mind. The enlightened physician's

34 This is in contrast to the heteroglossia (cf. Bakhtin) John Edgar Wideman creates through several black voices in the short story "Fever" (1989) and in the novel *The Cattle Killing* (1996).

stance represents a sanitationist view in light of a disease he believes to be non-contagious (from person to person) and of local origin. He advocates "cleanliness, reasonable exercise, and a wholesome diet" and argues against popular measures, such as "filling the house with exhalations of gunpowder, vinegar, or tar" (*AM* 5). Referring to the national implication of the disease, Cathy Davidson points out that Stevens puts his life on the line to "help his fellow Americans, to deny that yellow fever can represent his countrymen, his nation" (352). After his recovery in the Stevens household Mervyn is prompted to relate his tale to satisfy his hosts' curiosity, but mainly to defend himself against accusations. His account—in the form of moral autobiography—makes up the first part of the novel: from his venture into the city in an attempt to escape the bleak future in the country, to his involvement with the corrupt criminal Welbeck and his flight back to the countryside. There Mervyn finds work with the Hadwins, falls in love with their daughter Eliza and discovers 20,000 dollars of embezzled banknotes.

Mervyn's voice from his countryside retreat provides a first longer introduction to and description of the devastating fever in the form of a fever rumor.[35] The rumor that "gradually swelled to formidable dimensions" reaches Mervyn in the Quaker farmhouse of the Hadwins: "The city, we were told, was involved in confusion and panick, for a pestilential disease had begun its destructive progress. Magistrates and citizens were flying to the country. […] The numbers of the sick multiplied beyond all example; […] The malady was malignant and unsparing" (*AM* 99). A vivid and horrifying account follows, in which the social consequences of the disease are listed in detail: wives are deserted by husbands, children by parents, people are dying isolated in their houses or are "seized by the disease in the streets" and perish "in the public ways." A lack of nurses and undertakers produces "air with deadly exhalations" that adds "tenfold to the devastation" (*AM* 99). In fact, in the late eighteenth and nineteenth century yellow fever's horrifying symptoms together with a high case-fatality rate of 15 to 50 percent and higher created civic panic and fear incomparable to other diseases.

The 'epidemic of fear' (to use Martin Pernick's phrase), the rumors and tales Mervyn recalls having picked up, "distorted and diversified a thousand ways by the credulity and exaggeration of the tellers" (*AM* 99), precedes Mervyn's actual first-hand experience of the epidemic. Contagion does not only serve as metaphor, but contagious fear has reached the countryside, which is also reflected in the employment of disease-related terminology: the nearest neighbor of the

35 A similar description can also be found in Carey's *Account*: "the country people, are still alarmed with frightful rumours" (45).

Hadwins (where Mervyn resides), "though not un*infected* by the general panic persisted to visit the city daily with his *market-cart*" (102; first emphasis mine). We see a first dissolution of the previously clear dichotomy between city and country here; the contagion does not spare either location. It is at this point in the novel that Mervyn decides to go once again to Philadelphia in order to return the money he has found and to locate Wallace, the fiancé of the older Hadwin sister, Susan. Back in the city he contracts yellow fever, is almost buried alive, and again encounters Welbeck, who is in search of the banknotes. The deadly ill, but self-fashioned as virtuous Mervyn confronts Welbeck, burns the notes, and ends up almost dead on the steps of Medlicote's house, where Dr. Stevens finds him.

In the first part of the novel the city structurally remains a space of corruption: the two main sections describe Mervyn's two ventures into the city, he first experiences commercial corruption (chapters 2–12), then he experiences physical corruption during the yellow fever epidemic (chapters 13–23). Upon his first encounter with a person dead of yellow fever he smells "a vapour, infectious and deadly" (*AM* 111) before he actually encounters the sick foreign person.

> It resembled nothing of which I had ever before been sensible. Many odours had been met with, even since my arrival in the city, less supportable than this. I seemed not so much to smell as to taste the element that now encompassed me. I felt as if I had inhaled a poisonous and subtle fluid, whose power instantly bereft my stomach of all vigour. Some fatal influence appeared to seize upon my vitals, and the work of corrosion and decomposition to be busily begun. (*AM* 111)

Brown's yellow fever Philadelphia is described as "a city that smells of fear" (Orishima 12). Indeed people are constantly alert to invisible odors that seem almost tangible in substance; yet the alertness does not help them to avert the disease. Mervyn describes the effluvium as something that can be tasted and that subsequently "bereft[s] [his] stomach of all vigour" (*AM* 111). He ingests the fever, which infects him, but he is also invigorated by it: "This incident, instead of appalling me, tended rather to invigorate my courage. The danger which I feared had come. I might enter with indifference, on this theatre of pestilence. I might execute without faultering, the duties that my circumstances might create" (*AM* 111–12). At the end of chapter 16 when Mervyn knows that he "had received this corrosive poison" (*AM* 118), he is still able to succinctly express the spatial dichotomy and source of disease: "I wondered at the contrariety that exists between the scenes of the city and the country; and fostered with more zeal than ever, the resolution to avoid those seats of depravity and danger" (*AM* 118). Later in the novel, the farmer Hadwin also decides to leave the country, travels to the city in search of his future son-in-law Wallace, contracts the fever and dies.

The symbolic employment of the disease and contagion does not necessarily exclude newer readings of the fever as medical crisis widely discussed in information networks of the time (cf. Waterman; Arner). Brown, with the help of the medical knowledge available to him—through his friends and his involvement in contemporary medical discourses—assumes authority in *Arthur Mervyn* to interpret the disease, its origin and possible treatment in a literal medical sense. Like the writings of his "scientific friends," Brown's "novelistic enterprise" was based on "observational practices" (Waterman 240) and generated a wide audience and thus inevitably also informed the formation of identity in the new nation. Waterman cites as evidence the words of narrator-physician Stevens, who, at the beginning of the second part of the novel, recognizes that "[d]uring this season of pestilence, [his] opportunities of observation had been numerous, and [he] had not suffered them to pass unimproved" (*AM* 167). Furthermore, "Mervyn's ability to read his diseased environment transforms unself-consciously [...] into a desire to classify his diverse surroundings; self-government leads to social authority as his authoritative narrative drowns out competing voices" (Waterman 242). Mervyn dominates and takes control over the narrative in the second part of the novel. A distinct character development is discernible in that part. On the narrative level, he is no longer as easily deceived in the novel's second part. Yet, the overall tone is more skeptical than in the first part, and Mervyn's assessment of city and country becomes more complex (Kley 170). Once recovered from yellow fever, Mervyn resolves to learn the medical trade from Stevens and sets out to clean up the city's moral corruption and thus provides the means of the epidemic's eradication. His actions symbolically cure the disease that has occupied the nation. The process could easily be interpreted as a vision for the young nation (which symbolically is the same age as the novel's protagonist). Mervyn furthermore feels compelled to help Eliza Hadwin, who has lost her father and her sister to the disease: he takes her with him to the city. The country loses some of its innocence in the eyes of Mervyn after he learns that Eliza's uncle Philip Hadwin tried to deceive his niece of her rightful property (Kley 191). Furthermore, it is only in the city that he can improve himself by learning from Stevens. In this sense, Mervyn and thus Brown by the end of the novel does no longer believe in the Jeffersonian ideal of a nation based on industry performed on the farm. That is, he dismisses a mere pastoral longing for an era, but seems to promote a healthy combination of rural and urban. Jane Tompkins goes so far as to argue that "Brown's ideal reflects the Federalist concern with trade, manufacture, sound currency, credit, and generally, with a concept of America as a nation for which commerce within and without its borders is the lifeblood" (69).

In Philadelphia Mervyn finds Welbeck's mistress Clemenza Lodi in a brothel, and after Welbeck's death accommodates her with his friend Mrs. Wentworth. He also finds a new home for Eliza with his new friend Mrs. Achsa Fielding, the wealthy, rather dark-complexioned Portuguese Jewish widow of a French revolutionary fighter (Girondist). Dr. Stephens exposes Achsa's ethnicity in an attempt to provoke Mervyn to defend her: "But then she is unsightly as a *night-hag*, tawny as a Moor, the eye of a gipsy, low in stature, contemptibly diminutive, scarcely bulk enough to cast a shadow as she walks, less luxuriance than a charred log, fewer elasticities than a sheet pebble" (*AM* 320; emphasis in original). Mervyn notably follows her to the countryside—for one last time in the novel—where he confesses his love for her (*AM* 328). The novel concludes with the prospect of an inter-religious and possibly inter-racial marriage between Achsa and Arthur, who has reaffirmed his friendship and medical apprenticeship with Dr. Stevens and is now looking toward a happy future. This echoes both the Declaration of Independence's promise and Godwin's postulation that virtue—here pursued by Brown's protagonist Arthur Mervyn—is "any action [...] of an intelligent being proceeding from kind and benevolent intention and having a tendency to contribute to general happiness" (Godwin 185). Brown's novel thus supports nationalist formation by educating its readers in appropriate sentiment and a development of virtuous citizenship. Elements endangering this development in the formative years after the American Revolution, such as corrupt commercialism, racial destabilization, yellow fever, and Mervyn's country innocence, are textually curtailed by the symbolic education and development of the protagonist against those figurative crises. Furthermore, together with Achsa Arthur not only finds happiness, but she enables him to secure a property-owning future that in turn allows him to act benevolently.

Brown's novel denounces corrupt commercial practices as well as slavery. As cause of the national crisis and thus disease, it implicitly diagnoses American society's repression of the racial question, its economic reliance on slavery and its denial of a growing segmentation of mass society with free black and hybrid Caribbean/French subjects as future equals. It puts forward an alternative vision for a nation that is eagerly trying to define a distinct national identity against threats to a metaphoric and literal national health. The proposed therapy is the acceptance of a more diverse makeup of U.S.-American society. As a means to control the disease (a symbol for the crises within the new nation) the novel thus puts forward a vision of the post-revolutionary United States—already an imperialist power at this point (despite its own 'postcolonial' status)—to heed the impending social transformation. The development will be or is already triggered by the same process already prevalent in Caribbean societies and destined to spread to the United States (cf. Mackenthun 67). This will lead to an acceptance of a more hybrid societal makeup and cultural diversity of the nation which Arthur Mervyn professes in his own actions. In the course of the novel, the plot of which is largely based on Mervyn's coming of age, the protagonist develops from being an uneducated youth from a small farm in rural Chester County to becoming a medical apprentice and prospective husband of Jewish, previously married, and ethnically mixed Achsa Fielding. What could be read as conventional sentimental marriage plot becomes more complex through Achsa's hybrid identity and Mervyn's acceptance of it. The story thus becomes one of "cultural diversity, feminism, and class mobility" (Davidson 354), all of which are guiding themes envisioned for the society that is symbolically imagined in Achsa and Arthur's union. Tompkins has equally pointed for "social intermixture" to be the "key to stability and progress" (94). Even a cosmopolitan move from America to Europe is hinted at (*AM* 330), which would continue the reversed westward movement which Mervyn initiates when moving from country back to city.[36] With Mervyn's deliberate immersion in and determination to change the city in the second part of the novel, the qualities of health, virtue and freedom—formerly attributed solely to a rural lifestyle—also symbolically enter the city. Mervyn eventually re-qualifies his assessment of the city after his second visit by stating that if cities "are the chosen seats of misery and vice, they are likewise the *soil* of all the laudable and strenuous productions of mind" (*AM* 221; emphasis mine). Interestingly, Mervyn uses the metaphor of the agrarian *soil*, which can equally be found in the city where it fosters great inventions. Brown built on the intelligence and foresight of writers and leaders to continue to develop their national visions in the light of a health threat that gripped the nation in the last decade of the eighteenth century and was not likely to disappear any time soon. By equating his protagonist with the young nation whose journey and further edification is only beginning, Brown puts forward "a vision of geographical [and thus spatial], social, and political integration" (Birkle, *Literature and Medicine* 3), a concept—according to Carmen Birkle—which many authors of disease narratives in nineteenth-century America develop in their texts. Instead of a dichotomy of the rural and the urban, a more nuanced understanding emerges in the course of the novel: neither location emanates pure virtue or pure vice and both are essential for the national experiment to bear

36 "Our household, while we staid in America—in a year or two we hie to Europe—should be *thus* composed" (*AM* 330; emphasis in original).

fruit. Brown's novel also achieves a wider transnational meaning than those certainly present in Brown's orientation toward William Godwin's writing.

2.3 Political Dimensions: Matthew Carey's *Short Account* (1793) and Absalom Jones and Richard Allen's *Narrative* (1794)

In many ways Matthew Carey, Richard Allen, and Absalom Jones set the stage for *Arthur Mervyn*. Their writings served as blueprints for Brown's novel which then established a standard for the genre of the fever narrative, including its national dimension.

Matthew Carey was a successful Irish-Catholic printer and bookseller who had worked with Benjamin Franklin in Paris before settling in Philadelphia in 1784 (Barnard and Shapiro 380). His *Short Account of the Malignant Fever, Lately Prevalent in Philadelphia*, published on November 14, 1793, immediately following the decline of the fever, became the most popular overview of the epidemic, going through four editions in only a few months between November 1793 and January 1794.[37] An incentive for Carey was the counteraction of "the magnifying tongue of rumour" (qtd. in Otter 29) that damaged the city's reputation and its economy. An equal interest can also be detected in Brown's novel, in which he confronts his protagonist with rumors before the actual experience of disease (*AM* 99). Both men notice that it is mainly rumors that generate panic among the citizens and spread an epidemic of fear.

Despite his good intentions to disperse rumors and offer a balanced account, the antislavery and pro-Irish Carey solidifies the false belief in the lesser susceptibility of African Americans to the fever. Even in his improved fourth edition of January 1794 Carey informs his readers that although African Americans contract the fever, "there were scarcely any of them seized at first, and the number that were finally affected, was not great; and, as I am informed by an eminent doctor, it yielded to the power of medicine in them more easily than in the whites" (*Short Account* 63). Regarding the 'fear of contagion' Carey reports that "as soon as any one was taken ill, an alarm was spread among the neighbours, and every effort was used to have the sick person hurried off to Bush Hill, to avoid spreading the disorder" (*Short Account* 32). Carey's Bush Hill passages stirred immediate controversy among his African American readers. In his descriptions of African American conduct during the crisis, Carey accuses them of

37 Editions in French and German for Philadelphia's immigrant population were published in January 1794, and a European edition was published in London in 1794. Altogether, more than 10,000 copies of Carey's *Account* were sold (Brooks 167).

using their positions (as nurses and undertakers) to exploit and rob dependent whites. The paragraph that outraged the African American population reads:

> [T]he elders of the African church met, and offered their assistance to the mayor, to procure nurses for the sick, and aid in burying the dead. Their offers were accepted; and Absalom Jones, Richard Allen, and William Gray, undertook the management of these two-several services. The great demand for nurses, afforded an opportunity for imposition, which was eagerly seized by some of the vilest of the blacks. They extorted two, three, four, and even five dollars a night for such attendance, as would have been well paid by a single dollar. Some of them were even detected in plundering the houses of the sick. But it is unjust to cast a censure on the whole, for this sort of conduct, as many people have done. The services of Jones, Allen, and Gray, and others of their colour, have been very great, and demand public gratitude. (*Short Account* 63)

Carey's account makes black immunity sound like "providence" (Brooks 164), something that they were almost obliged to put to use for the community. Yet, at the same time, Carey constructs the service blacks provided as nurses and undertakers as "an affliction" (Brooks 164) rather than a help for the white community. In present scholarship Carey's account is most often discussed together with Richard Allen and Absalom Jones's pamphlet *A Narrative of the Proceedings of the Black People during the Late Awful Calamity in Philadelphia in the Year 1793* (1794). Jones and Allen's text borrows from several literary forms, among them "plague narrative, sentimental narrative, sermon, petition [...], protest pamphlet [...], and black idealist history" (Otter 40–41). Absalom Jones was born a slave in Delaware in 1746, and Richard Allen—born in 1760—experienced slavery in Philadelphia and later in Delaware. When both men were able to purchase their freedom, they became lay preachers and established the Free African Society in 1787, the first black mutual aid society in the city. With the help of Benjamin Rush and others, they founded the first independent African churches in the United States in 1794. Richard Allen opened Bethel African Methodist Episcopal Church and, in 1799, was ordained as the first black Methodist minister. Absalom Jones was associated with the African Episcopal Church of St. Thomas, of which he became a deacon in 1795 and a priest in 1804. As leaders of the Philadelphia African American community Jones and Allen organized black residents during the 1793 yellow fever crisis to serve as nurses, bleeders, purgers, carters, and buriers of the dead (Otter 5, 32). Their *Narrative of the Proceedings of the Black People* is based on that experience. Historian Joanna Brooks points out that the authors of the *Narrative* are merely identified by their initials "A.J. & R.A." on the frontispiece of their *Narrative* and explains that "this near-anonymity or pseudonymity was a literary formula for establishing an author's disinterested virtue and dedication to the common good" (167). In their pamphlet, written as a response to Carey's account, Jones and Allen implicitly demand a rectification of this unbalanced paragraph that includes an honorary mention of their personal involvement but discredits African American service as a whole. Allen and Jones's *Narrative* serves as a rebuttal to the false accusations made by Carey and strives to illustrate the service the free black people of Philadelphia had rendered to their mostly white patients. Philip Lapsansky has called it "the first account of a free black community in action" (61). Black laborers were among the first volunteers to organize relief efforts in the face of the epidemic in September 1793. Allen and Jones recall that "[w]hen the sickness became general" Benjamin Rush had called them "immediately to attend upon the Sick, knowing we could both bleed; he told us we could increase our utility, by attending to his instructions, and accordingly directed us where to procure medicine duly prepared with proper directions how to administer them, and at what stages of the disorder to bleed" (Allen and Jones 5). Rush—as we know today—ineffectively treated patients by bleeding. He referred to his method of aggressive bleeding and purging as "heroic" medicine and taught his students to not rely on nature and instead "wrest the cure of all violent and febrile disease out of her hands" (Rush qtd. in Workman 34). Pierce and Writer assess Rush's role and popular acceptance of his methods in treating the disease as generally positive, largely because other physicians did not fare much better: "For most Philadelphians, Rush's art was more acceptable than the others' performance. Despite the verbal and published fisticuffs, Rush's relentless war against yellow fever, unyielding faith in his treatments, and obvious concern for his fellow citizens endeared him to the populace, and he emerged the hero of the crisis" (45). Rush received help from members of the Free Africa Society, of which Jones and Allen were members. The society served as the major coordinator of African American volunteers during the epidemic.

Jones and Allen were outraged about Carey's passage discrediting the African American community as a whole, which they think is "splitting rather than joining residents in crisis" (Otter 37). They base their criticism on the fact that Carey had actually fled the infected city and published his account upon his return, suggesting that he lacks any firsthand experience or knowledge. In a public address Carey later justified his leaving the city for the greater part of September, but he also makes clear that he returned in October (*Address* 1–2). The accusation of Carey's desertion is thus one of the weaker arguments given by Allen and Jones. It remains without doubt, that—although there is no explicit dedication—Allen and Jones's document is addressed to Carey. Almost two hundred years later, author John Edgar Wideman rewrites the narrative of the two African American ministers in his short story "Fever" (1989). Wideman attributes a fictional epigraph addressed to Mathew Cary to his primary narrator Richard Allen. The fictional Allen accuses Carey of damaging the whole black race with his attack on the Philadelphia African Americans. He writes: "To Matthew Carey, Esq., who fled Philadelphia in its hour of need and upon his return published a libelous account of the behavior of black nurses and undertakers, thereby injuring all people of my race and especially those without whose unselfish, courageous labours the city could not have survived the late calamity" (Wideman, "Fever" 239). As Lisa Lynch points out, the mock 'dedication' of Allen and Jones to Carey, partially invented by Wideman and partially re-written after Jones and Allen, suggests that their pamphlet has been inspired by Carey's account (Lynch 784). The original, in fact, does not deviate significantly from the fictional rendition. Allen and Jones begin with a rather general observation and accusation: "We feel ourselves sensibly aggrieved by the censorious epithets of many, who did not render the least assistance in the time of necessity" (Allen and Jones 5). The wording also makes clear that Carey was not the only one who accused African American nurses and undertakers of profiteering. Yet Jones and Allen's criticism becomes more pronounced in the course of their narrative and is eventually directly addressed to Carey by citing his subjective denunciation of solely black people: "We feel ourselves hurt most by a partial, censorious paragraph, in Mr. Carey's second edition, of his account of the sickness, &c. in Philadelphia; pages 76 and 77, where he asperses the blacks alone, for having taken the advantage of the distressed situation of the people" (7). Allen and Jones point out that Carey left the city although he was an elected member of the relief committee. They acknowledge that he had the right to leave the city but no right to judge those who remained to help by "giving so partial and injurious an account of the black nurses" (8). If they or some of them had indeed taken monetary advantage of the public distress, which Allen and Jones admit, they also argue that Carey has reaped even greater advantage from the situation with the immediate publication of his economically quite successful pamphlet: "We believe he has made more money by the sale of his 'scraps' than a dozen of the greatest extortioners among the black nurses" (8). In terms of the service rendered by the African American population of Philadelphia after their solicitation through the relief committee, Jones and Allen write:

> Had Mr. Carey been solicited to such an undertaking, for hire, *Query*, "What would he have demanded? but Mr. Carey, although chosen a member of that band of worthies who have so eminently distinguished themselves by their labours, for the relief of the sick and helpless-yet, quickly after his election, left them to struggle with their arduous and hazardous talk, by leaving the city. 'Tis true Mr. Carey was no hireling, and had a right to flee, and upon his return, to plead the cause of those who fled; yet, we think, he was wrong in

> giving so partial and injurious an account of the black nurses; if they have taken advantage of the public distress? (8)

The idea of service is crucial for Allen and Jones, who explain that "[w]hen the people of colour had the sickness and died, we were [...] told it was not with the prevailing sickness, until it became too notorious to be denied; then we were told some few died, but not many. Thus were our *services* extorted at the peril of our lives. Yet you accuse us of extorting a little money from you" (15; emphasis mine).

Allen and Jones furthermore make their case by pitting black and white during the epidemic against each other: "We wish not to offend, but when an unprovoked attempt is made, to make us blacker than we are, it becomes less necessary to be over cautious on that account; therefore we shall take the liberty to tell of the conduct of some of the whites" (8). The authors implicitly differentiate between black and white conduct as almost half of the white population left the city whereas only ten percent of the black population did the same.[38] While the low percentage of black refugees given by Jones and Allen is probably correct, historians estimate that one in four white Philadelphians left the city (Klepp 167). By implication, however, this means that ninety percent of the black population and seventy-five percent of the white population did not want to or, most likely, were not able to afford a temporary move to the countryside—a circumstance that is not explicable by considering race alone; class issues play an equally important role. Finally, Allen and Jones also cite evidence against the common assumption of the time that blacks are less vulnerable to yellow fever than whites: "The bill of mortality for the year 1793 [...] will convince any reasonable man that will examine it, that as many coloured people died in proportion as others" (15).

That an exchange, and a willingness to change, was going on between Jones, Allen, and Carey becomes evident in the fact that Carey added an apologetic footnote to the criticized passage in his fourth (January 1794) edition. It reads: "The extortion here mentioned, was very far from being confined to the negroes: many of the white nurses behaved with equal capacity" (Carey, *Short Account* 63). Of course, as a footnote this clarification is subordinate to the text that still stands as it did in the earlier editions, but it does reflect a change in Carey.[39] And Rush acknowledges in his *Account* that

---

38 The city's two thousand black residents included African Americans, black West Indians, black Britons, and native Africans (Brooks 157).

39 A more elaborate change of the wording is not carried out by Carey until the very last edition published in 1830. The revised passage reads: "The great demand for nurses, afforded an opportunity for imposition, which was eagerly seized by some of those who acted in that capacity, both coloured and white" (68; also qtd. in Otter 54).

> [i]t was not long after these worthy Africans undertook the execution of their humane offer of services before the sick, before I was convinced I had been mistaken.[40] They took the disease, in common with the white people, and many of them died with it. I think I observed the greatest number of them to sicken after the mornings and evenings became cool. A large number of them were my patients. The disease was lighter in them than in white people. I met with no case of hemorrhage in a black patient. (*An Account of the Bilious Remitting Yellow Fever* 97)

Despite these (limited) rebuttals African Americans continued to be associated with the fever in popular culture, literature, and folk beliefs throughout the nineteenth century,[41] not only geographically—as refugees from St. Domingue—but also epidemiologically—as being innately immune, yet importing and profiteering from yellow fever. In this sense, I am less optimistic than Joanna Brooks who believes that "Jones and Allen's narrative functions as an immune system for Philadelphia's black community" (172) in the years to come. While Allen and Jones's text is certainly powerful in its construction of a collective African American subject by developing a story of shared resistance, and thus functions to strengthen the community against racism, it stands against many other writings and beliefs that continue to prevail.

Brown, for example, only includes his stance against slavery and racism on an abstract level. No substantial African American characters grace his novel. Two structural elements of his novel can already be found in Carey's narrative: firstly, the presence of universal fear, and, secondly, spatial dialectics. First, "an universal trepidation benumbed people's faculties, and flight and self-preservation seemed to engross the whole attention of a large proportion of the citizens" (Carey, *Short Account* 92). Second, the oppositional spatial movement of Brown's protagonist traveling to the city is described in Mathew Carey's *Short Account of the Malignant Fever, Lately Prevalent in Philadelphia*: "The removals from Philadelphia began about the 25th or 26th of this month [August]: and so great was the general terror, that, for some weeks, carts, wagons, coaches, and chairs, were almost

---

40 Rush and others from the Philadelphia College of Physicians had relied on John Lining's *Description of the American Yellow Fever, which Prevailed at Charleston in the Year 1748*. Lining describes members of the Charleston black population as not susceptible to yellow fever (7).

41 One such rumor—a dominant trope of slave revolts—had it that African Americans had poisoned the water wells and caused yellow fever in Philadelphia (Brooks 162, 163; Smith 327). Well poisoning has actually been used since antiquity as a wartime strategy. It was a major unfounded accusation against Jews during the Middle Ages when the bubonic plague (Black Death) was ravaging Europe and survivors looked for an explanation as well as someone to blame.

constantly transporting families and furniture to the country in every direction" (*Short Account* 16–17). The liminal status of those between city and country becomes apparent in another episode related by Carey:

> A servant girl, belonging to a family in this *city*, in which the fever had prevailed, was apprehensive of danger, and resolved to remove to a relation's house, in the *country*. She was, however, taken sick on the road, and returned to town, where she could find no person to receive her. One of the guardians of the poor provided a cart, and took her to the almshouse, into which she was refused admittance. She was brought back, and the guardian offered five dollars to procure her a single night's lodging, but in vain. And in sine [in time], after every effort made to provide her shelter, she absolutely expired in the cart. (*Short Account* 24–25; emphasis mine)

The plight of the servant girl also exemplifies the implications of class in times of disease. While "[t]he governor, who had been sick, had gone, by directions of his physician, to his country-seat near the falls of Schuylkill—and nearly the whole of the officers of the state had likewise retired" (30), the

> [p]oorer persons took refuge in hoys, smacks, and fishing boats; but these took the infection; others went up the river in boats, lodging by night in tents made of their sails, on shore; for though the country people would supply them with provisions, they would not receive them into their houses. The poor who ran abroad in their extremities into the country, were often ill used and driven back, which caused great exclamation against the cruelty of the country towns; but self-preservation extinguished humanity; and yet notwithstanding all their care, there was not a town within twenty miles but [sic] suffered more or less by the disorder. (Carey, *Short Account* 100)

It is also quite clear that Carey believes in a miasmatic origin, explaining that those who died in the country had been infected in the city: "Some others in different places caught the infection, and died. But the cases of this kind have been extremely few, considering the numbers, who carried the disorder from hence, and died with it in the country" (82). Carey points toward "the benefit of the country air," citing as evidence that those residing in the suburban western part of the city suffered much less (62).

The contagiousness of fear that reaches the countryside serves as a recurrent theme in Carey's *Short Account*. City dwellers who moved to the county and lost their relatives to the fever could not even count on their new neighbors' help in making coffins due to their fears (cf. 84). Consequently, "[m]any travellers from this city, [...] have fallen victims to the fears, not to the want of charity, of those to whom they applied for relief" (82). Only at one point does Carey relativize his condemnation of country residents by pointing out those who have offered acts of kindness: "The instances [...] have been very few; but they are therefore only the more precious, and ought to be held up to public approbation" (60). Despite this one mention of kindness, the country clearly loses its status as sole seat of virtue. One of his major aims remains to plead for solidarity between those who stayed in the city and those who fled for equally understandable reasons; Carey argues for a unified effort in "cleansing and purifying our scourged city" (*Short Account* 94). The assessment is echoed in Brown, who resolves the proposed dichotomy between city and country to some extent in the very end.

The written accounts and the fictionalization of the epidemic (by Charles Brockden Brown), and—in Carey's case—the near-endless list of the dead continue to linger and affect the emerging U.S.-American collective identity. Some examples of this will be treated in the following section.

2.4 Looking Back to 1793: The Philadelphia Epidemic in/and Cultural Memory

Philip Freneau's "Pestilence: Written during the Prevalence of a Yellow Fever" (1793) is also among the first literary responses to the epidemic. As indicated in its title, Freneau lived and worked in Philadelphia at the time. Tying his Democratic-Republican worldview to the journalism of the era, he was the editor of the bi-weekly *National Gazette* (published in Philadelphia) and worked as a translator for the State Department under the patronage of Secretary of State Thomas Jefferson. Freneau was a spokesman for the Jeffersonian political program and *The National Gazette* became the mouthpiece of the liberal politics promoted by Democratic Republicans. Although he was careful not to attack President Washington too fervently, he was less cautious regarding his representation of Alexander Hamilton and John Adams. His support of the cause of the French Revolution became increasingly unpopular because of the Reign of Terror in France and the effects it had on Philadelphia, for example regarding the influx of refugees (Krieg 54). In 1793, Freneau had to resign his appointment in the State Department as Jefferson was leaving his post. *The National Gazette* ceased publication in the fall of that year.

Freneau's yellow fever poem is an example of his critical neoclassicist political verse and far from the nationalistic and celebratory "The Rising Glory of America" (1772) on which he collaborated with Hugh Henry Brackenridge. Freneau addresses his newspaper readership, the common American:

> Hot, dry winds forever blowing,
> Dead men to the grave-yards going:
> Constant hearses,
> Funeral verses;
> Oh! what plagues—there is no knowing!

Priests retreating from their pulpits!—
Some in hot, and some in cold fits
  In bad temper,
  Off they scamper,
Leaving us—unhappy culprits!

Doctors raving and disputing,
Death's pale army still recruiting—
  What a pother
  One with t'other!
Some a-writing, some a-shooting.

Nature's poisons here collected,
Water, earth, and air infected—
O, what a pity,
Such a City,
Was in such a place erected! (230–31)

In the four stanzas of his poem Freneau touches on the issues most heavily discussed in connection with the yellow fever epidemic. He paints a bleak picture of nature and blames the city environment and the conduct of physicians and priests. As Tuomi Forrest has pointed out, Freneau thus presents "an anti-pastoral, anti-urban, and necessarily anti-social vision of the world" (n.pag.). The third stanza criticizes the doctors who are disputing about the right treatment of the disease while their patients are dying. Freneau is even more explicit in his critique of the medical profession in "On Dr. Sangrado's Flight," in which he condemns doctors who fled Philadelphia during the crisis (Krieg 54). In "Pestilence" the ministers are fleeing from their duties, leaving those they should care about behind. Freneau sides with those promoting a miasmatic-environmentalist cause of yellow fever, i.e. Democratic Republicans, who believed in its local origin. Freneau asks rhetorically why "such a place" was picked not just for any city but for the nation's capital. The line might also be read as a critical side remark to the District of Columbia, where at that time the future capital was being built in a very similar environment to Philadelphia, namely on reclaimed wetlands. As an all-out attack, it is understandable that the poem was not well received at the time. Freneau's view of nature is only revised in his later poems such as "On the Religion of Nature" (1815).

Although very different in tone from Freneau's political poem "Pestilence," John Searson's "poetic lines" (80) also call upon the frequent yellow fever epidemics in Philadelphia in the 1790s. Searson was an Irishman, who wrote and published poetry. Born in 1750, he served as a tutor in a New York family, later failed as a Philadelphia merchant and became a schoolmaster. Since 1796 he had tried to obtain a position in Washington, D.C., which we know from his correspondence with President Washington ("To George Washington" n.pag.). On May 15, 1799 Searson visited Mount Vernon and in 1800 he published a book of poems entitled "Mount Vernon: A Poem…" as an homage to the country seat of George Washington. On the title page, Searson describes his poetry as "rural, romantic and descriptive" (n.pag.). "On the Return of the Epidemic Fever to Philadelphia, in 1799" is the last poem of the series[42]:

> Ah! Philadelphia, I must mourn for thee;
> Because thy desolation now I see!
> Harass'd by sickness, and death walking round,
> We see our friends brought low unto the ground.
> Spare, gracious God, O! spare, for mercy's sake;
> And do not thine own heritage forsake;
> Tho' we have sinn'd, O! spare thy chast'ning rod!
> For, tho' we've sinn'd, we have a pard'ning God.
> Alas! How puzzled are our doctors here,
> To find whence is the fever—far or near!
> Some one thing says, some devise another,
> But the great first cause, from us, they smother.
> Some say, alone 'tis by infection;
> But ev'n so 'tis by God's direction!
> He that rais'd the dead and cur'd ev'ry fore,
> Is now in heav'n, and can our health restore.
> Let's cease from sin, and not provoke our God;
> He then will heal and take away his rod!
> Make Philadelphia, once again, to shine,
> So that we all may see his hand's divine.
> 'Tis from his hand we safety can obtain,
> And in our health and happiness remain!
> 'Tis in our God we walk and live,
> And to his own will ev'ry blessing give.
> Diseases, when they come, and threaten death;
> We'll look to heav'n with solemn praying breath!
> And should we, ev'n in death, our souls resign.
> We'll ever dwell with God, who's all divine.
> Father of all, our eyes are unto thee!
> O! give us of thy happiness to see!
> Whether in sickness, or life, or death,
> To thee, O! God, we'll e'er resign our breath! [82]

---

42 "On the Return" is followed by elegiac poems (85–88) which John Searson added late in 1799, upon the death of George Washington, when his book was essentially finished.

'Tis heav'n to be, where thou dost shew thy face!
O! give us happiness in ev'ry place;
So that disease and death, can't hurt our way,
For God will be our all in endless day.
It is the God of heaven we must implore;
For happiness on earth and evermore;
Who can disease and death keep far away;
If we love God and never from him stray.
If thousands fall at our left hand and right,
He's able to still to keep us up by his might;
No pestilence can hurt where he doth save,
Nor fever snatch us to untimely grave.
O! let us, then, this God of health pursue,
In all we act, in all we say or do!
We'll then be happy here and evermore,
Praising our God, whom heav'n and earth adore. (Searson 80–82)

Searson—like Freneau—reflects on the role of the doctors, who do not agree on the treatment nor the origin of the disease. Contrary to rational Enlightenment thought and medical reasoning, Searson's emphasis lies on the representation of the disease as symbol for divine providence. He interprets the frequent yellow fever epidemics in Philadelphia as God's punishment. In the end the means to control and cure disease lies solely with God, who saves those that pray and stay with him: "Diseases, when they come, and threaten death; / We'll look to heav'n with solemn praying breath! (81).

An exemplary list of Philadelphia yellow fever lyrical production must include one of the most influential and widely read poems of the nineteenth century which also ends with said epidemic. Henry Wadsworth Longfellow's epic poem *Evangeline: A Tale of Acadie* (1847)[43] includes a personification of the disease: "Then it came to pass that a pestilence fell on the city / […] Wealth had no power to bribe, nor beauty to charm, / the oppressor; But all perished alike beneath the scourge of his anger" (*E* 20). Saturated with cultural nostalgia, the dominant themes of the long narrative poem are romance and sentiment, which is most apparent in the star-crossed relationship between Evangeline and Gabriel. Set at the time of the expulsion of the Acadians from the former French colony Acadie (today Nova Scotia, Canada),[44] the betrothed lovers become separated. Gabriel is

43 In the following, I will use *E* for Henry Wadsworth Longfellow's *Evangeline: A Tale of Acadie*.

44 The so-called expulsion (1755–1764) of Acadians occurred during the French and Indian War and was part of the British military campaign against New France. Between 1755

forced to board a ship, while Evangeline is adopted by a family in Maryland. They are removed from the "forest primeval" of "murmuring pines and hemlocks" (*E* 1) to "lonely and wretched roofs in the crowded lanes of the city" (*E* 19) The name *Evangeline* refers to the Latin 'evangelium' (translating into 'gospel'), which can be divided into the Greek words 'eu' (good) and 'angela' (news). Evangeline—"with God's benediction upon her" (*E* 2)—searches for Gabriel but fails, becomes a Sister of Mercy and dedicates her life to the service of others in Philadelphia. The yellow fever-infected city of 1793 serves Longfellow as the "ideal romantic setting for the reunion of Evangeline and Gabriel" (Krieg 43). Signs of a dark nature invade the city of her ministry in the summer of that year, such as "wild pigeons, / Darkening the sun with their flight" and "death flooded life, and [...] [s]pread to a brackish lake" (*E* 20). In this atmosphere, while tending to those sick of yellow fever, Evangeline encounters her long lost love Gabriel on his deathbed; he dies and figuratively returns to "green Acadian meadows" (*E* 21). Despite the pastoral recurrence, the lovers remain "[s]ide by side, in their nameless graves, [...] / In the heart of the city, they lie, unknown and unnoticed" (*E* 21). The image speaks out against a diseased urban existence very similar to Charles Brockden Brown who speaks of the "loneliness and silence" of "perish[ing] in the public way" from yellow fever (*AM* 118). It is exactly this image of the yellow fever-stricken national capital that endures in American cultural memory.

At least three novels of the nineteenth and early twentieth century make use of the culturally symbolic setting of Philadelphia in 1793. In Catharine Maria Sedgwick's first two novels, *A New-England Tale* (1822) and *Redwood: A Tale* (1824), the epidemic occurrence seems initially to be used as a plot device, but also affects the configuration of the still young nation. S. Weir Mitchell's *The Red City* (1907) presents a political-historical tale of 1790s Philadelphia. In the words of Joann P. Krieg, Mitchell achieves a "demystification of the disease" (43).

Sedgwick's first novel, *A New-England Tale* was published in 1822 and was well received. Following her father who had converted from Congregationalism with its Calvinistic emphasis on eternal damnation to the more liberal rational Unitarianism on his deathbed in 1813, Sedgwick became a member of the Unitarian Society in New York City in 1821. She was dissatisfied with the conduct of the Calvinist elders at her Stockbridge church (Kelley 36–37; Maddox 95–98). While the Constitution did not give any significant rights to women, granting

and 1758, when the Acadians refused to offer allegiance and dencounce their Catholic faith, the British deported them to the Thirteen Colonies, and later also to France. Many also relocated to Louisiana. An estimated 11,500 Acadians were deported.

freedom of religion remained an exception. Still Sedgwick grappled with her decision of conversion and began *A New-England Tale* (1822)[45] as a Unitarian tract and justification. She ultimately promotes a "chaste disobedience informed by piety, reason, and decorum" while obedience remains "a conditional virtue for men and women alike" (Sweet 109–10). The plot revolves around Jane Elton, the heroine of *A New-England Tale*, who is orphaned at the age of twelve and adopted by her strict Calvinist aunt Elvira Wilson. What takes yellow fever above a mere plot device in the novel are the circumstances of Jane's father contracting it. As a wealthy merchant, he likes to show off his "pecuniary superiority" (*NET* 17). Yet when his business fails, and "after his pecuniary embarrassments were beyond the hope of extrication," he dies of the "violent fever" (*NET* 20). His wife follows him soon thereafter, although the cause of her death is not given. The narrative hints at her mental constitution, her "habitual passiveness" (*NET* 19) in never demanding for her husband to change his speculating practices, and thus attributes the father's financial demise and later death to the unquestioned submission of Jane's mother to Mr. Elton and passivity in "avert[ing] an evil" (*NET* 19). In this vein, Nancy F. Sweet has pointed out that "Sedgwick intends this meek and unthinking endurance of the wrongs of the world as an indictment of female acquiescence to husbandly authority" (113). Jane equally adheres to her aunt's strict regimen and respects her authority, but she also practices selective disobedience, for example, when leaving the house at night to help a young girl to give birth.[46] It is Jane's dedicated self-discipline that the novel promotes, yet also the right to dissent from intolerant church authorities, when she adopts the non-hierarchical Quaker tradition of her future husband Mr. Lloyd. Through her conversion and break with the Puritan conduct of her ancestors, as well as the strict religious practices of her parents and her aunt, Jane stands for national progress, representing "the promise of a new nation as it refashions its colonial and Calvinist legacy into a future of benevolent piety, toleration, and order" (Sweet 115). In recurrence to the yellow fever death of her father one may also interpret Jane's proposition to follow the "requisitions and restraints" (*NET* 180) of religion as the basis of virtue for men and women alike as a cure to disease and the advancement of a more tolerant nation and society (regarding religion and gender).

---

45 In the following, I will use *NET* for Catharine Maria Sedgwick's *A New-England Tale* and *R* for *Redwood: A Tale*.

46 Although one might be reminded of Anne Hutchinson's accusations against the authoritarian Boston ministers while preaching a 'covenant of grace,' the practice of selective dissent by Sedgwick's protagonist is much less revolutioniary.

The promotion of the equality of men and women is even stronger in Sedgwick's second novel *Redwood: A Tale* (1824) since its female characters are suggesting this course. Like *A New England Tale* the novel focuses on religious concerns and features a highly-principled protagonist named Debby Lenox. With regard to *Redwood* Sedgwick has been praised for the creation of "women characters who overturn typical nineteenth-century gender roles and make their own decisions, particularly about whom and even whether to marry" (Ross 246). Like Jane Elton, the protagonist of *Redwood* is orphaned at a very young age, and the culprit again is the yellow fever in Philadelphia: "My father was a lawyer, a man of talents, and rising rapidly in his profession, when he was carried off by the yellow fever, then raging in our city. I was but a month old when he died" (*R* 378). Debby Lenox, in other words, is born at the time of a major national crisis that extends financially, politically and socially beyond the epidemic then raging in the capital. As the one person of her family surviving this crisis—her mother dies two years later from the "fatigue of removal" (*R* 378)—Debby Lenox personifies a new course of the nation toward religious tolerance and gender equality.

The title of S. Weir Mitchell's historical novel *The Red City* (1907)[47] refers to Philadelphia with its many red brick buildings. Mitchell once lived at 1524 Walnut Street and spent his boyhood years in the city (Hayne 149). Set in the Quaker milieu, with its emphasis on the equality of men and women based on non-hierarchical relationships, the novel chronicles the events and political upheavals of the early 1790s, especially the relations between the United States and revolutionary France. The Philadelphia yellow fever epidemic of 1793 is at the center of the novel, which revolves around three main characters: René Vicomte de Courval, a recent Huguenot immigrant who has fled from the terror of the French Revolution with his mother; his friend and mentor, a German named Johann Schmidt who turns out to be a Count von Ehrenstein but does not presume upon this title; and Margaret Swanwick, the daughter of de Courval and Schmidt's Quaker landlady. The novel is driven by a revenge plot with de Courval pursuing the murderer of his father, a cruel Jacobin named Carteaux, who has been appointed to Philadelphia as the French consul-general's secretary. The novel ends with Carteaux—and the threat he poses—sailing back to France after having been irrevocably maimed in an assault by de Courval. With the legitimacy of his deed confirmed, De Courval is restored to his post in the State Department and is going to marry Margaret Swanwick. By the time he wrote *The Red City*

47 In the following, I will use *RC* for S. Weir Mitchell's *The Red City*.

S. Weir Mitchell was a popular writer and famous physician.[48] Already in *Doctor and Patient* (1887) Mitchell had warned his readers to be "careful when you come to test [the physician] by his ability to feel what you call sympathy" (qtd. in Boudreau 122). Addressing mainly women and a non-medical audience he clearly seeks to counter the narrative sentimentalism he sees present in his age. In her study on sympathy in American literature, Kristin Boudreau comments on Mitchell's and the commonly held nineteenth-century assumption that "[n]ot only did sympathy between a doctor and his patient threaten to interfere with the medical treatment, as many doctors believed, but a patient's attempts to gain sympathy could result in dissimulation and thus undermine medical authority" (122). The doctors in *The Red City* all have medical authority and believe that they are prescribing the right regimen. Sympathy is far from a guiding principle in the direct relationship between doctor and patient. Mitchell is quite critical and almost cynical in describing the conduct of his own profession, in particular with Benjamin Rush and his treatment of radical bloodletting and induced purging. To put this into perspective, we also have to consider that Mitchell is writing after the medical advancements and microbiological findings of the mid-nineteenth century. The vector of yellow fever transmission had been identified seven years prior to the publication of Mitchell's novel. In this way, de Courval's exclamation that he would hope the peaceful Quakers "would attend to the mosquitos" is an ironic side-remark. Mitchell presents both the contagionist and miasmatic schools of origin when he refers to the two theories prevalent at the time: firstly, that "[i]t had come from the Sans Culottes, privateer," a French merchant ship that had reached Philadelphia in July 1793, or, secondly, "because of damaged coffee fetched from he knew not where" (*RC* 202). Benjamin Rush especially defended the miasmatic theory of rotting coffee beans left on the docks as source of the outbreak. Many such historical details are fictionalized in the novel. After the non-fictional Dr. Redman, President of the College of Physicians (*RC* 202), confirms the prevalence of yellow fever, Schmidt, who has witnessed the fever in the West Indies, moves the Swanwicks as well as de Courvals out of the city. Schmidt stays in "the city to care for the sick" (*RC* 205), and when messages from him cease to reach René de Courval in his countryside retreat, he sets out for Philadelphia "dismiss[ing] his fears with a silent appeal for strength and support" (*RC* 208). De Courval qualifies disease as more appalling to man than war. This

48 It was Mitchell who prescribed the rest cure to the prominent feminist writer and editor Charlotte Perkins Gilman. She fictionalized her experience in her short story "The Yellow Wall-paper" (1892).

is due to the fact that the perceived "peril" or threat of disease overshadows the actually much lower "risk" of falling sick (*RC* 208). Fear and panic are, in other words, more dangerous to the public good than the actual disease. De Courval's statement speaks of a rational assessment regarding yellow fever on the part of Mitchell. After reaching the city and witnessing the yellow fever-death of a very young child, left alone by its mother out of fear of infection, de Courval is left to ponder the loss of humanity in times of great anxiety: he sits in "solitude and loneliness [...] as the night closed dark about him" (*RC* 210). Stephen Girard, a non-fictional fellow Frenchman, philanthropist, and responsible for organizing the Bush Hill hospital, helps de Courval to find Schmidt who lies sick with the fever. Girard recommends the so-called milder French treatment of providing lots of water, then milk and bathing the patient (*RC* 212). Pipe-smoke is equally given as capable of repelling the disease; it may indeed have been effective against the biting mosquitoes. When Dr. Rush—another non-fictional character in the novel—later also visits Schmidt, the German refuses Rush's regimen of Calomel and blood-letting ("Out with your drugs!" *RC* 213) and recovers nevertheless. The negative assessment and depiction of Rush's drastic methods is certainly informed by the medical experience of the early twentieth century. While Rush disqualifies himself as a hero in *The Red City*, the relief committee is represented positively in Mitchell's novel. Introduced by his friend Stephen Girard, the fictional René de Courval joins the historical group of notable men who stood together in times of crisis: Mayor Matthew Clarkson, "Carey, the future historian of the plague; Samuel Wetherill, the Free Quaker; Henry de Forrest, whom he had met; Thomas Savory; Thomas Wistar; Thomas Scattergood; Jonathan Seargeant" (*RC* 220).

The Red City is not merely a history of the origin, catastrophe, and right treatment of yellow fever, but the disease is used as part of the fictionalization of the political events during Philadelphia's era as capital of the United States and a reflection on the construction of a nation at crisis in the 1790s as well as its entanglement in French and British affairs. The latter critique might also be directed against a growing imperialism and internationalism in U.S. politics at the beginning of the twentieth century when the novel was written. In the end, the French aristocrat marries the simple Quaker girl, and thus accepts both the Quaker belief in the equality of men and women as well as the insistence on classlessness or unimportance of class in the United States. Furthermore, as a member of the State Department and continuing to serve Thomas Jefferson's successor Edmund J. Randolph, De Courval promotes the democratic principles on which the American nation is built.

2.5 Yellow Fever and the Nation

The examination and interpretation of the selected literary sources focusing on the 1793 Philadelphia epidemic show exemplarily how these fictionalizations of a health crisis were actually concerned with building and defining the nascent nation. While fiction became the "carrier zone" (Samuels, *Reading the Novel* 96) to construct the nation, Philadelphia became the microcosm to carry it out. Yellow fever needed to be controlled and overcome, and the national project was still in need of further interpretation and solidification. This interpretatorial work was taken up by writers in the 1790s. Charles Brockden Brown puts his version of a more hybrid makeup of U.S. society and political ideals against the outgrowth of disease. Taken together as texts conversing with each other, Mathew Carey's *Short Account* and Absalom Jones and Richard Allen's *Narrative* set an example of addressing questions of exclusion and agency and their connection to race and class for the nation. With his poem "Pestilence: Written during the Prevalence of a Yellow Fever" Philip Freneau critically approaches the fields of religion (ministers), medicine (doctors), and city versus country as areas of national impact.

The fact that the Philadelphia epidemic retained its significance as imagined space for the nation testifies to its metaphorical usability, of representing a "usable past" (Commager) throughout the nineteenth century. John Searson primarily celebrates the President in "Mount Vernon: A Poem…" and interprets the frequent yellow fever epidemics in Philadelphia as God's punishment and the love of God as the cure. Henry Wadsworth Longfellow's epic poem "Evangeline: A Tale of Acadie" personifies the disease and manifests it in the nation's capital. Catharine Maria Sedgwick's novels *A New-England Tale* and *Redwood* promote a humanist religion that provides an equal basis for men and women as a cure, which will lead to a more tolerant nation and society (regarding religion and gender). Finally, S. Weir Mitchell's *The Red City* (1907) fictionalizes yellow fever in Philadelphia in his political-historical tale. Since the vector of the disease is known at the time of his writing he is able to demystify the disease (Krieg 43) in his realistic descriptions. Yet he also employs it as a metaphor for a nation in crisis in the 1790s and entangled in international politics—a nod to the growing international and imperialist involvements of the United States since the late 1890s and early 1900s.

3 Displaying Disease: Yellow Fever Visualized

3.1 Picturing Yellow Fever

American studies scholarship and visual culture studies have never been mutually exclusive. To the contrary, Americanists have explored visual representations of 'America' and examined their cultural agency in the construction of 'American' identities and ideologies before the 1990s. The iconic or pictorial turn thus "marked less of a watershed for American Studies" (Hebel, "'American' Pictures" 401; cf. also Hebel and Moreth-Hebel 187; Orvell, "Cultural Studies" 88). Yet, a renewed emphasis on the agency, function, and historical as well as cultural embeddedness of pictures furthered the recollection of art historical approaches (Hebel 403), most famously conducted by Aby M. Warburg in his interdisciplinary research on the iconography of the antique imagery in the Renaissance (*Bilderatlas Mnemosyne*) and by Erwin Panofsky in his iconological interpretation (*Ikonographie und Ikonologie*). Nineteenth-century America has received particular scholarly attention with regard to the visual (cf. Burns; Colbert; *Early American Visual Culture*; Nemerov; Pyne; Rainey; Van Hook). In their entirety these publications point to a powerful relationship of art, visuality and culture during that time. In other words, studying American visual culture of the nineteenth century furthers "our understanding of the way in which American culture operates" (Cutrer 908). With regard to yellow fever representations, this chapter covers the period from 1800 to the early twentieth century, thus enabling an access to the period under scrutiny in this study in its entirety. This examination precedes the analysis of more specific issues, such as gender and race and its intersectionality, in connection with the disease (see chs. 4–5).

As early as January 1857, the *Cosmopolitan Art Journal* commented on the increasing number of visual representations in magazines and newspapers. With regard to the recently started enterprises of *Frank Leslie's Illustrated Newspaper* and *Harper's Weekly*, it stated that "[t]he 'illustration mania is upon our people" (qtd. in Mott, *1850–1865* 192). Nicholas Mirzoeff has aptly commented that "[t]he hyperstimulus of modern visual culture from the nineteenth century to the present day has been dedicated to trying to saturate the *visual* field, a process that continually fails as we learn to see and connect ever faster. In other words, visual culture does not depend on pictures themselves but the modern tendency to picture or visualize experience" (5).

In order to better understand what have become almost inevitable visualization practices, we need to take a look at the nature of the visualized experience.

It is nothing new or modern that these experiences often pertain to extremes, i.e. the most basic human needs and anxieties, which are triggered by fears of disease, death, and war. In the case of epidemics, the perceived risk of transmission and the spread of panic very often accompanies their appearance. In medieval and Renaissance art, for example, the iconographic 'Dance of Death' or 'Danse Macabre' accompanied the plague years in Europe (e.g. Hans Holbein's piece from 1538). The "multifaceted relationships between culture and transmissible disease" (Wald, Tomes, and Lynch 618) are also evident in nineteenth-century pictorial representations of yellow fever epidemics. Illustrations from the early and late nineteenth century, as well as photographs taken during and after the Spanish-American War, the so-called 'splendid little war' in Cuba in 1898 and 1899, lend themselves to the recognition of the processes producing the disease experience as well as the affective responses to it. While early nineteenth-century lithographs established a visual rhetoric of yellow fever, the pictures in the post-bellum illustrated newspapers *Harper's Weekly* and *Frank Leslie's* enabled readers to gaze at the disease from afar. Keeping the (pictorial) distance, late nineteenth-century military photography directed the focus even more on witnessing other people's pain.

The pictures of diseased and dead bodies, which frequently sensationalized the epidemics for American readers and viewers, constitute complex sites of tension: viewing them generates disgust that might also be accompanied by a morbid delight. Miles Orvell has called this feeling of fearful awe the 'destructive sublime' (Orvell, "After 9/11"). The visualization of the yellow fever experience furthermore serves as a form of control and normativization. The contradiction between revulsion and pleasure provides a point of entry for critical engagement with the politics of aesthetic expression and the process of identity formation in delimiting disease and embracing health. If we are to understand more fully the processes of medical and imperialist power formation in the United States, we need to explore these pictures that rely on emotion and affect—ranging from sympathy and compassion to fear and revulsion—to control disease (cf. Gessner, "Epidemic Iconographies"). The productivity of applying affect theory to visual culture has not only been proven by the editors of *Feeling Photography* (Elspeth H. Brown and Phu) but is also taken up in Christof Decker's proposition to study pictorial media in "how they work and create meaning, and how they tell stories and affect audiences" (123).[49]

49 In the proposal for their "Affect, Empire and Photography" panel (ASA 2012), the organizer Elspeth H. Brown points to the affective turn in photography, an understanding of emotion and feeling as one of the key sites through which power relations—including imperial rule—are produced. "Whether emphasizing specific affects (melancholy, for example [or sympathy, one might add, with regard to yellow fever depictions]), the

In order to define power relations, the images destabilize notions of ethics or moral obligation and aesthetic expression, such as an understanding of what can and should be represented. Do the depictions stimulate complicity or resistance; or, in other words, do they involve the reader or do they provoke confrontation and abhorrence, both as a means of control?

3.2 Establishing an Etiology and Iconography of Pictured Disease

A rhetoric of yellow fever representation was established with illustrations from the early nineteenth century onwards. Yellow fever has an even longer history in the United States; Cotton Mather's nephew John Mather died of yellow fever in Charleston, South Carolina in 1699. A watercolor print created by Abraham James and published by William Holland in London on October 1, 1800 critically exemplifies the early nineteenth-century understanding of the disease in poster size (30.4 x 47.7 cm) (fig. 3). It was published at the same time as Charles Brockden Brown's *Arthur Mervyn* (see chapter 2).

Fig. 3. Abraham James, "The Torrid Zone, Or, Mixed Blessings of Jamaica." London: William Holland, 1 Oct. 1800. Wellcome Library, London.

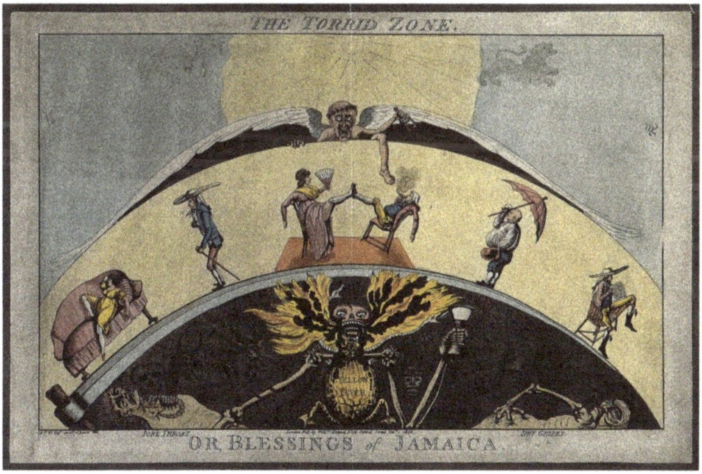

circulation of emotions between bodies, or the significance of feelings in public life, the scholarship on affect offers new approaches to thinking through the relationship between bodies, images, and publics." The proceedings of the ASA panel were partially published in *Feeling Photography* (2014), edited by Elspeth H. Brown and Thy Phu.

The print is a comment on the mixed "blessings of Jamaica" or, in other words, imperialist practices. "The torrid zone," or the tropics, is defined in the zodiac as situated between crab and lion in the Northern hemisphere, or the tropic of Cancer. The signs of the zodiac with the sun in the middle also signify the summer months between June and August when yellow fever was most aggressive. It is a parodic and caricaturesque cosmological diagram that represents the dichotomy of colonial life in Jamaica, suspended between languorous, careless living—including napping, dancing, and smoking—that is bordering on debauchery, and the horrors of disease lurking underneath. The bottom sphere is circumscribed by a scythe which the skull-faced beast of yellow fever is holding with its right hand. The conspicuously yellow-colored demon which has "yellow fever" written on its abdomen is an allegorical depiction that follows in a long line of representations of disease in the form of serpents, skulls, monsters, and thieves.[50] In its left hand, it holds an empty hour-glass, clearly signifying death in the form of the Grim Reaper. The flames emanating from the skull represent the high body temperature of the fever victim, or hell raging below. The ghoulish figure on the left is being attacked by a scorpion which has inserted its tail into his neck, about which the lettering tells it to be a "sore throat." On the right, the bony hand of the mustached ghoul, suffering—as the lettering tells us—from West-Indian dry gripes, clutches his side with sharp talons. The upper sphere is circumscribed by an angel's wings; however, with its aged complexion it resembles more a Father Time figure, which is holding a bottle of opium (to alleviate pain or sedate the colonialists). Underneath his fierce, white-eyed visage, the colonialists swoon, between blissful unawareness of the fever that rages below and an active repression of the underlying potential for racial upheaval. The print ironizes this form of controlling the beast of disease, suggesting that it cannot be kept repressed for long. Like its literary companion *Arthur Mervyn* the illustration criticizes colonial practices gone astray.[51]

In the early 1800s British medical writing consolidated its belief in the climate of the West Indies as the main agent in causing the disease. Yellow fever was

50 The microbiological revolution of the nineteenth century inspired new visual metaphors for disease such as anthropomorphic germs and grotesque bacteria ("Visual Culture and Public Health Posters").

51 *Arthur Mervyn* criticizes the merchants who prosper from slavery's benefits and a society that allows this. The threat of black revolution spreading to the United States as a direct result of slavery's aberrations is also broadly associated with a "fever." Charles Brockden Brown's abolitionist stance is even more emphatically expressed in his non-fiction writings, e.g. *An Address to the Government* (1803) (cf. Christophersen 108).

thought to be the result of heat on persons who were not yet acclimatized to the tropics. British military surgeon Robert Jackson, who had served during the American Revolutionary War, attributed it to the "principle of vegetation" which he described as extreme in the tropics (Jackson, *Outline of the History and Cure of Fever* 107). It depleted the body of its vital power. The effect was described as the oppression of the circulation, a distension of the blood vessels, and the secretion of bile. Consequently, the restoration of vitality was the prime aim of any treatment, and bleeding was seen as the preferred initial treatment for yellow fever by Jackson (Charles Powell 6–7; Harrison, *Medicine* 180).

Yet as early as 1760, a shift away from bloodletting had also occurred in the West Indies. By questioning the efficacy of bleeding, many overseas practitioners broke with European medical authority, arguing that bleeding was unsuitable in hot climates. Instead chemical remedies such as calomel and mercury, and also botanical remedies such as small quantities of bark in a glass of wine, gained in popularity (Harrison, *Medicine* 126–29). Mercurial treatment became increasingly popular in the West Indies after 1790 and after the devastating yellow fever epidemic on St. Domingue in 1793. In particular British surgeons practicing on St. Domingue, among them Colin Chisholm and army surgeon James Clark, were among its advocates (Chisholm, *An Essay on the Malignant Pestilential Fever* 163).[52] By the 1800s treatment with mercury was well established in the West Indies. It was recommended by James Clark and also by Benjamin Rush of Philadelphia who was probably introduced to the treatment by West Indian practitioners (Harrison, *Medicine* 155).

Yet Rush, during the devastating 1793 Philadelphia yellow fever epidemic, also relied heavily on the practice of bleeding. Although he drew far less blood than his contemporary Robert Jackson recommended and did not consider himself a follower of the British military physician, his practice strengthened the Englishman's case in Great Britain (Harrison, *Medicine* 183; Jackson, *Outline of the History and Cure of Fever*). In fact, in the 1810s and 1820s Edinburgh MD dissertations, often written by surgeons after returning from the West Indies, argued in favor of bleeding as the preferred treatment for yellow and other fevers, followed by "purgatives, emetics, and bark" (Harrison, *Medicine* 184; e.g. Steel). Bleeding again became the preferred treatment of the British and was to be accompanied by hot baths (e.g. M'Cabe 26–27, 32, 34).

---

52 At the same time the French still employed bloodletting extensively.

Spanish physicians who had encountered yellow fever in Seville in 1800 and Alicante in 1804 advocated cold baths as most effective (e.g. Arejula 211); and French physicians followed their lead (see Moreau de Jonnès 130). Interestingly, bleeding seemed to lose its attraction with French practitioners at the same time as its popularity was rising again with the British (Harrison, *Medicine* 188). While less intrusive and radical treatments generally seemed to get the upper hand in the course of the nineteenth century, the origin of the disease remained a mystery and object of speculation and imagination throughout the century. As early as 1848, physician Josiah Clark Nott published papers in which he proposed some connection between animalculae (Latin for little animals, in this context possibly insects) and disease. Writing at a time before the germ theory of disease had taken hold, Nott made no clear distinction between insects as pathogens and as vectors of pathogens (see also Humphreys, *Yellow Fever* 20) and thus cannot be credited as the originator of the mosquito theory. Interestingly, in a comic and highly ironic illustration in *Harper's Weekly*, mosquitoes are anthropomorphized as a nuisance; they are planning their attack, leaning over the globe, and practicing on their fiddles for their "summer campaign" (fig. 4). One might even argue that the sun emerges as an anthropomorphized trope—looking at the emerging catastrophe—in a repertoire of illustrations of nuisance and disease (cf. fig. 3). The tragic irony of the illustration only becomes apparent in retrospect. The year 1873 saw one of the worst yellow fever epidemics, yet the mosquito as its culprit was not yet known.

Fig. 4. Frederick S. Church, "Latest from the Front—Our Friends the Mosquitoes Preparing and Off for the Summer Campaign." Harper's Weekly *21 June 1873, 532.*

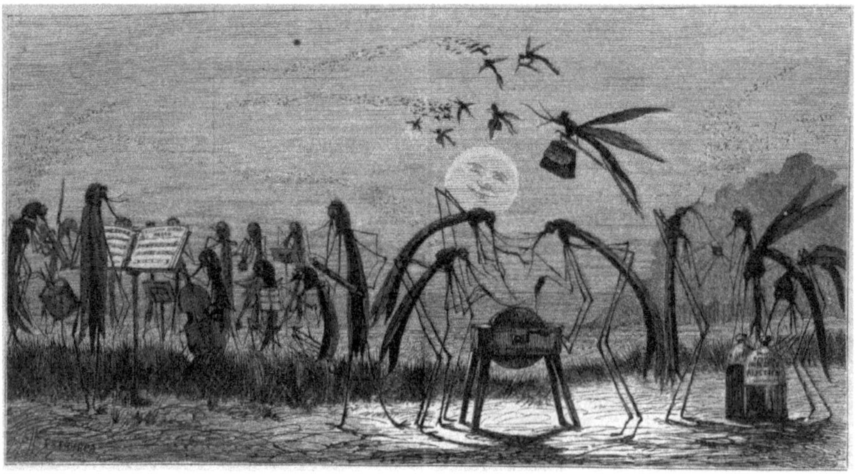

Beyond medical and literary discourses of origin and treatment, depictions of yellow fever are a favorite product of nineteenth-century culture in which the visual gained more and more prominence. The fascination with disease and its visualization was not a new phenomenon in the nineteenth century. The earliest European depictions of disease in the Americas probably date back to the sixteenth-century *Historia general de las cosas de Nueva España*, a collection of materials and information on Aztec and Nahua history collected by Fray Bernardino de Sahagún (fig. 5). The illustration created by an unknown author shows Nahuas infected with smallpox and is accompanied by a text in the Nahuatl language.[53]

Shortly after the smallpox illustrations by Sahagún, a painting of indigenous people treating their sick originated during René Goulaine de Laudonnière's expedition to Florida (fig. 6). Jacques Le Moyne de Morgues depicts three methods with which native people treated their sick (Le Moyne de Morgues and Bry). Theodor de Bry later produced the engraving. The sick Indians were placed on wooden benches lying on their back or on their stomach, depending upon the nature of their illness. The sick person on the left bench has the skin of his forehead cut with a sharp shell in order to collect the blood. A nursing woman with an infant in her arm stands behind the bench waiting to receive the blood to strengthen her child. For the sick person to the right, lying with his face downward, a fire is prepared onto which seeds are thrown, for the man to inhale. The idea is to purge possible poisons from the body and thus cure disease. A third treatment is depicted in the middle background. A man is holding a long pipe to his mouth and nose in order to cure an infection, while a woman is handing him dried leaves, called petum by the Brazilians and tapaco by the Spaniards.

53 An English translation of Sahagún's description is provided by James Lockhart and reads in part: "[The disease] brought great desolation: a great many died of it. They could no longer walk about, but lay in their dwellings and sleeping places, no longer able to move or stir. They were unable to change position, to stretch out on their sides or face down, or raise their heads. And when they made a motion, they called out loudly. The pustules that covered people caused great desolation; very many people died of them, and many just starved to death; starvation reigned, and no one took care of others any longer. On some people, the pustules appeared only far apart, and they did not suffer greatly, nor did many of them die of it. But many people's faces were spoiled by it, their faces were made rough. Some lost an eye or were blinded" (181–85).

An illustration, probably dating to the seventeenth century, shows the effects of European diseases, notably smallpox, measles, and typhus, upon the native population in a North American context (qtd. in Vogel n.pag.). Cut by colonial craftsmen illustrations such as this one are early examples of American graphic art (Reilly xiv). The round-houses pictured in the background help trace the engraving to a smallpox outbreak among Massachusetts Indians (fig. 7). The pathos of the gestures of the two standing women—raising their arms and tearing their hair—communicates desperation and fear. Two women and two children are spread at their feet: the children dead or almost dead, the women twisting in agony in front of their huts. In all three illustrations the focus is on the diseased Other. While the devastating effect of European diseases on the native population is depicted in the Sahagún and the North American engraving, de Bry's engraving shows foreign and cruel—i.e. savage—methods of healing. European explorers are absent in the three instances. Besides white curiosity and fascination, the visual rhetoric follows that of the superiority of the invaders and serves to justify their right to the land. Another engraving supports this reading: it depicts Edward Winslow's famous healing visit to Chief Massasoit of the Wampanoags in March 1623 (fig. 8). Winslow offered the sachem, who was most likely suffering from typhoid fever, "a confection of many comfortable conserues, &c. on the point of [his] knife. [...] then I washed his mouth, and got an abundance of corruption out of the same. After which I gaue him more of the confection, which he swallowed with more readinesse" (28). The presence of the colonial leader nursing the sick Indian leader prevails as a visual demonstration of superior European medical practice and treatment methods as well as the Europan leader's relationship to divine forces that caused disease—despite the fact that modern scholarship doubts Winslow's successful cure of Massasoit but attributes it equally to the Wampanoag's medical knowledge of local herbs and their properties (Priewe 87–88; Wisecup 78–79).

Fig. 5. Bernardino de Sahagún, Florentine Codex. *1540–1585. Book XII folio 54 [detail]. In: Sherry Fields,* Pestilence and Headcolds: Encountering Illness in Colonial Mexico. *Gutenberg-e series, e-book ed. New York: Columbia UP, 2008. Reproduction from the Ms. held at Biblioteca Medicea Laurenziana, Florence.*

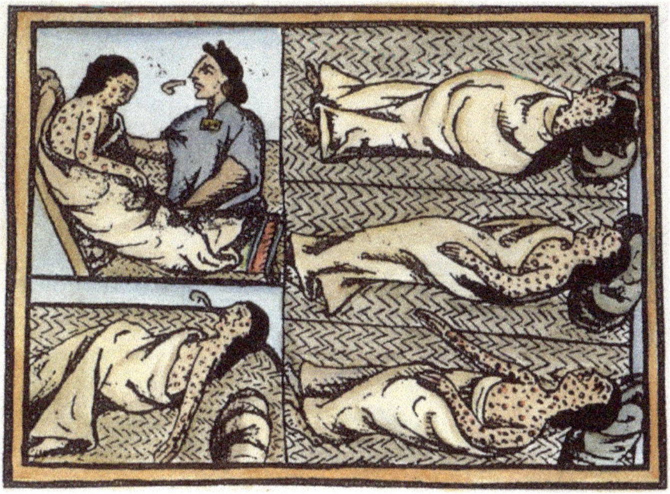

Fig. 6. How the Indians Treat Their Sick. *Theodor de Bry engraving, woodcut made after a painting by Jacques Le Moyne de Morgues (died 1588) while on the Laudonnière Expedition in Florida, ca. 1564.*

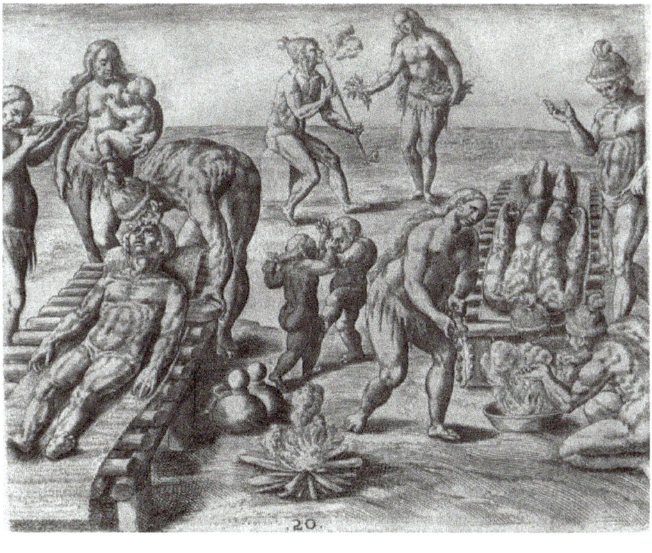

Fig. 7. "Smallpox epidemic among Massachussetts Indians." In: Virgil J. Vogel, American Indian Medicine. *1970. Norman: U of Oklahoma P, 1990. N.pag.*

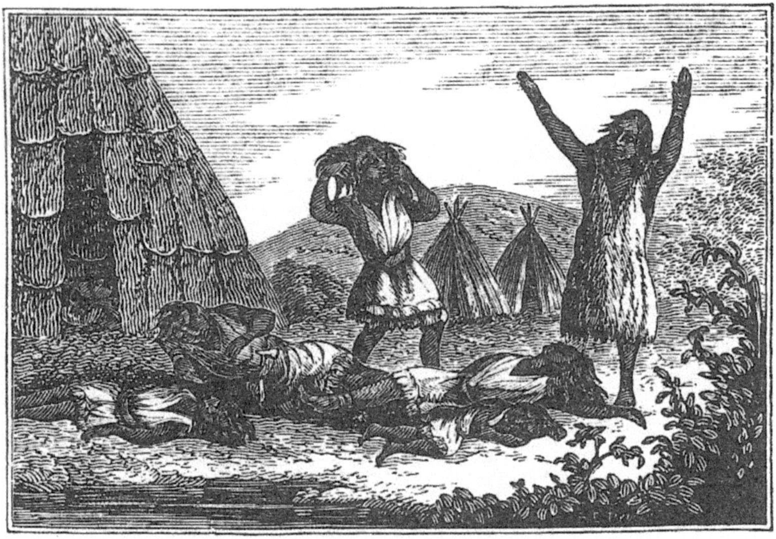

Fig. 8. "Edward Winslow's visit to Chief Massasoit of the Wampanoags." In: Virgil J. Vogel, American Indian Medicine. *1970. Norman: U of Oklahoma P, 1990. N.pag.*

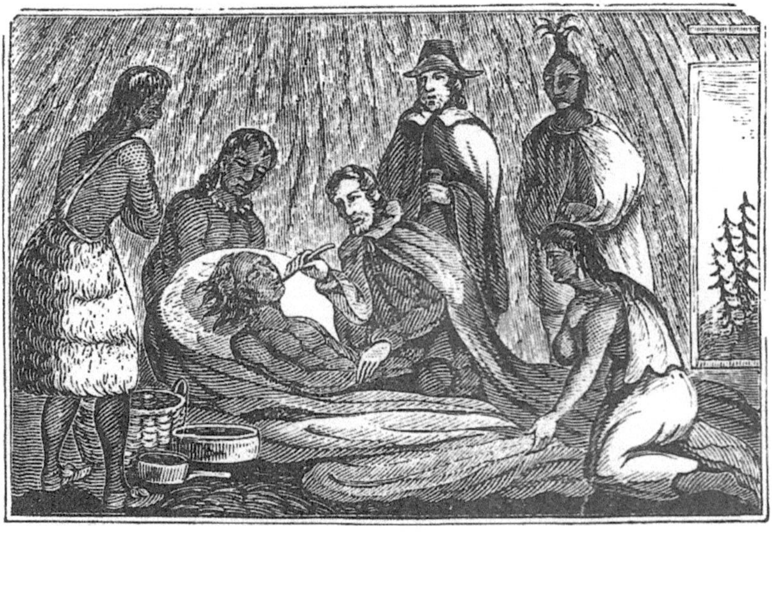

Another particularly memorable incident feeding into the culture of fear and disease imagination is the gift of the smallpox-infected blankets to Native American in what must be termed bio-medical warfare[54]. Stories of disease-infected blankets deliberately given to Native Americans have their roots in poison-garment tales of classical antiquity, most notably the Nessus shirt, the poisoned garment that killed Heracles. The plan of Lord Jeffrey Amherst to infect Indians with smallpox-infected blankets, taken from the corpses of British soldiers at Fort Pitt in 1863, is documented in a letter to Colonel Henry Bouquet. However, whether there was a direct command issued by Amherst is part of an ongoing controversy. Historians only agree that a smallpox epidemic did indeed rage that summer (cf. Mayor 54–55, 57–58).

Invisible adversaries continued to stir anxieties in the nineteenth century, for example through 'undetected' immigrant carriers of disease such as the infamous Typhoid Mary. Yellow fever, in turn, was known as 'strangers' disease' in the nineteenth-century United States because 'unacclimated' newcomers to the region seemed much more vulnerable to infection than longtime residents. This, in turn, led to the stigmatization of those groups.

Disease topics were naturally taken up by the leading illustrated newspapers of the second half of the nineteenth century. There had been some illustrations in magazines for nearly a hundred years, when *Leslie's* and *Harper's* first appeared in 1855 and 1857 respectively (Mott, *1850–1865* 36–38, 208–10, 519–24). Yet the illustrations in the two pictorials—first with woodcuts and later with half-tones from daguerreotypes and photography—set new standards in illustrated publishing in the United States.[55] *Frank Leslie's Illustrated Newspaper* was first published on December 15, 1855 as a small sixteen-page weekly illustrated with large, striking woodcuts, selling at ten cents an issue (or four dollars a year). The pictures usually followed the events portrayed by two weeks. Such a quick preparation

54 Laurence Hauptman, Francis Flavin, and Constance Cappel even speak of a Native American genocide in their studies (Hauptman 4; Flavin 1; Cappel; see also Banerjee, *Ethnic Ventriloquism* 180–81).

55 Many American magazines, in fact, were modeled closely after British periodicals. *Harper's Weekly* drew on the *Illustrated London News*; and Henry Carter, alias Frank Leslie—who had even worked on British illustrated papers—copied their characteristics for his own endeavors (Mott, *1850–1865* 130). Leslie had come to New York in 1848. Originally from England, he was an engraver on wood and became first associated with Gleason, Strong, and then P.T. Barnum in a publishing venture before he became involved in the publishing business himself. He started several periodicals, among which *Frank Leslie's Illustrated Newspaper* was the greatest.

and publication of pictures was a novelty and made possible by a woodcut technique introduced by Leslie. He divided a block into as many as 32 sections and gave a section to each of his many engravers. The joins would sometimes show as white in the printed picture, but were deemed negligible (cf. Mott, *1850–1865* 454). The method also allowed him to produce larger pictures. The pictures were mostly of the sensational kind, including murders, prizefights, and disasters (such as the war in Nicaragua, prize fighting in Kansas, or the Burdell murder; cf. Mott, *1850–1865* 454).

Soon after its introduction in 1857 *Harper's*, whose weekly was also referred to as their "illustrated Bible," dominated the market because it produced the best pictures (Mott, *1850–1865* 192).[56] To emphasize its pictures even more, *Harper's*—soon after its inception—moved the editorials to the second page in order to create more space on the first page to feature pictures (Mott 2: 471). Pictures became more and more important, and the technique of producing sections that were then put together was copied from *Leslie's*.[57] Another model for *Harper's* was the *London Illustrated News* (especially the typography is similar) (Mott, *1850–1865* 470).

Subtitled *A Journal of Civilization*, *Harper's Weekly* was marketed as a "family newspaper" and "a first-class newspaper" (qtd. in Mott, *1850–1865* 470–71) toward an educated audience that resembled an emerging middle class. As such, *Harper's* had a distinctly higher quality than *Leslie's* and was better edited and better printed (Mott, *1850–1865* 44–45). An 1860 advertisement for the newspaper also points to its superior picture quality. The ad was printed in *The Diary of a Samaritan*, written by William L. Robinson (1860), a narrative journal published by Harper & Brothers that details the experiences of a male Howard's Association worker (who is hierarchically positioned between nurse and physician) during the 1853 New Orleans yellow fever epidemic; a book which does not include any illustrations of the epidemic:

> Every Number of HARPER'S WEEKLY contains all the News of the week, Domestic and Foreign. The completeness of this department is, it is believed, unrivaled in any other weekly publication. Every noteworthy event is profusely and accurately illustrated at the time of its occurrence. And while no expense is spared to procure Original Illustrations, care is taken to lay before the reader every foreign picture which appears to possess

56 *Harper's* (1857–1916) was stronger editorially and more dignified than *Leslie's Weekly*. Frank L. Mott ranks Harper's as of "distinctly higher quality than *Leslie's*" (*1850–1865* 44) and speaks of *Leslie's* "freshness and freedom," while *Harper's* is "better edited and better printed" (*1850–1865* 45).

57 The first major pictures were of President Buchanan and his cabinet (April 11, 1857) and a double-page picture of the steamship *Leviathan* (March 6, 1858) (Mott, *1850–1865* 471).

general interest. In a word, the Subscriber to HARPER'S WEEKLY may rely upon obtaining a Pictorial History of the times in which we live, compiled and illustrated in the most perfect and complete manner possible. (Robinson n.pag.)

Harper's was undoubtedly a serious competitor of *Frank Leslie's*, which criticized the younger paper in several bitter paragraphs and introduced aggressive price policies to regain the upper hand (4 Feb. 1860, qtd. in Mott, *1850–1865* 455).[58] Gib Prettyman concludes that *Harper's* "subject matter blended aesthetics and news. Its purpose combined politics, education, and entertainment" (26). *Leslie's* content, on the other hand, was highly miscellaneous; it published serial fiction, travel sketches, and also crusades against local abuses.

An example of the political influence of disease-related pictorial representations and one of the most memorable episodes in the early history of *Frank Leslie's Illustrated Newspaper* was the campaign against the "swill milk" abuse (cf. Moore). In May 1858, the paper attacked the shocking conditions in the dairies that supplied most of New York City with milk. Cows were fed on distillery waste, which stimulated milk production until the poisoned cow's death. The cows developed sores and their tails rotted off. It was exactly those images of "diseased, stump-tailed, dying cows" (Mott, *1850–1865* 456) that *Leslie's* artists created that proved to be more effective than the sharp editorial comments (fig. 9). A cover illustration from May 22, 1858, shows the dissection of a diseased cow and accompanies an article on "Our Exposure to the Swill Milk Trade." The caption of the larger illustration names the location, the Offal Dock, at the foot of Forty-Fifth Street, East River, N.Y., to which the cow was brought from the 16th Street swill cow stables. The putrefied upper right side of the cow is visible, and the dissection is witnessed by health wardens, Frank Leslie, and his corps taking notes. Lewis J. Kirk, the dissector, is portrayed as soldierlike in the smaller illustration. The continued visual and textual attacks of the paper (which became deeply involved in city politics) eventually prompted the corrupt city government to appoint an investigating committee from the New York Academy of Medicine. The report, made public in spring of 1859, "fully justified Leslie's every contention" (Mott, *1850–1865* 457). However, it took another two years until the sale of milk from distillery-waste to feed cows was forbidden (in the spring of 1861). The *American Medical Times* wrote on May 17, 1862, that "the delineations of Mr. Leslie, horrible as they were,

58 The older paper reduced its price (to six cents a number and two dollars a year) and increased its circulation to 164,000 before the war. Production costs brought the price back, by degrees, to ten cents a number and four dollars a year; by 1865 circulation was down to 50,000 and leveled out at 70,000 after the war and before the depression of the later seventies, when it declined to 40,000 (Mott, *1850–1865* 460).

fell short of the truth" ("Finale of Swill Milk" 278). The paper's yellow fever reporting, albeit ten to twenty years later and with a somewhat different agenda (to inform about the epidemic, to prompt public donation, and to secure the paper's circulation in economically dire times), again applied the—by this time—successful sensationalist formula with regard to medical concerns.

Fig. 9. "Our Exposure to the Swill Milk Trade." Frank Leslie's Illustrated Newspaper *22 May 1858, 385. Library of Congress Prints and Photographs Division, LC-USZ62-121642.*

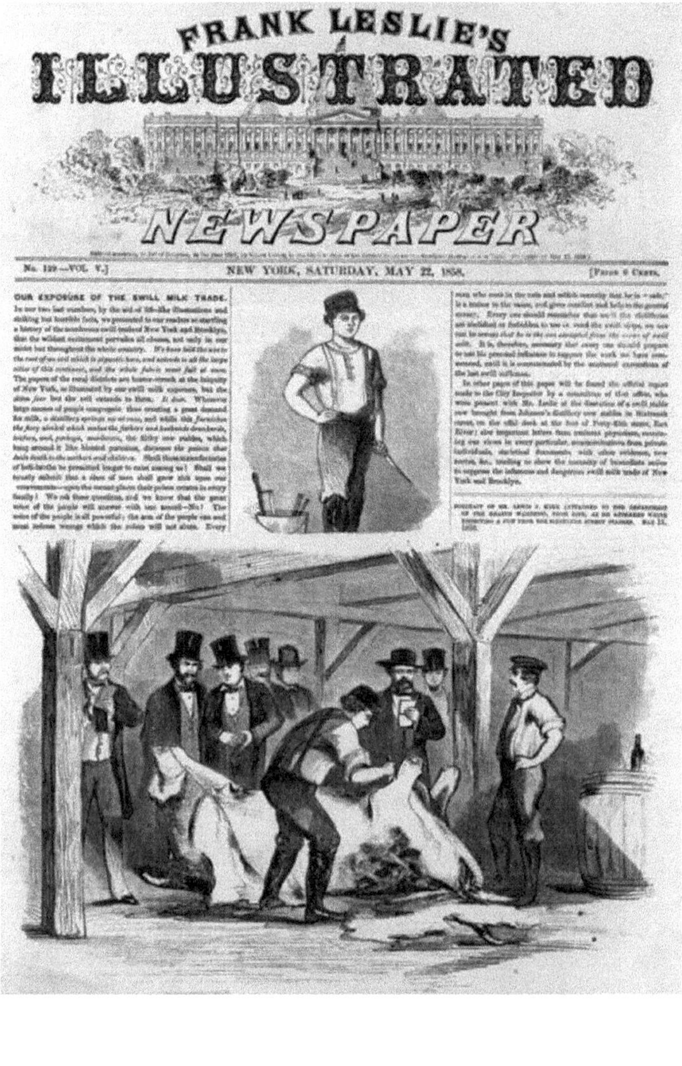
FRANK LESLIE'S ILLUSTRATED NEWSPAPER

NEW YORK, SATURDAY, MAY 22, 1858.

OUR EXPOSURE OF THE SWILL MILK TRADE.

Sensationalist pictorials were also very much sought after when the war broke out in 1861. *Harper's Weekly* took the lead in reporting (in pictures and articles) about the war[59]; *Frank Leslie's* probably ranked second (cf. Mott, *1850–1865* 150). By 1865, *Harper's* was the most important weekly in existence because of George William Curtis' editorials and Thomas Nast's news pictures and political cartoons, both of which proved to be important shapers of national public opinion.[60] Illustrations remained an important part of the *Weekly's* content, and it developed a reputation for employing some of the most renowned illustrators besides Nast, notably Winslow Homer, Granville Perkins and Livingston Hopkins.[61] *Frank Leslie's* newspaper was equally elaborately illustrated, yet its character in editorship was much less pronounced and circulation went down during the war, while that of *Harper's Weekly* was going up (Mott, *1865–1885* 40).

By the 1870s pictures had become a large part of the contents of the *Weekly*, including illustrations of events, places, and persons in the news, and social cartoons, as well as fashion plates. Despite the financial crises of the 1870s and fluctuating markets, *Harper's* (both *Monthly* and *Weekly*) upheld a circulation of over 100,000 in the period between 1865 and 1885 (Mott, *1865–1885* 6), reaching 160,000 in 1872, whereas *Leslie's*—whose circulation had again improved after the war—had to file for bankruptcy in 1878. It recovered, and a later success of the paper was its excellent pictorial history of the Spanish-American War. However, no drawings or half-tones from photographs that depict yellow fever patients in Cuba were published.[62]

---

59 The war circulation of *Harper's* was larger than ever: 120,000 by the end of 1861 (Mott, *1850–1865* 475) and above 100,000 throughout the conflict (an unusual circulation for that time).

60 The twenty-two year old Nast "who had worked on *Frank Leslie's Illustrated Newspaper* and the *Illustrated News*, the two competitors of *Harper's Weekly* in the field of illustrated journalism" joined in 1862 and lead *Harper's* into a new epoch (Mott, *1850–1865* 474).

61 *Harper's Weekly* "was distinguished for the quality and quantity of its illustrations at a time when the laborious process of woodcut engravings made pictures expensive and journalistically cumbersome" (Prettyman 26). Engravings were first (and until 1865) mostly based on steel and copper as proper mediums (Mott, *1850–1865* 192). Later, pictorial weeklies, such as *Leslie's Illustrated* and *Harper's Weekly*, and *Gleason's Pictorial* used wood cuts (Mott, *1850–1865* 193).

62 Artists such as F. Cresson Schell, B. West Clinedinst, and G.A. Traver were responsible for the drawings, correspondents: Gilson Willets, Edwin Emerson, George Edward Graham, Teresa Dean. *Leslie's* at this point was able to publish half tones from photographs as a special feature (and also published many personal stories of the war) (Mott, *1850–1865* 464).

The United States saw a rapid development of mass-market periodicals at the end of the nineteenth century when large-circulation periodicals emphasized journalistic prose and included plentiful illustrations. The period also marked the shift from wood-engraved illustrations to half-tone reproductions and publication of photographs that allowed more newspapers and magazines to include illustrations. In 1892 the *Chicago Graphic* commented that numerous new magazines engaging "every field of human thought" transformed the medium not only into "a school of literature but of science, art and politics as well" (qtd. in Mott, *1885–1905* 12). Gib Prettyman points out that "[i]n this capacity as explorers of new territories and educators of new audiences, American magazines seemed not just democratic but positively transformative" (25).

3.3 Yellow Fever under the Touristic or Distant Gaze: An Aesthetics of the Destructive Sublime

> It is by [sympathy] that we enter into the concerns of others; that we are moved as they are moved, and are never suffered to be indifferent spectators of almost anything which men can do or suffer. For sympathy must be considered as a sort of substitution, by which we are put into the place of another man, and affected in many respects as he is affected.
>
> (E. Burke 44)

In the 1870s and 1880s, *Frank Leslie's* and *Harper's Weekly* turned their journalistic gaze to yellow fever victims and their circumstances. In contrast to the medical gaze theorized by Foucault in a French cultural context, which separates the patient's body from the patient's person, the yellow fever illustrations rely more on a 'touristic' gaze in the sense of providing insights into the culture of disease from a safe distance. The pictures represent a virtual tour of diseased America and enable viewers to participate in the journey the illustrators and reporters undertook to document the epidemic.

An often pictured experience in yellow fever illustrations is not only the suffering of the sick body but also the moment of death or dying. In this way, the illustrations depict the experience of disease, sometimes at the sublime moment of death or shortly after it. Barbie Zelizer examined the journalistic practice of of suggesting, yet not showing death. What he states with regard to news photography of insinuated death can also be applied to yellow fever illustrations, adding "impulses of implication, contingency, conditionality, play, imagination, emotionality, desire, supposal, hypothesis, hope, liminality, and (im)possibility to the supposed certainty of visual representation," which proves their usefulness "in the unsettled times associated with war, terrorism, natural disaster, epidemic, torture, and planned violence" (14; cf. Leikam 42). Sara Blair speaks of "afterlives" of popular, but controversial pictures and their "agency in competing narratives" (692). The images conjure up a feeling of the 'destructive sublime' (Orvell, "After 9/11"). They may also be read under Edmund Burke's contemporaneously revived and adapted paradigm of an 'aesthetics of the sublime,' a theory that had defined artistic impact with regard to its effect on the viewer, calculating that through the viewer's dissociation from the perceived pain there is enjoyment to be found in suffering. In other words, Burke carefully distinguished the sublime from the beautiful and instead associated the feeling of terror with it (Gasché 25). With reference to Burke, Oliver Jehle explains that:

> [t]his aesthetic affect that arises when contemplating a tragic image leads to the paradoxical phenomenon that the enjoyment received by the viewer of the tragic object increases in proportion to the vehemence of the existential threat with which he is visually confronted. [...] [T]he viewer experience[s] pleasure because he believes himself to be secure and able to withdraw from the aesthetic horror and return unscathed. (91)

In regard to fictional representations, this rational operation—to compare one's own condition to that of the recipient—has been described as a delight at a distance (*Distanzlust*).

While these nineteenth-century illustrations fictionalize the experience, the degree of their fictionalization (*Fiktionsgrad*)—or their relative representation of reality—also determines their moral and political implications. In the case of the yellow fever illustrations, the reason for their creation is not in the first degree aesthetic but aimed at sensation as well as economic success of the paper. Matthew Rubery explains that "the sensational elements of the press were a crucial means by which audiences engaged with the world through sentimental narratives designed to elicit an emotional response" (504). The newspaper reporters and illustrators from *Frank Leslie's* and *Harper's Weekly* were explicitly sent to New Orleans and Memphis during the epidemics to illustrate moving scenes from the yellow fever devastation. They created pictures that 'tell a story' and as such strive to represent a version of the suffering experienced in the Southern United States (at the location of yellow fever epidemics), and the readers reacted to it.[63]

63 See fig. 33 in Orvell's *American Photography*, a cover illustration from *Frank Leslie's Illustrated Newspaper* showing the horrible treatment of prisoners at Andersonville. The original photographs were translated as engravings to make "them less shocking than the actual photos" (*American Photography* 65).

In 1878, a double-page spread series of dramatic yellow fever illustrations in *Frank Leslie's* represented graphic depictions of suffering ("Yellow Fever Visitation" 56–57). In some of these chaotic scenes, readers beheld sick and dying people on park benches and in the shrubs beside railroad tracks like wounded animals, with physicians refusing to go near or people fleeing the scene (figs. 10–11).[64] *Frank Leslie's* "Two Tramps Dying in Jackson Square, New Orleans" is a highly theatricalized representation of the yellow fever scene. The inclusion of a man fleeing from the dying acts as an implied spectator to the staged scene. Signifiers of disease that are graphically depicted within the accompanying text—"the horrible black vomit"—are absent in the lithograph. The picture bears witness not primarily to the ravages of yellow fever but to its sentimental response and its re-representation for bourgeois consumption. As the implied spectator flees the scene in disgust, not to get help, but to preserve himself, removal is depicted as a strategy to evade the disease. Interestingly, the subordination of the image of disease to sentimental norms is not conducted by the 'sayable'—the accompanying text is quite specific about the disease—but by the 'seeable,' which sanitizes the graphic newspaper text for media consumption.[65] However, these sentimental pictures, with people dying in the squares or in "out-of-the-way places" ("Yellow Fever Visitation" 59), also destabilize ethical notions of how the sick should be treated. By examining other people's cruel and gruesome experiences, readers and viewers also become more conscious of their selves. The newspaper texts and the illustrations confronted readers with the documentary intensity of direct observation and at the same time presented a wide variety of yellow fever experiences of different classes, genders, and ages (cf. Prettyman 29). They provide visual evidence of the epidemics and produce coherent narratives for public consumption. In this sense, the pictures serve as a means to bearing witness, symbolized on some of the illustrations by the presence of the reporter. He is, for example, carefully approaching (with his head drawn) the dying woman beside the railroad tracks, and he is entering a sick room on Jefferson Street. He is, as such, taking over a role similar to the examining physician (who in the case of the woman beside the tracks refuses to go near), yet the reporter's examination of the scenes—because of its intended publication—takes on a wider public dimension.

---

64 The accompanying news report further explains: "Of course, there are some cases of inhumanity in the more rural districts, where the scare is greatest. A correspondent recently, in journeying by rail, saw at Grand Junction, Tenn., a lady from Memphis alone in the weeds by the side of the track, dying of yellow fever, and three doctors within fifty yards, who refused to go near" ("Yellow Fever Visitation" 59).

65 I am grateful to Christopher Lukasik for his astute comments regarding the illustration.

Fig. 10. *"Two Tramps Dying in Jackson Square."* Frank Leslie's Illustrated Newspaper *28 Sept. 1878, 57.*

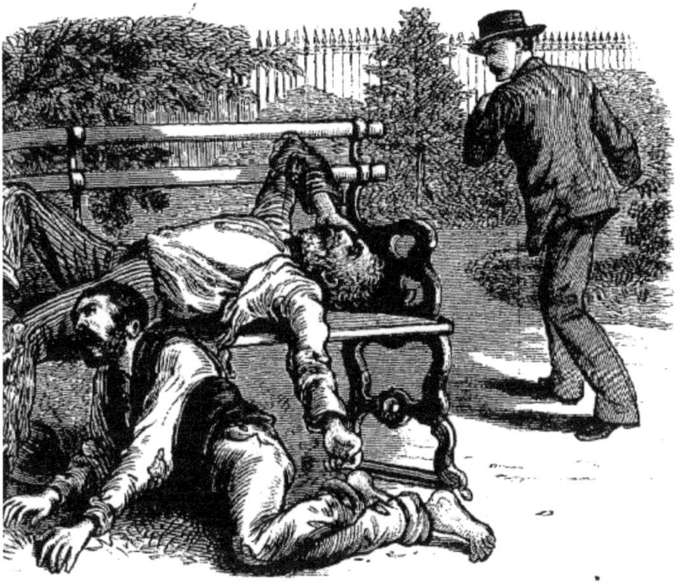

Fig. 11. *"Woman Dying Beside the Railroad Tracks."* Frank Leslie's Illustrated Newspaper *28 Sept. 1878, 56.*

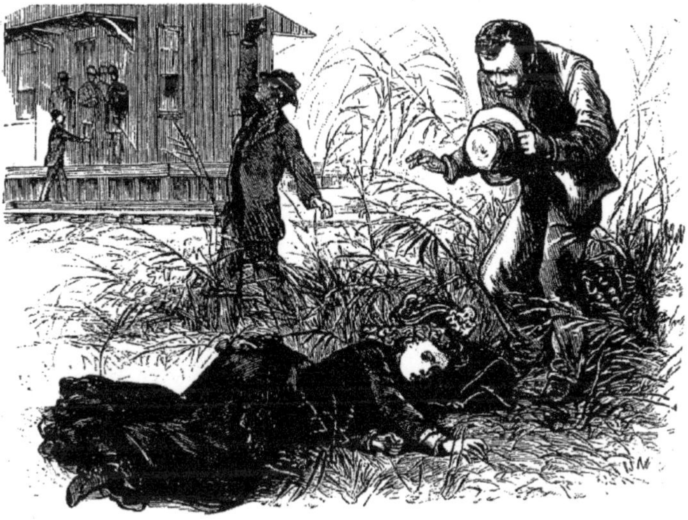

The pictures, often surpassed in pictorial detail by the accompanying texts, are revolting and—as such—satisfy voyeurism; yet, they are mainly effective in arousing public (communal) feeling. This is similar to nineteenth-century sentimental fiction, whose cultural work Jane Tompkins has asserted as "an act of persuasion aimed at defining social reality" (141) by "presenting an affective alternative that not only gave political actions their emotional significance, but beyond that, intimately linked individual bodies to the national body" (4). This is also a testament to just how visualized sentimental literature had become. In their composition, *Frank Leslie's* pictures build on the habits of the viewers, employing the familiar forms of emotional style and sentimental formulas with mainly children and women suffering and domestic settings in complete disarray representing a loss of order. Pictures of childhood were popular for their ability to arouse feelings of affection and protectiveness of a state perceived as separate and innocent. Deathbed scenes equally drew from the sentimental storehouse and allowed for the exploration of pathos. Since strong or exaggerated physical gestures—pathos formulas in aesthetic representations—are recognized by most viewers, they enable an easy identification of the expressed emotion (cf. Schulz 52).

On one tableau a woman twists in agony, her husband and at least two of her six children are dead and spread across the bed and floor, while one child seems to pray and a boy looks to the doorway where help in the form of a reporter is entering (fig. 12). The absence of any other help and the imploring look of the boy intensifies the reporter's presence, the only option left to them in order to not die unnoticed and unseen. The visual narrative is even surpassed by the graphic description of the reporter, who professes himself "sick to think of [the sight]." The copious black vomit, which takes on a stigmatic function[66] that marks the diseased individual, is only mentioned in the copy text: "[T]he black vomit spattered all over the bed and the room. The mother was dying, and the horrible black vomit—it looks like coffee grounds—was running out of her mouth into the face and breast of one of the children that lay on the floor by the bed. Ugh!" ("Yellow Fever Visitation" 59). Avoiding any kind of medical jargon, the analogy quite visually describes the yellow fever experience to those who have never seen the disease. Yet it remains absent from the visual representation.

66 "[S]tigma exists when elements of labeling, stereotyping, separation, status loss, and discrimination occur in a power situation that allows them" write Bruce G. Link and Jo C. Phelan (Link and Phelan 363) referring to sociologist Erving Goffman's work.

Fig. 12. "A Sad Scene in a Jefferson Street Dwelling, Memphis." Frank Leslie's Illustrated Newspaper *28 Sept. 1878, 57.*

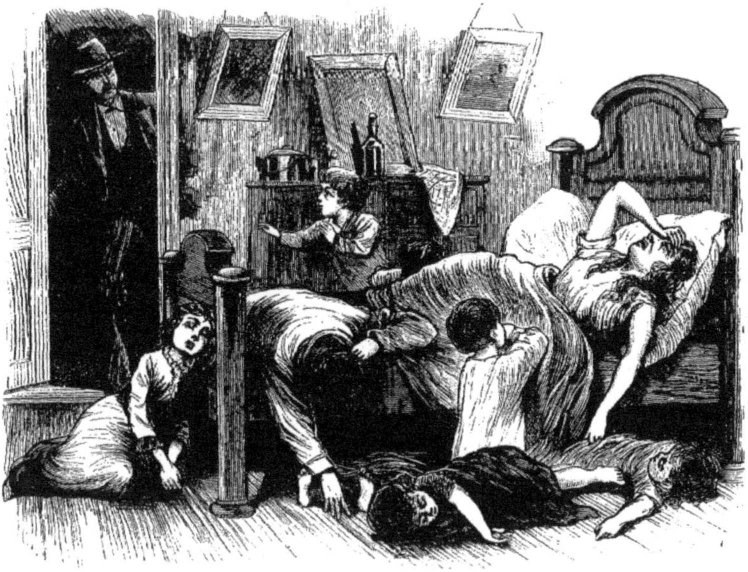

A more stately (and aesthetically more pleasing) deathbed scene is portrayed in another lithograph (fig. 13). A seemingly well-off but nevertheless sick woman lies in bed, bemoaned by her husband and children, and attended to by a physician and a black servant. From the accompanying text we learn that the woman, identified as Mrs. Zonane, was not told by her doctor about her yellow fever plight until shortly before her death. Her five children were discouraged from kissing her good-bye but did so nevertheless. The text describes their lips as "stained with that horrible stream of death" ("Yellow Fever Visitation" 59), yet none of them caught the fever—following the conventional narrative of redemption. The deathbed scene—widely used as a cultural trope at the time—and employed here in *Frank Leslie's*, presents a "version of the ethic of sacrifice [...] that the highest human calling is to give one's life for another" (Tompkins 128).[67] The appropriation of the deathbed iconography retains the focus on women and children and cites the salience of a body in agony.

67 Tompkins elaborates: "The power of the dead or the dying to redeem the unregenerate is a major theme of nineteenth-century popular fiction and religious literature. Mothers and children are thought to be uniquely capable of this work" (128).

Fig. 13. "The Five Children of Mrs. Zonane, of Memphis, Kissing Their Dying Mother." Frank Leslie's Illustrated Newspaper *28 Sept. 1878, 56.*

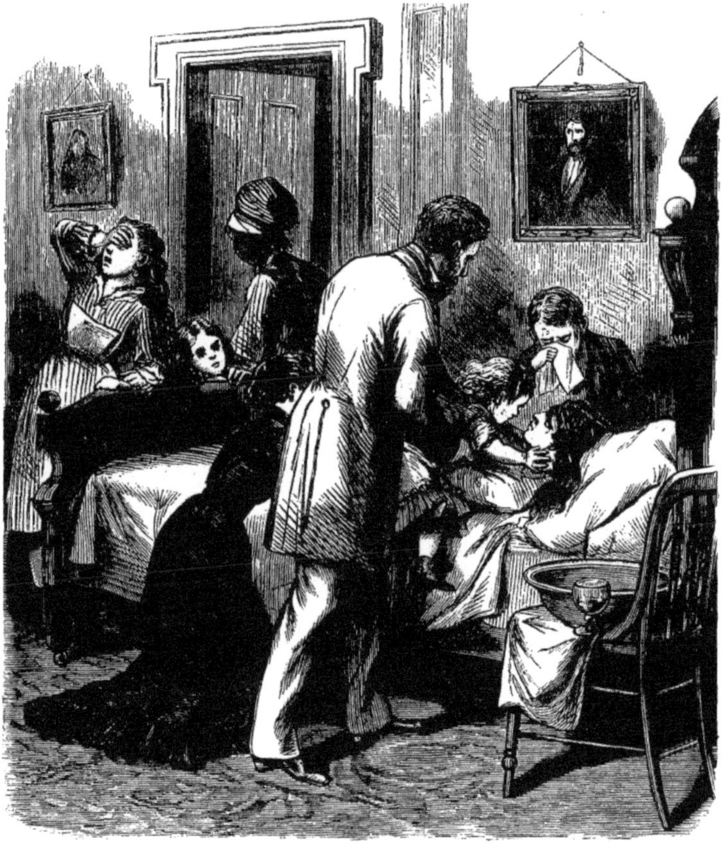

In New Orleans, the Sisters of Charity took care of those sick and dying of yellow fever (fig. 14). One picture shows them in attendance of the most innocent victims, the children at St. Vincent's Infant Asylum, many of whose parents had already died from the fever. The large hall-like room full of little cots represents the extent of the calamity, and the accompanying report gives the number of the sick: seventy out of 200 children. Their pinched bodies and grotesque black-rimmed eyes are marked by the disease. The picture focuses on the nursing care of the nuns: feeding, fanning, rocking, and hand-holding are represented, a physician talks to a child in the background. There's solace in the illustration, yet also desperation in light of the many suffering children.

Fig. 14. "Children in St. Vincent's Infant Asylum." Frank Leslie's Illustrated Newspaper *28 Sept. 1878, 56.*

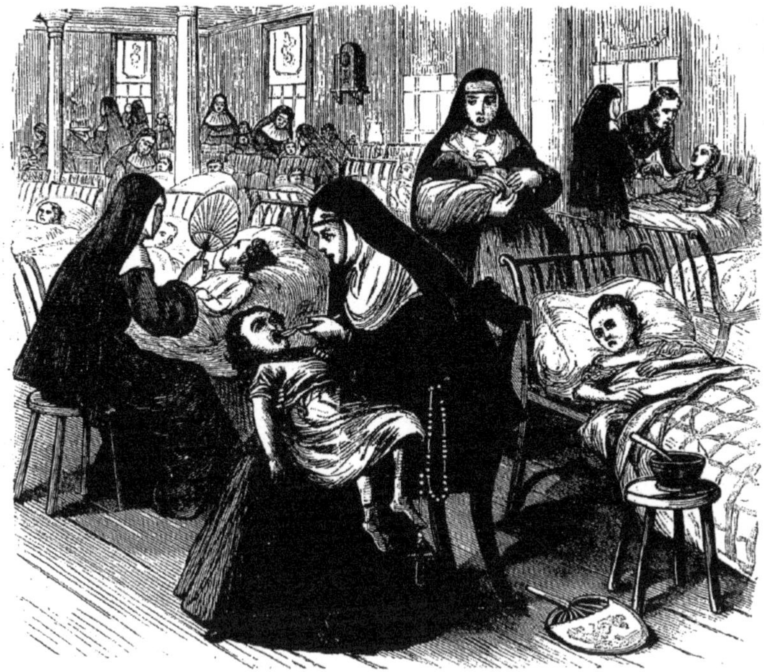

One year later, a front-page illustration from *Frank Leslie's* on September 20, 1879, confronted its readers with a shadowy, bare room in which a sick man writhes in pain while an equally worn-out woman, with a barefooted little child clinging to her apron, opens the door to admit a Sister of Charity (fig. 15). This lithograph from a sketch by D. B. Moise is a typical threshold situation employing the familiar forms of emotional style and formulas used in Christian art, such as the nun's blessing hand reminiscent of a guardian angel figure. The package in her other hand speaks of sustenance and relief. Moise's illustration is structured along the binary opposition between inside and outside, darkness and light; the sick are contrasted with the healthy savior. Interestingly, the figure of hope is a female nurse and not a male physician as in some of *Leslie*'s critical depictions of representatives of the profession, e.g. of doctors who refuse to go near the infected, as in the picture of the woman dying beside the railroad tracks (fig. 11). The candle on the table is blown out and illustrates the fading life of the sick man; the shadows equally portend death. The visual impact, the 'story' the front-page illustration tells, is enhanced in the accompanying article which, first of all, establishes it as "a scene from real life" ("Memphis Under Quarantine Rule" 43). The reader learns that the family had to sell their possessions for the provision of food and medicine, since the unfortunate sick man could no longer work. An illustrated book seems to be one of the items left; yet the once reliable written work lies discarded on the floor.

Fig. 15. "Sisters of Charity Administering to Sick and Dying Victims of Yellow Fever." Frank Leslie's Illustrated Newspaper *20 Sept. 1879, 33.*

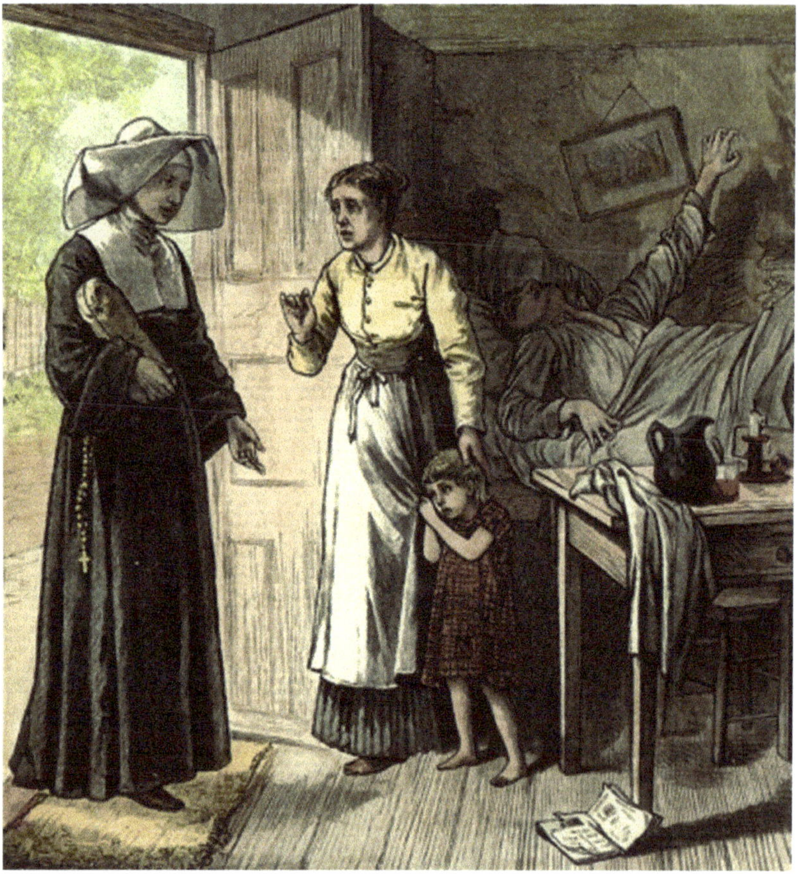

The terrible shadow of a terrible death is in that apartment. The wife now fears for her child, her famine-stricken child, who, already in the nausea of sickness, has ceased to clamor for food. Her husband dying, her child stricken—what a picture of utter desolation, of utter despair! A timid knock comes to the door; it remains unheeded. A second

> knock, and the crushed woman drags her tottering limbs to the portal. A ray of God's sunlight leaps into the room. In the doorway stands the messenger of consolation, the gentle messenger who will pour oil upon the bleeding wounds, and who will repeat the great grand lesson of the Good Samaritan. ("Memphis Under Quarantine Rule" 43)

The description—like the illustration—also provides an example of sentimental and religious pathos. It hardly comes as a surprise that an outpouring of sympathy, concern, and aid was stimulated by these illustrations, as documented in the picture with packages for yellow fever victims piled up (fig. 16).[68] Evidence of a Northern popular consciousness and willingness to donate is also given on the front page of the issue that contains a variety of reactions to the yellow fever crisis (fig. 17). It shows women and children, including a black woman, throwing money into a contribution box. Men are not contributing and are sketched only in the background. The compassionate sentiment is mirrored in the captions and the accompanying news reports.

Fig. 16. "New York City—The Organized Collection of Supplies for the Yellow Fever Sufferers at the South." Frank Leslie's Illustrated Newspaper *26 Oct. 1878, 128.*

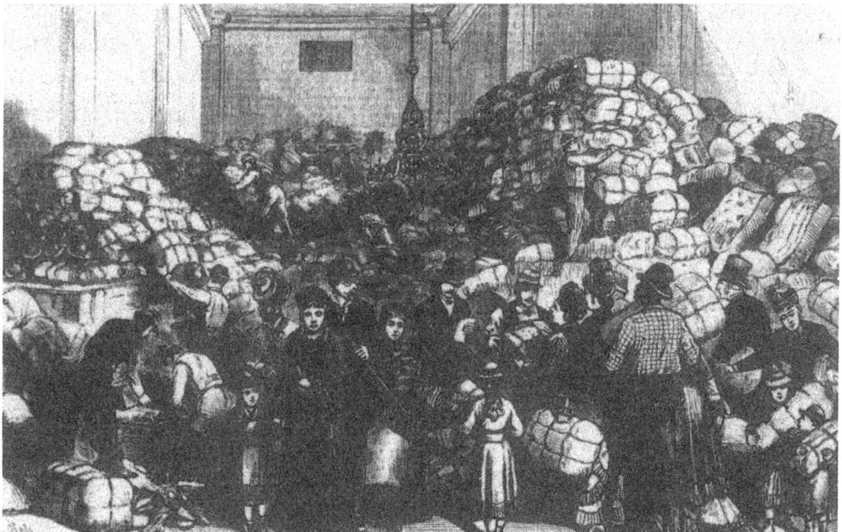

68 Two popular novellas of the 1870s by Wesley Bradshaw have the respective heroine read about yellow fever victims in the news to stimulate their rushing to the rescue (see ch. 4.3).

Fig. 17. "New York City—The Great Metropolis Heeding the Cry of Distress from the Fever-Stricken South." Frank Leslie's Illustrated Newspaper *28 Sept. 1878, 49.*

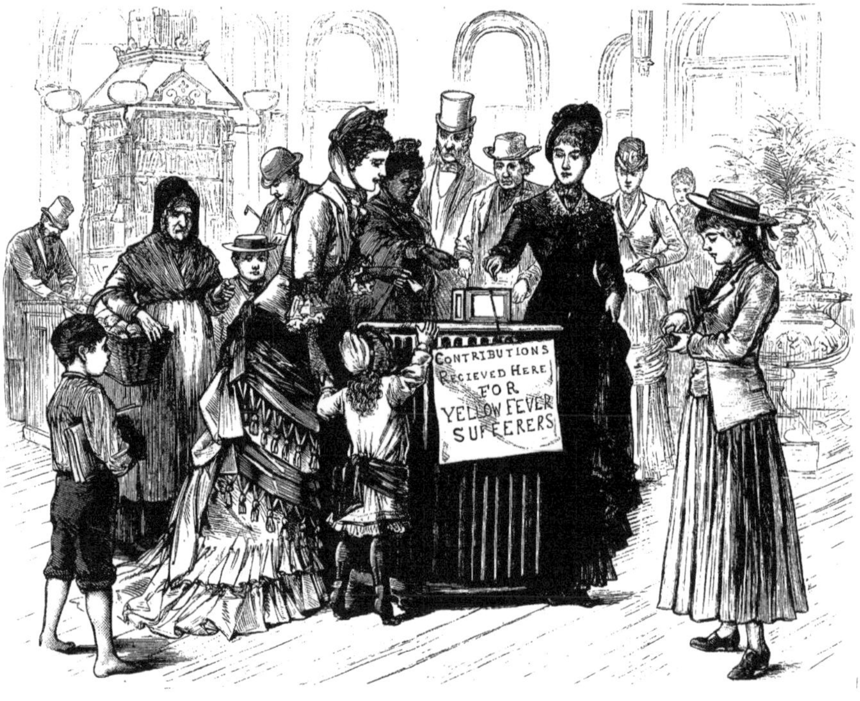

While the somewhat religiously inflated but realistic-sensationalist depictions presuppose the empathy of the readers to control the disease, two prints from the late 1880s use a different strategy and represent disease in a metaphorical way. Matthew Somerville Morgan's (1839–1890) drawing illustrates the 1888 yellow fever epidemic in the Jacksonville area of Florida (fig. 18).[69] The personification

69 The Jacksonville area experienced a devastating epidemic in the summer of 1888. Patterson estimates the deaths in the hundreds (858). The epidemic came from Cuba and had raged in Key West in 1887, the following year it moved up the west coast to Tampa and across to Jacksonville. *Frank Leslie's* frequently published reports on the epidemic between August and October of 1888 ("Yellow Fever in Florida"; "The Yellow-Fever Ravages"; "The Plague-Stricken South"; "Memphis Under Quarantine Rule"; "Under the Shadow of the Plague"; "Ancient and Modern Plagues"). The American Red Cross, established by Clara Barton in May 1881, offered relief during the 1888 Jacksonville epidemic (Jones 29).

of yellow fever dragging down Florida as Columbia rushes to the rescue was published in *Frank Leslie's*. The yellow fever demon with "Yellow Jack" written across his chest follows the visual language of allegorical representations of disease. Given the skull-like features of the beast one is also reminded of the British print of "The torrid zone, or, blessings of Jamaica" (fig. 3). The full lips allude to those known from blackface minstrelsy and as such point toward the constructed blackness of the disease (black vomit; presumed black immunity; African/Caribbean source of the disease). Furthermore, the animalistic legs and talons turn Yellow Jack into a hybrid non-human figure symbolizing evil. The demon clutches Florida's throat and her crotch with sharp talons. The sexualization and metaphoric curtailment of the reproductive organs add to the sensational character of the picture. Regarding the sexual connotation, it seems interesting to note the relatively low inhibition threshold (*Peinlichkeitsschwelle/Schamschwelle*) (cf. Elias) of the picture. In the case of yellow fever images, the borderline between what could be depicted and what might have been unseemly is somewhat hard to pinpoint, with the exception of a general avoidance of nakedness or explicit sexuality at least in the realist newspaper illustrations. Patients—even if in pain—are mostly tucked underneath sheets. However, the graphic depictions of the painful yellow fever experience seem to point toward a comparatively low threshold regarding appalling illustrations. Sensationalist detail, such as distorted suffering figures, satisfies voyeuristic enjoyment, but also stirs the capacity for empathy.

The triangular, pieta-style arrangement of the group relies on a dichotomous arrangement of good against evil. The shadowy demon is contrasted with the bright whiteness of the good 'mother' Columbia, the female personification of the American nation, who is wearing the Phrygian cap of freedom. As the once-beautiful Florida is gliding from her lap, Columbia seems to be waving toward help outside the frame. It is not clear whether her foot is caught in the thorny brush, where a broken "Trade" box lies on the ground and is about to be overgrown by thorns. 'Trade' furthermore represents the assumed reason how yellow fever reached Florida and also shows that traffic became a victim as well. Vile vapors ensue from the demon's mouth; they ominously try to reach and grab those fleeing the epidemic (in the right background). The odors emanating from the yellow fever beast are deadly, which points toward a belief in atmospheric transmission and contagiousness of the disease (miasma theory). The hope lies in the nation or a national effort personified in Columbia, who still hovers on top and above the vapors.

Fig. 18. Matthew Somerville Morgan, "Personification of Yellow Fever Dragging Down Florida." Frank Leslie's Illustrated Newspaper *ca. 1888.*

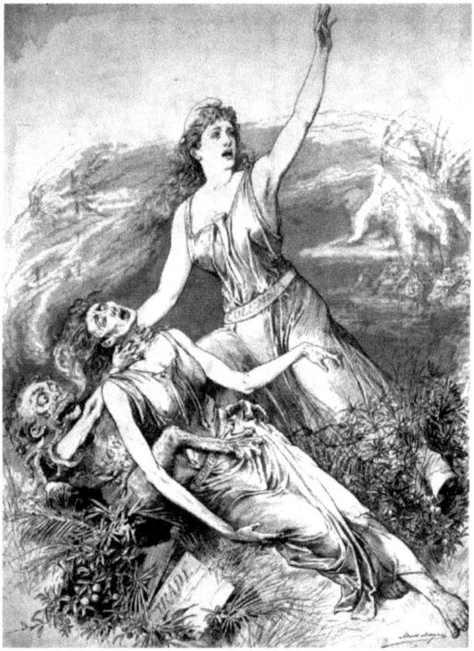

An equally national agenda underlies the wood engraving "At the Gates," which was published in *Harper's Weekly* in 1885 (fig. 19). The picture is another example of a metaphorical representation of disease that employs a simple good versus evil dichotomy. In this case, the shrouded specters representing cholera, yellow fever, and smallpox recoil in fear in the shadows of the gate. Their being caped and hooded as well as their crouched posture marks them as secretive, sick, and foreign. A radiant and bright angel approaches the evil group. With a star above her head, she represents the United States, holding a sword and a shield emblazoned with the word "cleanliness" and blocking their way through the quarantine barrier at the Port of New York.

"At the Gates" suggests a liminal situation with quasi-religious undertones: the gates might symbolize those of heaven and hell, of 'living' and 'death,' of 'sick' and 'healthy.' The shadow cast by the angel connects the figure with the personified diseases, thus seemingly dissolving the binarism. The threshold situation also points to the demographic contexts of the United States, which had become an immigrant nation at the time of the illustration's publication and had to deal with a growing xenophobia. In this sense, the subtitle "Our safety depends upon official vigilance," a clear call for more control, might also allude to the developments of the Public Health System or Ellis Island medical inspectors.

Fig. 19. "At the Gates." Harper's Weekly *5 Sept. 1885. Images from the History of Medicine (NLM).*

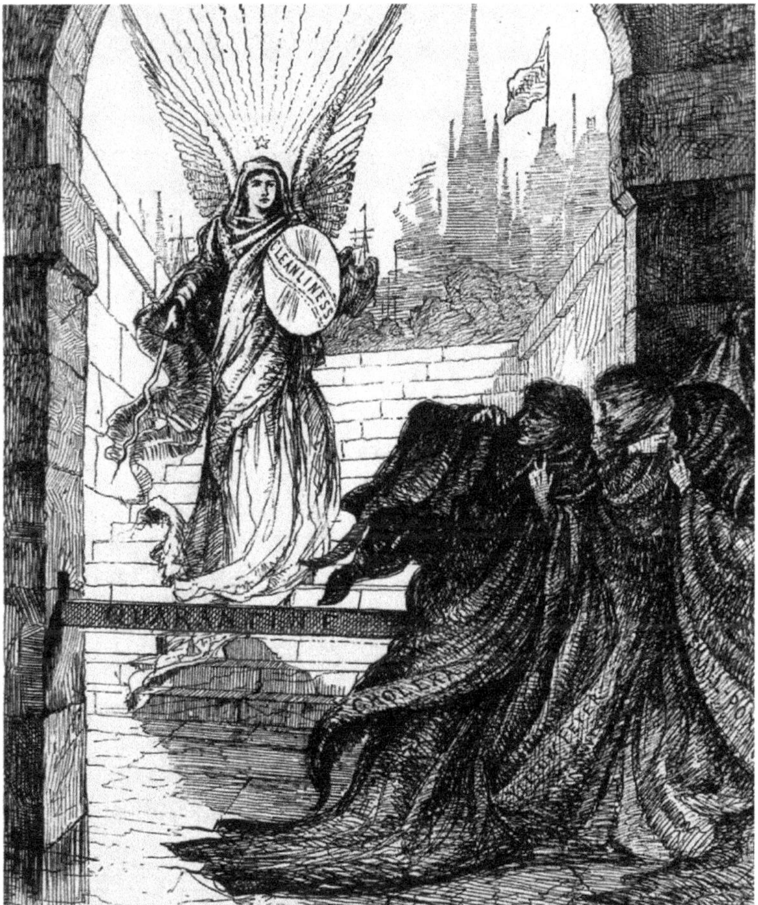

Although the technique and quasi-religious connotation is different, the means to control disease that is suggested in the two latter lithographs is also reminiscent of earlier medieval understandings of disease and death, i.e. as Grim Reaper. The (figurative) disease is controlled by banning it "at the gates" and burying it underneath. Yet, another means to control disease is also promoted in the "At the Gates" engraving, namely hygiene or cleanliness. Already by mid-century the local origin theory of yellow fever was seriously doubted by the majority of southern medical authors when the earliest cases of yellow fever in East Coast cities during the 1850s "could all be traced to ships arriving from yellow fever-infested Caribbean ports" (Humphreys, *Yellow Fever* 24). The paradigm of yellow fever's transportability subsequently became more and more widely accepted—especially in the last two decades of the nineteenth century when research on other diseases helped formulate a "germ theory of yellow fever" (Humphreys, *Yellow Fever* 25). Since the role of 'filth' in the evolution of the disease remained to be proven, sanitarians often failed to convince legislators that sanitation could help eradicate the disease; sanitary reform remained second to quarantine management (Humphreys, *Yellow Fever* 54, 57). In this respect, it is interesting that the illustration promotes both measures: quarantine as well as the more unpopular calls for better sanitation.

3.4 Capturing Yellow Fever on Camera

Compared to illustrations, photographs are often automatically grouped into a category of higher verisimilitude. Or, as Susanne Leikam has aptly pointed out, "[r] egardless of their cultural constructedness, photographs have the ability to capture the beholder's attention and appear 'reliable' witnesses of historical events, which makes them powerful discursive tools (41). Few photographic examples depict the human dimension of the yellow fever experience. The Louisiana State Museum owns a rare daguerreotype, made in New Orleans in 1855, of a stern-looking boy suffering from yellow fever (fig. 20). According to Roland Barthes's conceptualization of the linguistic message to construe the meaning of traumatic images such as this one, "the text replies—in a more or less direct, more or less partial manner—to the question: *what is it?* The text helps to identify purely and simply the elements of the scene and the scene itself" (39). The caption then merely identifies the boy as being from an Irish immigrant family, the Harrises. This mention of his Irishness' marks the boy as a 'stranger' and as such more susceptible to a disease to which—it was believed—acclimatization was possible. The fact that he is photographed in bed, which is against the prevailing conventions, and his feverish, glassy eyes mark him as diseased. He is gazing directly at the viewer with his right eye seemingly more in focus than the left, which also lies in shadow. Apart from his face and his tensely hunched bare shoulders his body is not visible, as he is neatly tucked into ornamentally patterned sheets. We can only speculate about the production history of this daguerreotype, whether his family wanted a memento of the still living boy instead of a post-mortem portrait, also quite popular in the nineteenth century. Disregarding the uncertainty, we are—similar to the illustrations discussed earlier—faced with a deathbed scene that contains all the sentimental stock elements including the suffering innocent child dying, competing for our attention and affection. The supposedly higher verisimilitude of photography is countered by a temporal distance; the moment of death has probably passed by now.

Even in the late nineteenth century, when a larger corpus of photographs is available, yellow fever photography remains scarce. In the pictures that include people, the hospital setting seems to be the location of choice. Stemming from a period when research on other diseases helped formulate theories of the origin of yellow fever, and taken shortly before and after the vector in transmission could be proven, they provide interesting evidence of a transitional period in medicalization practices and understanding of epidemic disease. Similar to the sentimental newspaper illustrations, they mostly convey a rather sanitized and non-infectious version of yellow fever allowing viewers to regard—at a safe distance—other people's pain.

With reference to photography, Susan Sontag has reflected on the "innumerable opportunities a modern life supplies for regarding—*at a distance*, through the medium of photography—other people's pain" (*Regarding the Pain of Others* 11; emphasis mine). Jay Prosser notes that photography has also "kept pace with atrocity, not only by chronicling it but also by developing the technology to capture atrocity in all its new forms" (7). In *Regarding the Pain of Others*, Sontag thus describes the enduring ethical dimension of photography and pleads for the atrocious images to haunt us: "Even if they are only tokens, and cannot possibly encompass most of the reality to which they refer, they still perform a vital function" (102).[70] I follow Sontag, who has insisted that "[s]omething becomes real by being photographed." It becomes real "to those who are elsewhere, following it

70 Sontag rejects iconoclastic perceptions of images as mere spectacles and discards assumptions that what can be seen by means of photographic imagery only appears to be real. Judith Butler has further qualified Sontag's view in some of her recent writing (Butler, "Photography, War, Outrage"; Butler, *Frames of War*, especially in her chapter "Survivability, Vulnerability, Affect"; Butler, *Krieg und Affekt*). She points toward the increasingly interpretive character of photographs—including those with a documentary character—with regard to choice of subject, camera angle, focus, and lighting. According to Butler, photos do not automatically include facts or truths, even if an inherent moral claim seems to suggest otherwise. Butler argues against Sontag that specific modes of representations and culturally determined practices of reception define what becomes fact (cf. also Meyer 365–66).

as 'news'" (*Regarding the Pain of Others* 19). Marita Sturken and Lisa Cartwright have expressed it similarly: "The meaning of a photograph is thus derived from the belief that it has a referent in the real." The "cultural meaning" of photographs, they write, "is derived in large part from their indexical meaning as a trace of the real" (Cartwright and Sturken 140). In other words, the experience and narratives of the individual viewer determine the photograph's cultural meaning.

Fig. 20. A boy from an Irish immigrant family, the Harrises, shown suffering from yellow fever in New Orleans in 1855. Daguerreotype. Louisiana State Museum.

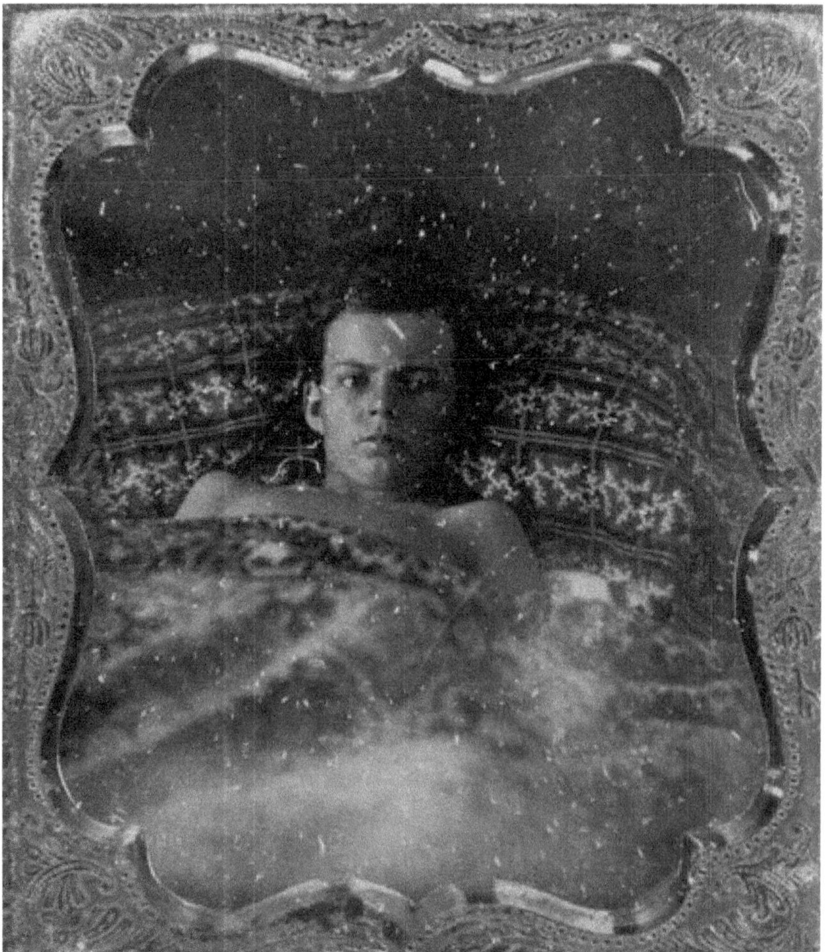

Yellow fever pictures were also taken by U.S. Army photographers to record treatment and prevention efforts in Cuba and Panama. A photograph taken during the Spanish-American War shows a yellow fever patient sleeping on an army cot in a makeshift tent hospital in Siboney, Cuba (fig. 21). With his pinched face and emaciated arms, a deathbed connotation is plausible. Yet the typical disease symptoms are absent. Light shines through the tent from outside behind the patient's head; his face is turned away from the viewer in a somewhat unnatural position that draws attention to his dominant nose and open mouth.[71] The drink on the table to his side is covered (against mosquitoes), while his body is not. The militaristic context of the photograph taken during a war, in which more people died of diseases than under enemy fire (cf. Cirillo), speaks for a scientific-didactic approach to control yellow fever, namely by recording the cases.

Fig. 21. "Yellow Fever Patient in Hospital at Siboney, Cuba, July 1898." Images from the History of Medicine (NLM).

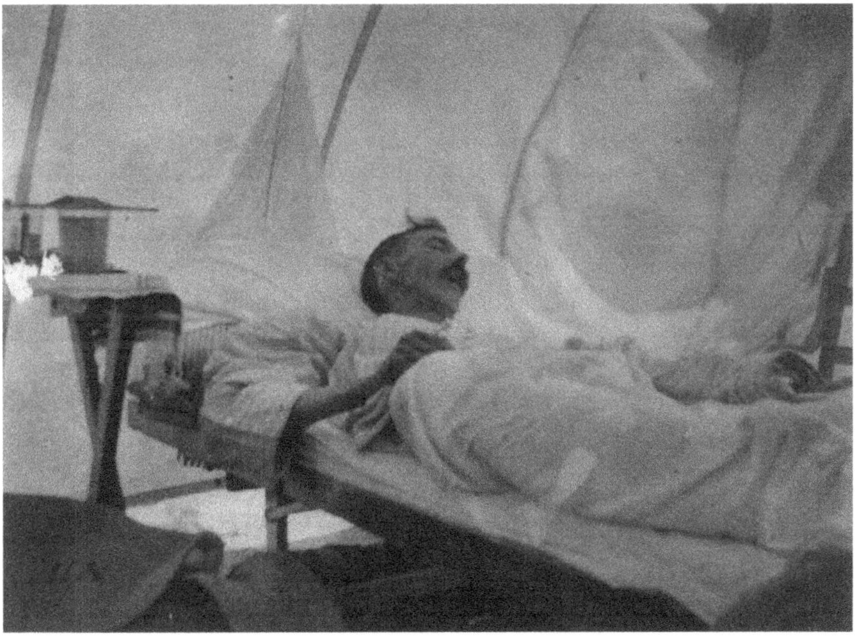

71 The head's position forming a triangle may also allude to what is known as a death triangle (*Totendreieck*) underneath the nose and around the mouth, which points toward a soon approaching death.

It is worth considering whether the distance generated by the sanitized depiction of the disease and the sentimentalization of the sight as a deathbed scene informs the presumably more 'real' photographs of the disease. In other words, this gaze generates precisely the distance that photography—by virtue of its medium—reproduces. The distance of the photograph is temporal, the knowledge that the situation the image depicts has already passed, and that the figure in the bed is undoubtedly dead by the time the picture was published. The evidentiary impact of the 'real' here is mitigated by its distance, and the photograph is inevitably imparted with the notion of a "memento mori" (Sonntag, *On Photography* 15).

Compared to the previous one, the photograph from a yellow fever hospital in Havana, Cuba, (taken one year later, in 1899) is striking for its de-individuation of the patients, who are arranged in a seemingly endless row of cots (fig. 22). The fact that only few patients are reclining and most patients are sitting on their beds points toward the convalescent status of most hospital inhabitants.

Fig. 22. "Patients in Yellow Fever Hospital, Havana, Cuba ca. 1899." Library of Congress, LC-USZ62-101537.

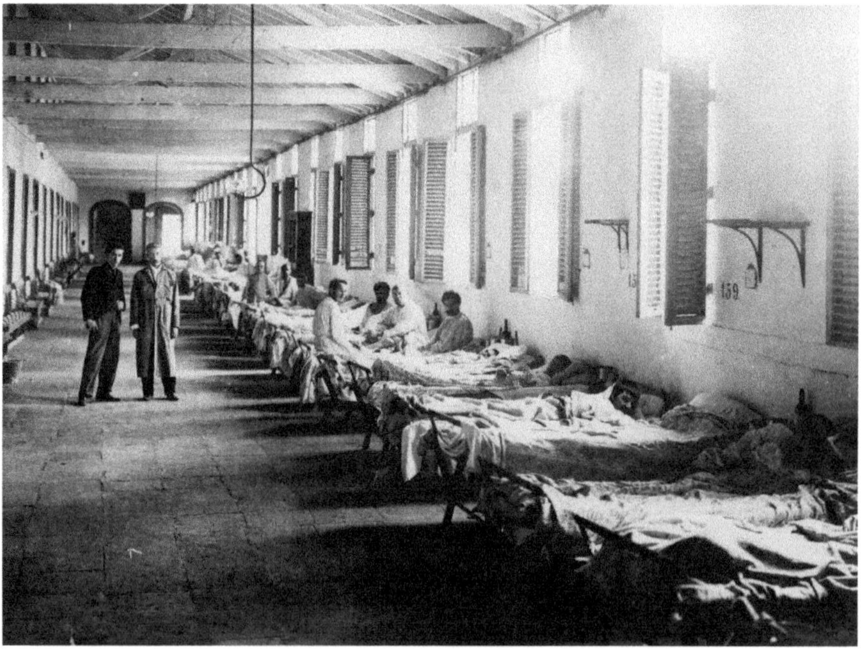

This is in stark contrast to a photograph, which shows an individual patient locked away in a mosquito-proof cage (fig. 23). Although no date for the photograph is given, it can be dated to the early 1900s, that is after Reed's discovery of the yellow fever vector that initiated measures such as the use of mosquito netting and systematic elimination of mosquito breeding grounds. It was taken at Gorgas Hospital, Ancon, in the Panama Canal Zone.[72] The ominous black cage that contains the patient is contrasted to the smoky white light to the left of the picture. It both speaks for a stigmatization of the diseased patient and illustrates the fear of infection. The netted cage prevents transmission as mosquitoes are barred from feeding on the infected patient. Considering the effort involved in building the cages, it also again puts more emphasis on the individual sufferer. Yet, it does not help or save the victim, who lies imprisoned. While the patient's face rests in the shadows and is hardly discernible, the crossed arms behind the head point toward a rather relaxed state of someone who is clearly not lying on his deathbed. While still a threat with the need to be locked away, yellow fever has finally been conquered, yet still needs to be contained physically.

Fig. 23. "Gorgas Hospital, Ancon, Canal Zone Screening Method of Segregating Yellow Fever Patients in Old Hospital." Images from the History of Medicine (NLM).

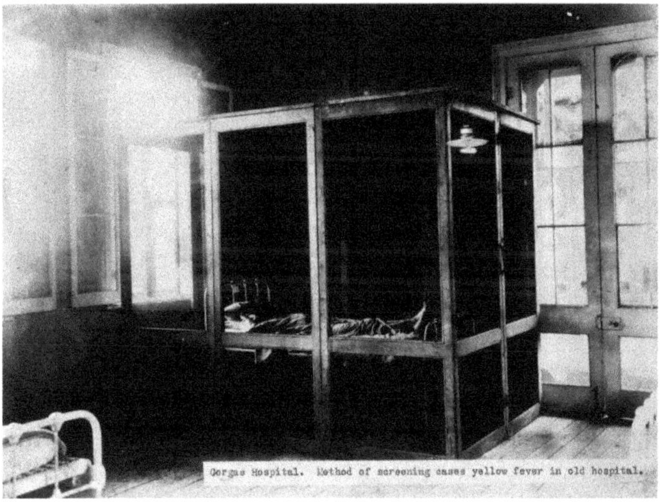

72 According to Stephen Greenberg from the History of Medicine Division (National Library of Medicine) the picture could not have been taken before 1904, since that is the year the United States took over the French hospital in Ancon. The hospital was extensively rebuilt in 1915, creating an 'old' hospital and and 'new' hospital. The name was actually only changed to Gorgas Hospital in 1928, so I think we should conclude that the picture was taken after 1928 (Greenberg n.pag.)

3.5 Visual Functionalizations of Yellow Fever

In order to make sense of visual practices and patterns of pictures that do not as easily lend themselves as material for creating a unifying myth, looking at yellow fever illustrations from the perspective of affect studies proves valuable. On a general level the nineteenth-century newspapers turn yellow fever victims into an object of attention, making the yellow fever experience accessible and understandable for wide audiences. Offering means to control the epidemic in the sense of curtailing it were primarily relegated to metaphorical depictions, some of which harbor underlying educational intentions, such as promoting quarantine and "cleanliness." The allegorical yellow fever demons or specters of other diseases are horrifying and repulsive and play with contagious fears as well as xenophobic tendencies to control disease. The images of actual sufferers, on the other hand, have the capacity to arouse sympathy for the victims. Oscillating between pity and disgust, sympathy and antipathy, viewers experience their own vulnerability by means of medially transmitted pain. Illustrations and accompanying text enable readers to empathize with the victims and generate a spectatorial self-consciousness about caring for the diseased and encouraging acts of benevolence. Despite possible tendencies toward self-protection or because of varying degrees of capacity for empathy, readers at least familiarize themselves with the experience of yellow fever through what I have termed the touristic or distant gaze. The military photographs of yellow fever victims also convey—*at a distance*—other people's pain. The pictures do not show heavily distorted victims or the characteristic black vomit, but sleeping or reclining patients. The invisible origin of the scenes—the disease—remains unseen, perhaps unrepresentable. It is replaced by the indexical nature of the photographic medium itself.

The representations from the yellow fever epidemics of the nineteenth century furthermore embody striking contradictions between the aestheticization of what could be put in the category of the abject—the suffering but still beautiful mother and the deeply vulnerable sick man—and the moral implications emerging from voyeuristic engagements with disease, death, and suffering that continue to call for close examination. As witnesses to abjection and calamity, they demand a political rather than an aesthetic response. W.J.T. Mitchell has equally insisted on the political task of visual culture "to perform critique without the comfort of iconoclasm" ("Showing Seeing" 170). Already in *Picture Theory* (1994) he postulated an alertness to examine the power of images "that is capable of discriminating the variety and historical specificity of their uses" (2–3). Jacques Rancière has equally pointed toward understanding "the image as discourse encoding a history" (11). Just because these epidemic pictures are in an odd way attractive (and had mass appeal), we should not discard them as merely sensational, commercial, or sentimental but as political and continue to engage with them and the emotional and political processes they stimulate.

4 Gendered Accounts of Yellow Fever

4.1 Women, Writing, and Yellow Fever

The nineteenth century, with increasing vigor in the antebellum and Civil War periods, was marked by a debate on woman's roles and her place in the private and public sphere. The same period witnessed the emergence of the womens' rights movement, starting with the first influential convention held at Seneca Falls in 1848, and its manifesto "A Declaration of Sentiments." A growing number of women entered the public realm of education and the workplace (including the medical) in the second half of the nineteenth century. The social and political development was mirrored in writing, both by and for women. An ever stronger female literary presence in white middle-class American culture established itself in the course of the nineteenth century. Mid-century popular novels by Susan Warner (*The Wide, Wide World*, 1850), Maria Cummins (*The Lamplighter*, 1854), and Fanny Fern (*Ruth Hall*, 1855) demonstrate the growing presence and agency of women writers. The emergence of new publication formats enabled ever more women to become writers and publish their work, reaching and influencing wide audiences. The formats included short stories, essays, sketches and poems, as well as novels, especially in a serialized publication. Since the mid-nineteenth century women writers dominated the literary marketplace. Novels by women made up forty percent of those reviewed in journals and newspapers in the antebellum period. This number increased together with the print explosion after the Civil War, and by 1872, as Susan Coultrap-McQuin has documented, "women wrote nearly three-quarters of all novels published" (2). Not surprisingly, the perception of novel writing as a female business intensified after the war (cf. Leverenz 4; Ammons 26). On the side of critical scholarship, the recent *Oxford Handbook of Nineteenth-Century American Literature* (Castronovo) makes a visual statement and significant nod to women as readers with its cover illustration of American painter Frederick Carl Frieseke's *Girl Reading* (ca. 1903–04) (fig. 24). Influential studies reappraising women's writing of the nineteenth century have appeared since the 1970s (A. Douglas; Baym, *Woman's Fiction*; Tompkins; Davidson)[73] and several new critical anthologies of

73 Women's writing of the colonial period and early republic has been the focus of Annette Kolodny's *The Land Before Her* on female frontier fantasies, experiences, and creativity from 1630 to 1860 and Linda K. Kerber's *Women of the Republic*.

recovered and newly discovered women's writing have followed since the 1980s (Fetterley; White and Freibert; Kilcup; Bennett).

Fig. 24. Frederick Carl Frieseke, Girl Reading *(ca. 1903–04). Wikimedia Commons. Web.*

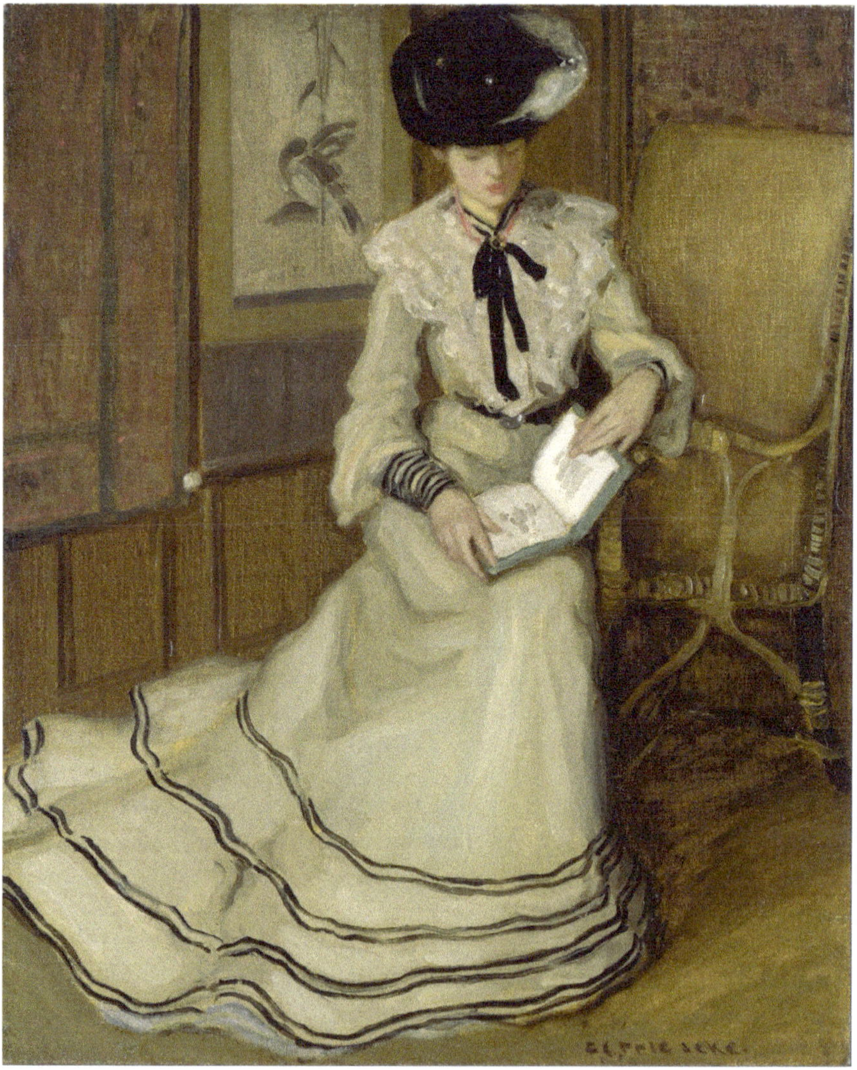

Shorter forms seem to have been favored by women writers as the time available to them to engage in writing was broken into smaller increments due to traditional female occupations of child rearing and housework (see Fetterley; Pryse and Fetterley; Samuels, *Reading the Novel* 157). The ideology of separate spheres, together with the cult of domesticity situated within a "culture of sentiment" (Samuels, *Culture of Sentiment*) and the paradigm of true womanhood have provided tools to understand the nature of most literary work of women in the nineteenth century. Ideology stipulated the protection of bourgeois white women in the domestic sphere and their separation from the economic and political corruption of public life. Since its introduction in 1966 by Barbara Welter, the paradigm of true womanhood has been called into question and was challenged by subversive and alternative models that also existed as well as the many ideologies of gender at work (cf. Rupp; Laffrado 6; see also Saulsbury). The permeability of the borders between the so-called separate spheres has equally been shown (Baym, *American Women Writers*).[74] In an ironic commentary on July Fourth celebrations in 1859 Sara Willis Parton (better known under her pen name as Fanny Fern) described the restriction of nineteenth-century U.S. middle-class women to the domestic sphere by pointing toward the public as well as medical domain, also desired and finally attained by women: "Can I go see anything pleasant, like an execution or a dissection?" (Warren 315; also qtd. in Laffrado 1).[75] That sentimental fiction performs important cultural work as "an act of persuasion aimed at defining social reality" (141) has long been pointed out by Jane Tompkins and others; it presented an "affective alternative that not only gave political actions their emotional significance, but beyond that, intimately linked individual bodies to the national body" (Tompkins 4). Amy Kaplan has similarly shown that "the

---

74 See Baym on the "inadequacy of current gender-based distinctions between the public and private spheres, of beliefs that cults of true womanhood or ideologies of domesticity confined female literary behavior to overtly celebrating or subtextually undermining women's domestic incarceration" (*American Women Writers* 4). See also Cathy Davidson and Jessamyn Hatcher's collection of essays, *No More Separate Spheres!* (2002).

75 In *Fresh Leaves* (1857), Fanny Fern draws an analogy with yellow fever: "As well might she have said, that it was none of her business that her neighbor's house was in flames, or that they had the yellow fever or the plague" (81). That New Orleans is symbolically connected to yellow fever is wittily commented on by Fern in *Rose Clark* (1856): "A stiff breeze, captain; we shall soon be in New Orleans at this rate. Talk about yellow fever; it can not be worse than sea-sickness. If a good appetite does not come to my rescue, on reaching land I shall pass for a live skeleton" (189).

concept of female influence [is] so central to a domestic discourse and at the heart of the sentimental ethos" (599).

This chapter looks at works of the postbellum and post-Reconstruction period, including one set in New Orleans during the Gilded Age; all texts use a female perspective to fictionalize yellow fever crises. Based on the online version of the bibliography *Wright American Fiction 1851–1875* (referencing 2,887 volumes by 1,456 authors), 205 fictional texts (or seven percent) mention yellow fever at least once in their narratives. Of those 205 texts 76 (or 37 percent) can unmistakably be identified as written by women writers. In the more detailed analyses offered in the following a female lens is applied to both the production of the works and the narrative focus. Showcasing three works by women writers, I additionally include two yellow fever novellas by Charles Wesley Alexander who published more than twenty books anonymously or under the pseudonym Wesley Bradshaw.[76] He took his middle name as a unisex first name in a move allow for the possibility of a female authorship. His crime confessions and historical fiction fall in the sentimental-sensationalist category. In his yellow fever fictions one can see that the dramatic events, crises, and catastrophes which are functionalized in gothic fiction also lend themselves to evoking the desired affect in sensationalist fiction. Furthermore, his and the yellow fever narratives by Mary Faith Floyd, Elizabeth Stuart Phelps, and Mollie E. M. Davis all focus on the figure of a medical practitioner (nurse or physician) who symbolically acts to resolve the crisis situation.

In terms of categorization of sentimental romance, domestic novel, and realist fiction, I rely on Alexander Cowie's differentiation: the conclusion of the sentimental romance is the death of the heroine, while the domestic novel relies on the marriage plot (9–21).[77] In 1871 Southern writer Mary Faith Floyd includes in her domestic novel *The Nereid* the description of a yellow fever epidemic on the Georgia seaboard in the late 1850s.[78] Introducing herself as "witness" and "sufferer" of that epidemic in her preface Floyd claims authority for and authenticity of the

---

76 Since for the purpose of this study, I will be concerned with the fictional output of Charles Wesley Alexander, a small Philadelphia publisher, he is identified here and in the following under his pen name Wesley Bradshaw (cf. Mills).

77 Many nineteenth-century novels end with marriage, which not only satisfies the heterosexual romance plot but also recognizes that "a woman's life will so much alter as she becomes a mother that her very identity as a character will be transformed" (Samuels, *Reading the Novel* 123).

78 The region witnessed severe yellow fever epidemics throughout the 1850s, Charleston and/or Savannah were affected in the years 1852, 1853, 1854, 1856, and 1858 (Patterson 858).

episode, although she admits the fictitiousness of the place, Brunswick, where she situates the outbreak. Yellow fever serves as a representation of the unspeakable Civil War experience and functions as a plot device to turn the fate of the central female characters of the novel and also enables their gradual emancipation.

In his mostly sensational and often sentimental fiction, Wesley Bradshaw employs female protagonists who not only transgress conventional gender roles, but find themselves outside of mainstream white American middle-class femininity (in his Civil War fiction) and thus do not necessarily function as role models. Bradshaw ventures in a different direction with his yellow fever fictions where his protagonists succumb to fatal illnesses rendered as punishment for female independence. His popular sentimental novella *Angel Agnes or, The Heroine of the Yellow Fever Plague in Shreveport* (1873), and his fictionalization of the story of *Mattie Stephenson: The Sweet Young Martyr of Memphis* (1873) both narrativize the 1873 epidemic when Northern physicians and nurses went South to offer relief (cf. Gessner, "Contagion, Crisis, and Control").

The 1878 yellow fever epidemic that overtook many southern states is represented in Elizabeth Stuart Phelps's short story "Zerviah Hope" (1880).[79] "Elizabeth Stuart Phelps was a writer with a central cause—women" begins Carol Farley Kessler's study on Phelps (Preface n.pag.). This assessment may even fall too short, since Phelps did more than criticize American patriarchy. Indeed Phelps, who lived from 1844 to 1911, worked to dismantle gender identity in her realist fiction. She destabilized "the seemingly sure category of gender, showing that the 'natural' behaviors ascribed to men and women are not natural at all," writes Lisa A. Long (266). Phelps's writing, together with other female writing of the period; was only critically rediscovered with the resurgence of interest in late nineteenth-century women writers in the 1960s. "Zerviah Hope" features the first of Phelps's actively and successfully practicing female doctors, who is partnered with a male nurse serving as title character.

Bradshaw's and Phelps's texts follow doctors and nurses from Pennsylvania, Illinois, and New York as "volunteers to the fever district" ("ZH" 78). While *Angel Agnes* and *Mattie Stephenson* rely on a conventional male doctor/female nurse setup, the sex of physician and nurse are reversed in Phelps's story, thus inverting the conventional pattern of male dominance and female subordination (cf. Gessner, "Of He-Nurses and She-Doctors"). In her study on the *Romance of Reunion*

79 In the following, for simplicity's sake, I will use *AA* for *Angel Agnes, or, The Heroine of the Yellow Fever Plague in Shreveport*, *MS* for *Mattie Stephenson: The Sweet Young Martyr of Memphis* and "ZH" for "Zerviah Hope."

Nina Silber has observed that northerners in the reconstruction period "began to fashion an image of reunion that built upon sentimental values and developed an explicit vision of gender and power" (64).[80] Silber's findings regarding this 'image of marital reunion' that is tied to the 'language of romantic and sentimental reunion' offer themselves to be tested in the three texts under discussion, as Silber asserts that "the yellow fever epidemic prompted repeated expressions of the sentimental view of reconciliation" between North and South (65). Following the rhetoric of sentimental fiction; the nurses in all three texts die a martyr's death. Agnes Arnold, weak from exhausting caregiving, accidentally falls and dies of a broken spine; Mattie Stephenson succumbs to the fever, and Zerviah Hope dies after aiding a freedman. I will show how *Angel Agnes*, *Mattie Stephenson*, and "Zerviah Hope" represent and (re)define existing social power structures of racism and patriarchy as well as present "human fellowship—food, physician, purse, medicine—that spoke from the heart of the North to the heart of the South" ("ZH" 81) as strategies to heal a nation still divided, yet united by the common threat of yellow fever. In all three narrative enactments the role of the medical woman as an "agent of healing between the North and South" (Wegener 2) becomes apparent

Mollie Davis's novel *The Queen's Garden* (1900) came out in the year in which the arthropod vector in yellow fever transmission was confirmed. It fictionalizes one of the last great yellow fever epidemics in New Orleans, in the late 1890s. Despite its much shorter form, romantic overtones, and indebtedness to a realistic fashion, the novel's uncanny and gothic elements provide a reading experience similar to Charles Brockden Brown's *Arthur Mervyn,* written one hundred years earlier. *The Queen's Garden* is the story of an orphan, Noel Lepeyre, who travels to New Orleans to meet her long-lost aunt, only to find her ill with yellow fever and herself caught in a terrifying atmosphere and confined to a house emanating death and decay. While the novel features a male physician, the focus of the story is on the young female protagonist Noel Lepeyre, who experiences a rite of passage classically encountering both death (her aunt's and her own illness) and love. In the succession of works discussed in this chapter, it could be aligned with Phelps's short story and its focus on a central woman character. Yet Noel Lepeyre is neither as professionally independent, self-reliant, nor as mature as Dr. Marian Dare in Phelps's short story. Davis resorts to the traditional marriage plot that has been so successfully subordinated in Phelps's story. However, both

80 Although many Northerners—in light of the political chaos and turbulence of Reconstruction—"remained skeptical about the likelihood of a genuine reconciliation," the 'bonds of matrimony' or the 'image of inter-sectional romance' (real and imagined) seemed to offer one way to stabilize the bond of union (Silber 40).

heroines survive the yellow fever, scarred by the crisis, but enabled to begin or continue independent lives.

4.2 Between Nostalgia and Women's Rights: Mary Faith Floyd's *The Nereid* (1871)

The central episode in Mary Faith Floyd's novel *The Nereid*, published in 1871 by J.W. Burke in Macon, Georgia, focuses on one of the yellow fever epidemics of the mid-1850s that gripped the Southern seaboard. *The Nereid* is a nostalgic portrait of pre-Civil-War times, published at the height of the Reconstruction period. Although yellow fever occupies a relatively minor role in *The Nereid* compared to the other texts discussed in this chapter, I am including the novel as an example of the functionalization of disease in general and yellow fever in particular, especially in its effect upon women. The disease serves, as what I have earlier called an empowering agent (between *deus ex machina* device and means to take one's life into one's own hands) in a society still deeply permeated by the ideology of separate spheres and the paradigm of true womanhood. Yellow fever also possibly stands in for the Civil War experience that is purposefully omitted from the narrative. Instead, Floyd—as she states in her preface—wants to present "a picture of life on the Atlantic seaboard of the Southern United States as it existed anterior to the late great 'Rebellion'" (*N* 5). She openly despises "the Scandinavian drafts of horrors [...]. The red mine of War and Bloodshed which recent writers have so thoroughly 'developed'" (*N* 5).[81] Emphasizing the 'developed' nature of much sensational literature, Floyd blames historians and novelists for misusing the power of their pens and for cashing in on the "[t]he literary taste of the day, in all sections of the Union" (*N* 5). In *The Nereid* Floyd instead conjures up the nostalgic moment, presenting a "faithful portraiture of that refined phase of life that existed fifteen years ago, among the highly-polished and educated inhabitants of the Southern seaboard" which she believes she can pin down to stand as a "fixed and immutable Past" (*N* 5). Yet, because she also mentions the "Rebellion" and the "rude hand of War," the conflict hovers over the narrative as an absent and impending presence, signified through the diseases, including yellow fever, and other disasters the fictional characters of *The Nereid* experience and face. Yellow fever represents the central metaphor of *The Nereid*. Other calamities—such as tuberculosis (Charlotte Elson), the cancer of the nineteenth century, and

81 Regarding Scandinavian immigrant authors, Dorothy Burton Skårdal evaluates them a ranging "from second- and third-rate down to absolutely horrible, producing doggerel verse, far-fetched plots with stock or wooden characters, and using a terrible style" (240).

hysteria (Blanche Ravenel), a horse-riding accident (Ralph de Coy), a boat- and a shipwreck (Ralph and Leda de Coy)—are subordinate to the meaning of the epidemic.

Mary Faith Floyd (1832–1913) was born into a family of military leaders and politicians, such as her grandfather John Floyd (1769–1839) and her father Charles Rinaldo Floyd (1797–1845), who also wrote poetry as we know from Mary Floyd's diary (Floyd et al.).[82] Orphaned in early girlhood she took over charge of the household and had to discontinue the formal education her parents would certainly have provided for her.[83] After her first husband, Randolph McDonald, died of yellow fever in Savannah in 1854, she married attorney William Gibbs McAdoo (1820–1894). During the war, the McAdoos lived near Marietta, Georgia, where their son William Gibbs McAdoo, Jr. was born on October 31, 1863. After the war the family moved to Knoxville, Tennessee. The family papers of the Floyd-McAdoo families are held by the Manuscript Division of the Library of Congress. They contain Mary Floyd's diaries from 1870 to 1891 and thus do not include the years of her own yellow fever experience in Savannah, on which she bases her description of a devastating epidemic in *The Nereid*. In *The Nereid's* preface, Floyd constructs herself as "a witness of [yellow fever's] ravages, and a sufferer," claiming authority and authenticity of the corresponding passage in her novel and excusing her fictional (mis)placement of the outbreak in Brunswick. Floyd's first diary notebook ends with entries from April 1871 and on the last two pages includes newspaper clippings from March 1871. For example, *The Rome Weekly Courier* (Rome, GA) commends Floyd on securing the serial publication of her novel *The Nereid* in the newspaper *The Farm and Home* (Senoia, GA). Mary Floyd's second major book *Antethusia*, which has disappeared into complete obscurity, is based on her experience living in Eastern Tennessee. She published poetry and pieces in magazines and papers, as well as the chapters "Journalism" and "Literature" in *Goodspeed's History of Tennessee* (Herringshaw; Knight). One reviewer calls her longer writing "original" in "style and matter, and being located in fields hitherto unexplored by the busy legion of fiction writers" (Tardy). In the 1880s Mary Floyd

82 John Floyd was the leader of the Georgia forces against the Creek Indians in 1813–14 and a general in the War of 1812. First a representative of the Georgia House of Representatives and later the U.S. House of Representatives, he was a close friend of Andrew Jackson. Charles Rinaldo Floyd (1797–1845) was a marine officer and commander of the Georgia state forces that removed the Cherokee Indians from the Okefinokee Swamps ("Floyd-McAdoo Families Papers" 3).

83 Biographical information on Mary Faith Floyd McAdoo was garnered from the following sources: "Floyd-McAdoo Families Papers"; Tardy; Herringshaw; Knight.

became an early member of the Ossoli Circle, a women's literary society founded by the director of the East Tennessee Female Institute, Lizzie Crozier French, in Knoxville.[84] Active in obtaining economic and educational opportunities for women in Tennessee, and later also promoting women's suffrage and the passage of the 19th Amendment, the name of the first federated women's club in the South is a nod to writer and women's rights advocate Margaret Fuller Ossoli, more commonly known as Margaret Fuller.

Despite her later membership in the women's club and its emancipatory activities, Floyd seems quite reluctant in her 1871 novel to promote what she referred to as "doctrines of woman's rights (so-called)" actively. An 1872 article on Mary Faith Floyd stresses her successful occupation as a housewife with her public literary success almost an afterthought, stating that she managed a large household from which her "literary labors" do not detract her (Tardy). In the preface to *The Nereid*, Floyd writes quite seriously: "Whosoever expects to find in the following pages elements of political sectionalism, religious dogmatism, irreligious free-thinking, philosophic theorizings, or doctrines of woman's rights (so-called), political or otherwise, may proceed at once in its perusal, being sure of obtaining a merited reward" (*N* 5).[85] While implicitly catering to the mentioned demands, including so-called women's rights, Floyd also promises to still "better please" (*N* 1) those readers who are looking for a description of life at the antebellum Southern seaboard. Although economic changes at the time were already turning the tide for women, *The Nereid*, although alternatives are offered, is still very much in tune with what Catherine E. Beecher wrote in *Harper's Monthly* in 1865: "Woman's *distinctive profession* includes three departments—the training of the mind in childhood, the nursing of infants and of the sick, and all the handicrafts and management of the family state" (710).

---

84 The members of the Ossoli Circle published their club's history as *History of Ossoli Circle, Knoxville, Tenn. Founded November Twentieth, Eighteen Hundred Eighty-Five.*

85 Sectionalist thoughts are expressed by the character of Ralph de Coy in the novel: "If our people had the energy of their Northern brethren to build railroads, all converging to this point, we could have a city and send our exports direct to Europe, instead of shipping them on a small scale to New York" (*N* 47). A more reconciliatory tone is struck by his wife Leda Elson (which is also in tune with the sentiment around the publication of the novel): "I feel a pride in the growth of New York. We are one great nation, and as such should enrich each other. We, of the South are an agricultural people, they are commercial. We furnish the crude material; they supply our wants in manufactories; what more ought we to desire" (*N* 47).

The Nereid is the story of Leda de Coy, née Elson, who is referred to as his nereid by the painter Paul Howard, whom she eventually marries. In Greek mythology Nereids are sea nymphs or friendly spirits of the sea, helpful to sailors caught in perilous storms (Grant and Hazel 292–93). Almost at the end of the novel, a ship accident off the Georgia coast reverses the mythical story of the nereids when Howard saves Leda by helping her into a life boat: "Leda's constitution, already impaired by yellow fever, felt the shock of the catastrophe very severely, and she was too ill to be removed soon from the kind refuge she had found" (70). Before the reader learns of these circumstances, Howard's story frames the novel, which begins in London in the year 1854. Paul Howard is residing in Europe (London and later Rome) to train as an artist, and only returns to the southern United States two years after the yellow fever episode that serves as the turning point of the narrative.

The novel follows the conventional wedding plot of sentimental fiction. At the beginning of the story, the first-born Leda Elson and her younger sister Florence seek the advice of an old mulatto, called Polydora, who promises to tell their futures. At the time Leda is seventeen and her sister Florence fifteen years old. The older sister is described as a classical beauty of medium height with a slightly rounded figure, and, among other features, a nose that "expressed all that firmness and pride of character which gives strength in suffering, and incites us to the accomplishment of great deeds" (*N* 14). Her younger sister was tall and slender with somewhat plainer features. Not only different in looks, Florence displays a more joyous character. It is she who convinces her older sister to visit Polydora under the pretext of delivering an ointment against rheumatism, but mostly to have their futures read. Possibly to tone down the slavery question, *The Nereid* relies on a relatively small set of black characters of which the free African American Polydora is the only one referred to by name. Moreover, her racial affiliation is downplayed, or rather, she is described as mentally superior to most blacks—a fact that exposes the author's attitude toward her: "[u]nlike most of her race her features had that Caucasian prominence indicating astute mental capacity" (*N* 16). She welcomes the two sisters by saying that "[i]t isn't often the rich come to see the poor" (*N* 15). Although the Elson sisters do not belong to the property-owning upper class, the societal and racial difference thus becomes apparent.

Polydora is not very specific in her divinations with regard to Florence, who is happily in love with her childhood sweetheart. The fortune teller only figuratively alludes to the yellow fever death of the two young lovers with a biblical comparison which entails more than their personal fate but that of their community as well "'Tender plants wither soon, more's the pity. The pestilence shall overrun the land worse than Pharaoh's plagues'" (*N* 16). Polydora refers to the ten plagues sent as punishments upon the Pharaoh and on Egypt for not allowing God's people, the Israelites, to go free from their slavery (Ex. 7–12). After this quite ominous and threatening prophecy Polydora has happier news for Leda. She will supposedly meet her future husband within a week, only to lose him and find a second husband for whom she will keep all her heart and who will take her across the seas. Ths glimpse into the future provides the blueprint of the evolving plot: while the doubt of reliability remains, the search for clues to prove the prophecy's truthfulness moves the story forward. Leda continually, yet guiltily and anxiously cross-checks the course of events with the prophecy. The marriage of Leda's parents is an entirely unhappy union, and she seems to do everything in her might to revolt against the marriage plot laid out in front of her by Polydora. Mr. Elson had married Catherine Courcy for the money the union was supposed to grant him, only to find his economic expectations ill fulfilled. He lets his wife as well as their children suffer under this disappointment and acts as a cruel and oppressive patriarch at home. The closeness of the two sisters, who are "attached by cords stronger than steel," is described as "the antidote to the subtle poison of their lives," which is only hinted at as a "long arctic winter of affliction" (15) and can only later be traced to their father's tyrannical presence.

Within a week of Polydora's prophecy, two suitors present themselves to Leda. She, however, eventually rejects the proposal of the "gifted and superior" Professor Porter and also remains reserved against Ralph de Coy's advances (*N* 24). She does not 'feel' anything for Professor Porter. Their intimate friendship rests on the proficiency of their intellectual exchange, which—as the narrative makes clear—does not suffice to warrant a marriage. To the contrary, the intellectual emancipation Porter stimulates in Leda disqualifies her as a wife according to the common assumptions of the time. One might read Leda's explanation to Porter as a regret or criticism of the current system as well as consent to it: "I have never carved out any career for myself. A woman's sphere is confined within the narrow limits of home life, and she wields little or no influence beyond it. Any step outside of the prescribed bounds proscribes her as trespassing on masculine territory." Porter understands and admires Leda and encourages her to aspire for more: "Ah! Miss Leda, if you are ever thrown on the world, I see the germ of a glorious career for you." Not long after the conversation Leda officially rejects Porter's proposal since love did not "enter [her] heart" (28). The reader learns that Porter retained a friendship with Leda Elson, but he is written out of the novel at this point. Matters are a little different with Ralph de Coy, who is training to become a physician. An orphan at a very young age Ralph had been brought up by a tender grandmother, which had made him "a most passionate boy," who first prefers Florence's happy spirit over Leda's contemplative nature. In fact, he is unable to relate to her character: "Mr. de Coy was mentally her inferior. Prosperity of the affections and disembarrassment in pecuniary matters left undeveloped his capacities and gave him an elasticity and fullness of spirits which could little understand the gravity in Leda's character, and which appeared to him perfectly unnatural" (44). In her dreams Leda contemplates Polydora's prophecy of the future husband who will take her across the seas, "where she reigned queen over the heart of one, who knew no joy, save that found in her own smile" (*N* 25). This husband has not yet appeared, and while she is not generally disinclined and perceives Ralph de Coy as "noble and good; [...] he was nothing to her" (*N* 24):

> She liked Mr. de Coy the best of all the gentlemen she had ever met; but if her sensations were those of love, they, as yet, were of the passive order, and she was too conscientious to give encouragement to a lover merely to gratify that idle vanity which unfortunately pervades the hearts of so many women. (44)

Reading Ralph's courtship as an allegory of the mythological tale of the god Zeus's seduction of Leda—daughter of the Aetolian king Thestius—seems anything but far-fetched. To win her heart Zeus, who admires Leda, approaches her in the form of a swan. Their daughter Helena's birth from an egg was a well-known story in ancient times. In *The Nereid* Ralph de Coy, whose name alludes to Zeus as decoy bird, courts Leda under false pretenses. It is only through a riding accident, which triggers Ralph's subsequent illness (his disguise), that she consents to a marriage: "There was no coquetry, no vanity in Leda's heart. She was a true woman; and in all good faith she left Ralph's claim an open question, feeling that she could make no better selection for a partner. Love only was wanting" (46). His recovery from the accident is uncertain, and the wedding is quite a modest one, with Ralph having to recline on a lounger. He eventually recovers which the narrative largely attributes to Leda's nursing care and to love as "a great healer of disease" (54).

> Both day and night Leda flitted like an angel around his bed anticipating every want, soothing every pain. How could he do otherwise than bear his ills with fortitude, as he watched that fair uncomplaining girl, in her unselfish devotion? And how could he help being happy when he felt that she was all his own? The only pang the expectation of death brought was the thought of leaving her-his lovely bride. As he daily saw new exhibitions of her pure, unassuming, unobtrusive piety, which tempered her every thought and action, he despised his own worldly character, and prayed God to change his heart and make him, too, a true living child of Christ. (54)

In her piety and devotion Leda is constructed as the ideal true woman. The narrative presents the new middle class that emerged since the early republic and produced what became known as Republican Motherhood as still largely intact.[86] The four ideals that comprise the 'cult of domesticity' and 'true womanhood,' purity, piety, submissiveness, and domesticity, are embodied in its idealized form by the heroine of the novel.

Back in the days in her family's house Leda had become a teacher by monetary necessity "to supply her own wants" but also to help her mother as her father grew more and more stingy. Her hard work without recreation and "[t]he constant tension upon her nerves affected her health, and she often felt a fainting weariness of flesh and spirit" (*N* 45). But her teaching also provides her with a professional occupation that imbues self-worth through being helpful to others. Yet Ralph makes very clear that there will be no need for such an occupation as her place will be the home: "You have no need of such exertion, and can find enough to do at home if you are determined to have an occupation" (*N* 45). Even when Ralph slowly recovers and Leda wishes to return to school, her husband does not consent.

The encrusted societal structures are shaken by yellow fever invading the town. The episode is at the center of the narrative and serves as its turning point. In the novel, yellow fever is imported from Savannah when a family which moves from the diseased city to Brunswick brings it with them. Floyd probably anchors her account in the 1854 Savannah epidemic during which a startling 6.9 percent of the population died (Patterson 858). In Brunswick yellow fever soon generates "a dread, a fearful horror, [that] thrilled every pulse" (*N* 59). The description of the fear the impending disease generates precedes the description of the actual cases: "Fright, like a devouring element, spread its torturing flames equally around the rich, the poor, the great, the small, levelling all to an equality—a panic stricken mass" (*N* 60). Leda's husband, physician Ralph de Coy, is far from being presented as an expert on the disease. To the contrary, he had no knowledge regarding the treatment of yellow fever except what he had read about it, and in contrast to his fellow practitioners he did not even have much experience in curing local fevers. While he does not cease to fulfill "his professional duties" (*N* 60), it is Leda who, as a nurse to the little daughter of the pastor, administers the greatest

86 While men spent more time in the work space, women and the monetary gains of their work were removed from the economy, and the family as the primary economic unit disappeared. The ideology of the separate spheres evolved: home was seen as a shelter and home and family became a separate sphere from work and the public realm occupied by men. While these boundaries should not be understood as rigidly defined absolutes, but often fluid delineations, they have provided tools to understand nineteenth-century literature (especially by women) set within white middle and upper class culture.

service. Although little Mittie dies—in what is obviously reminiscent of Harriet Beecher Stowe's description of Little Eva's death—Leda's presence through "all day and all night" (*N* 61) alleviates the child's agony. Since Mittie is too weak to give away strands of her hair like Little Eva in *Uncle Tom's Cabin*, "Leda, with her own hands prepared the child for her coffin. She cut off several of her golden curls, and put them aside for the poor mother" (*N* 61).

The disease not only deeply affects Brunswick, which loses a third of its population, but the protagonist Leda's fate is determined by the outcome of the epidemic: "The thirst of yellow fever is insatiable, and each day saw new victims swell the number who had already perished. Not until the middle of November did the delayed frost drive back this devastating foe. Long will its ravages be remembered, for each household had to mourn links rudely broken from the family chain" (*N* 64). Leda's very energetic younger sister Florence succumbs to the fever (together with her fiancé), as well as Leda's brother and her father who is "reformed" before his death. Enhanced by the twist of Mr. Elson's moral change, Leda's mother, Charlotte Elson, will not suffer under her tyrannical husband anymore. Structurally, the epidemic also represents an attack against the shelter of home in the separate spheres ideology. Caring and the safe haven of home are not sufficient to safeguard and control the home sphere, into which the disease equally intrudes. Consequently, it prompts Leda to leave that sphere. In the aftermath of the fever, and as the first-born after the death of her sister, brother, and father, Leda takes care of the education of her younger brother. In a quite ironic twist, Leda is empowered by the fever—through the work she is able to contribute as a nurse during the epidemic and later as a teacher. Like her mother after the death of Leda's father, the death of her husband Ralph de Coy sets Leda free. Ralph drowns on the way to visit a patient shortly after the epidemic's demise. Yet Leda is also weakened, psychologically and physically: she does not dare to fall in love. Accommodating herself to the role of an extremely young widow, she tries to adhere to and fulfill unspoken expectations of remaining unmarried. The loss of husbands and sons is a fate many women shared in the Civil War period, and one to which readers could relate. Adding to her grief Leda is physically weakened by the yellow fever she has also suffered from but survived.

While there is no detectable sign in the novel to speak of the formation of a women's movement—neither enlightenment thought nor the antislavery movement are behind the novel's female activities—the women's accomplishments demand further attention. Since the first half of the nineteenth century, moderate advantages to a socially approved female isolation presented themselves in the organization of religious and social activities (such as tea parties, church circles, and bazaars), as women were able to spend time exclusively with each other. They carved out a niche in which men had little or no influence. Correspondingly, at the beginning of the novel, the search for and later the accommodation of the new pastor and his family occupy the women of Brunswick. Notably the women decide on their new pastor. Besides the formation of a women's club to support the new priest, the closeness of women is emphasized through the intimacy between the two Elson sisters and through the freedom of female companionship their mother Charlotte Elson experiences after the death of her husband with her friend Bab Snubb. As survivors of the epidemic, the women of the novel rely on each other's support. And although the novel closes with a conventional turn towards marriage, a sense of community among the surviving women is retained. It remains however up to a man, Leda's second husband Paul Howard, to lead the women—Leda, whom he saves during a ship accident, her mother and Bab Snubb—into a new life and different society to Europe. The plot device of a return to Europe is shaking American cultural narratives of the Promised Land, of God's chosen people, of westward movement and Manifest Destiny. Howard furthermore displays traits conventionally seen as feminine, both in the sensitivity related to his profession as a painter and in his actions, such as quite superstitiously believing in Polydora's prophecy and joining in song with his future wife. Their musical harmony may also point toward a partnership on equal terms.

4.3 Yellow Fever and the Nursing Experience: Wesley Bradshaw's *Angel Agnes* (1873) and *Mattie Stephenson* (1873)

> May God protect you, reader of this book, from all manner of sickness; but above all, from that thrice dreaded pestilence, yellow fever. Of all the scourge ever sent upon poor sinful man, none equals in horror and loathsomeness yellow fever.
>
> Wesley Bradshaw, *Angel Agnes* (1873)

Yellow fever—and in this way Charles Brockden Brown's words in his preface seem prophetic—became something of a constant in nineteenth century America, with "periodical visitations of this calamity" it produced "change in manners and population [...] in the highest degree memorable" (*AM* 3). When yellow fever retreated to the South after the last major outbreaks in northern port cities in 1820 (Baltimore and New York in 1819, Philadelphia in 1820), it became more and more known as a scourge that affected the South. It was the reason for most of the medical reform activity and public health action in the South, and quarantines were the most popular measure in Southern efforts to control it. This was mainly due to the fact that the 'concept of transportability' had (re)emerged in the South since the 1840s (Humphreys, *Yellow Fever* 47, 53). The strictness and rigidity of quarantines, and sometimes even shotgun quarantines that were enforced by armed patrols, varied with the level of public anxiety accompanying an epidemic. For example, when in 1878 yellow fever spread as far north as to affect the Midwestern states of Indiana, Illinois, and Ohio, the "dramatic images of panic and death [...] generated a nationwide sentiment in favor of federal enforcement of a strong quarantine" (Humphreys, *Yellow Fever* 61). Yellow fever, despite its primarily Southern manifestation, affected the economy of the whole nation and thus remained a national problem. An increased reliance on the importance of quarantine measures dominated federal public health involvement in the late nineteenth century.[87]

Several yellow fever epidemics gripped the South in the 1870s. In 1873 the comparatively small Louisiana city of Shreveport on the Red River was struck. Less than half of Shreveport's population of approximately 10,000 people remained in town during the epidemic. About 3,000 or two thirds of the remaining population experienced attacks of yellow fever and at least 759 died. The Shreveport epidemic, during which at least 16.5 percent of the city's population perished, still ranks as one of the worst yellow fever outbreaks in the United States.[88] Its devastating progression was covered (not always accurately and often with a sensationalist bend) in newspapers across the nation, as well as extensively in *Frank Leslie's Illustrated Newspaper*. Several reports show that contributions to relieve the situation in the Louisiana city came from all over the nation (for example, "The Yellow Fever: Subscriptions for the Aid of Shreveport"; "Yellow Fever: Relief Contributions"). Historian Jo Ann Carrigan concludes about the Shreveport experience that "[w]ithout

87 Humphreys contends, that "[a]nalogies likening yellow fever to an invading army, or to an imported commodity such as bananas or coffee, emphasized those characteristics of the disease that made it a national, and not merely a state or regional, calamity. From this perspective, it was an easy step to the conclusion that protection from yellow fever should be in the hands of the federal government, just as military security and international diplomacy were constitutionally reserved for federal jurisdiction" (*Yellow Fever* 12). Besides yellow fever quarantines, cholera and bubonic plague quarantines were common at the end of the nineteenth century (cf. J. Brown, "Purity and Danger" 103).

88 I am basing the mortality rate of 16.5 percent on Patterson, who lists 759 yellow fever deaths (858) and on the 1870 Census that lists 4607 Shreveport residents (*Statistics of Population*, Table 3: 155). According to another source, the city lost between 20–25 percent of its citizens because, additionally to the deaths, many fled Shreveport during the epdidemic never to return. Carrigan estimates the case fatality rate for the Shreveport epidemic at 26 percent (*Saffron Scourge* 106; 111).

regard to the bitter struggles of Reconstruction then in progress, the northern 'enemy'—civilian and military—again responded with benevolent impulses and material assistance to a southern population afflicted by epidemic disaster" (*Saffron Scourge* 107). She cites President U.S. Grant's reply to General W. H. Emory, commander of the United States troops in New Orleans, to send 5,000 rations to the Shreveport victims at once, as a case in point.

In this calamitous atmosphere of 1873 Wesley Bradshaw wrote and published the sentimental novella *Angel Agnes, or, The Heroine of the Yellow Fever Plague in Shreveport* that presents the story of Agnes Arnold, the daughter of a wealthy Philadelphia businessman, who reads about the devastating yellow fever epidemic and decides to go to Shreveport to offer her assistance. This echoes the real presence and assistance of Northern volunteers, many of whom fell victim to the disease and were buried at Shreveport. Another cultural image resonating with volunteer nursing is the one embodied by Florence Nightingale who resembles the paradigmatic figure of the female nurse, primarily in a military context. Her writings based on her Crimean War experience *Notes on Nursing* (1859) and *Notes on Hospitals* (1859) informed and encouraged female nursing (in the United States especially in a Civil War-context and the post-Civil War period) as well as writing about it (Laffrado 87; Schultz, "Inhospitable Hospital" 364, 390; Schultz, *Women at the Front*; Vicinus 85–120).[89] The Civil War and wartime disorder served as a great leveler between the sexes; especially women's nursing practices during the war paved the way toward the subsequent "cultural acceptance of the female nurse" (Laffrado 104). "Nursing," as Shirley Samuels rightly asserts, "becomes the path to enter into the world"—a world, however, that lies in chaos, in which the bodies of wounded young soldiers arrive daily in the hospitals (*Reading the Novel* 139).

In Bradshaw's novella not the war, but yellow fever functions as a testing ground for virtue, dedication, and goodness, exemplified in the character of the volunteer nurse; in other words, morality is offered as a means to control yellow fever. A future female emancipation might be hinted at with the strong protagonist, but is not finally redeemed. The disease is also employed as a formula of danger to feed into a culture of fear, and thus also enables an at least imaginative reunion of North and South under the epidemic's threat.

89 In more recent scholarship a discussion of Florence Nightingale is rightfully paired with the story of Mary Seacole, a Jamaican free woman of color who worked as a nurse in the Crimean War providing a counternarrative to the Nightingale myth (see Birkle, "Traveling Nurses"; Dallmann, "Popular Icons, Transnational Nursing Narratives"; "Fish 64).

Earlier popular historical fiction and crime confessions by Bradshaw also feed into this culture of fear, mainly with themes of the Civil War, or the hardships of the Mormon trek to Utah (*Brigham Young's Daughter*, 1870). His brand of sensational writing (*Pauline of the Potomac, Or General McClellan's Spy* 1862; *Maud of the Mississippi*, 1863; *General Sherman's Indian Spy*, 1865; *The Angel of the Battlefield*, 1865) democratized society during wartime. Distinctions in rank, class, or between men and women did not exist in his fiction that featured female heroines with access to high-ranking generals. In his pulp fictions Bradshaw introduced female soldiers or spies and often imbued his armed women characters with magical powers. His literary debut *Pauline of the Potomac* (1862) features such a heroine, whose father on his deathbed sends her off to the Civil War and thus symbolically dedicates his daughter's life to save the union.[90] In *Angel Agnes*, Bradshaw employs the successful formula of his Civil War narratives with an initial family disruption that leaves an orphaned heroine destined to fight, in this case, yellow fever. Analogies with the Civil War are inserted early in the narrative: "During the late war, fond fathers sent their sons to the battle-field, not that they wished to have them slaughtered, but willing that, for the sake of their cause, they should take the risk" (*AA* 7). It is by the same reasoning that Mrs. Arnold, Agnes's mother, approves of her daughter's wish to go to the diseased city of Shreveport. Her action also stands in line with fiction which opens with mothers saying goodbye to their daughters (Baym, *Woman's Fiction*; Samuels, *Reading the Novel* 123).

Besides the sentimental pattern, the narrative addresses veteran readers directly, and even puts the female heroine's emotional strength above that of the veterans:

> Reader, if you are a man, possibly you have been in the army, and then possibly you have been in a column, to which has been assigned the task of storming a well-served battery of pieces. If so, you may remember the feelings that were within your heart as you left the last friendly cover of woods [...]. To Agnes Arnold going into Shreveport, the emotions must have been very much like yours in front of that battery. Yet there was no fluttering of her pulse. (*AA* 8)

Following up on Bradshaw's Civil War successes and feeding on the attention the fever received in the 1870s, it is not surprising that *Angel Agnes* became a national best-seller and was re-issued in 1878 during the yellow fever epidemic that affected several southern states and cities (Memphis in particular). The novella follows in the tradition of sentimental fiction with its focus on marginalized disenfranchised groups, such as mothers, children, and blacks, who are

---

90 See Fahs (241–45) for a brief analysis of Bradshaw's Civil War writings.

symbolically empowered to serve as social models while true emancipation is withheld. Sentimental strategies furthermore include suffering (sick or dying) children and infants[91]; partings (Agnes leaving her mother) and reunions (with her ex-fiancé, who later dies); domestic settings mirroring moral settings; and a litany of values (of Christian piety, loyalty, solidarity) which are also represented in the novella by the Sisters of Mercy Agnes meets on the train and who stand by her until her death.[92] Both the reunion of the two lovers on the fiancé's deathbed and the presence of the Sisters of Mercy conjure up parallels with Longfellow's *Evangeline* (1847).

The saintlike, 'angelic' Agnes[93] seems to operate on a higher moral level than her patients with regard to the disease; she is never infected by the fever. This points to a notion that disease and character are connected. Representing a typical sentimental novel's protagonist, Agnes—who is merely twenty-two years old—"seeks a kind of spiritual and emotional calm by faithfully adhering to [...] moral absolutes" (Crane 111). Like her namesake she is chaste and also becomes a virgin martyr like Saint Agnes, who is frequently depicted with a lamb at her side (*agnus*). Agnes's work ethic, her superior moral goodness—merely helped along by the power of the treatment she administers to her patients—is offered as a means of controlling the disease. The narrative reverts to the notion of character as the main notion of redemption and control, and Agnes is "not a mere fancy nurse. Far from it. Up went her sleeves, and for the next two hours she worked with her four patients like a Trojan" (*AA* 10).[94] She ignores official measures to control the epidemic, such as quarantine, and boards a train to Shreveport despite the regulations.

> A little short of the stricken city they were all stopped, and it required the positive statement of the Sisters of Mercy that their youthful, lovely companion was really going into the place for the purpose of nursing the sick.
>
> "Miss," asked an elderly gentleman, "were you ever acclimated here? Because if you were not, we cannot let you pass, for you would only get the fever yourself, and become a

91 In reality children were less likely to be struck by yellow fever or suffered from milder cases.

92 What has been described as innate capacity for fellow feeling in sentimental fiction can be traced to the eighteenth-century moral sense philosophy of the Earl of Shaftesbury.

93 Apart from the title, we learn from the sick Sister Theresa that Agnes's patients call her 'Angel Agnes'; Theresa prays that "God and the saints keep [her] an angel, as [she] is now," which also foreshadows Agnes's untimely death (*AA* 19).

94 Brown's contemporary and friend, Benjamin Rush, had held sympathy as essential to a physician's success "sometimes so powerful, as to predominate over the fear of death" (Rush qtd. in Haakonssen 218).

> care instead of a help to us. Not only that, but you would surely be a corpse inside of twenty-four hours."
>
> Agnes explained to the firm but kind gentleman, her New Orleans experience, and he relaxed and said: "In that case, Miss Arnold, I sincerely welcome you, and in the name of the sick and dying people here, pray God that you may be spared to help them. Pass through, and heaven bless your brave and noble heart!" (*AA* 8)

When the train is stopped and Agnes is interrogated, it is through her earlier experience in yellow fever-stricken New Orleans that she is admitted into the diseased city. The passage also refers to the medical opinion of the time that not all residents were equally vulnerable when yellow fever struck and that one could become 'acclimatized' (in the terminology of the time, or 'acquire immunity' in today's terminology) (Patterson 860). An 1856 report in the *New Orleans Medical Surgical Journal*, for example, noted the extreme vulnerability of—what the journal referred to as—"unseasoned" newcomers to the local "climate" of New Orleans in contrast to the immunity of its native citizens (qtd. in Patterson 860). Patterson points out that "it was believed well into the 19th century that new residents could become 'acclimatized' to local fevers without a life-threatening illness and could gradually acquire the immunities conveyed by native birth" (860).

The city's efforts of burning tar and pitch as disinfectants are dismissed by Agnes as ludicrous. At one point, she "would have laughed at the silly man [...] who had nearly choked himself by thrusting his head into the dense black fumes" (*AA* 9). Her attitude seems to echo the sanitationist view of a Doctor Stevens in *Arthur Mervyn* who promotes a healthy living and diet over the burning of gunpowder or tar. Agnes's actions indicate that she does not believe in or fear a person-to-person communicability of the disease. Her treatment of the sick Sister Theresa shows "how little she dreaded the pestilence, for, instead of going to another room, she lifted Theresa further over the bed, and laying herself down beside her, placed her arm over her" (*AA* 18). Agnes strictly adheres to her own "design and method" to keep herself in "perfect health and spirits" (*AA* 22) and apparently defies the risk of infection. Agnes, we are told, in her "treatment of the sick victims [...] would not interfere with the medicine they [her patients] were taking" (*AA* 11). However, the narrative also suggests that "during the whole epidemic, it seemed as though mere medicine was of no avail whatever, and that really the methods and means used by the natives, independent of the doctors, did all the good that was done" (*AA* 11). When the district's physician pays a visit to the house under Agnes's care (and, one might add, control), he is astonished in light of the recovery of the fever victims. He also attributes the recoveries to Agnes's "faithful and intelligent nursing" and admits to the ineffectual modes of treatment his own profession employs. These treatments fail "in nearly eighty per cent. of every hundred" (*AA* 14). He also advances the view that it was not the medicine offered by the doctors but "the methods and means used by the natives" (*AA* 11), in this sense a Southern treatment, which made the difference in disease control. Prompted to elaborate on the efficiency of what the physician terms "grandmother remedies" (*AA* 14), Agnes rejects this denotation and instead attributes her treatment to a Spanish gentleman from Havana:

> "This is not a grandmother's remedy, Doctor," smilingly replied Agnes. "It was told to me some years ago in New Orleans." She here concisely narrated to him the history of her experience when she helped to nurse her father in the latter city. "Who was it told you, Miss Arnold? was it Dr. Robinson? He was noted about that period for his success in treating bad cases of the fever. Once in Vera Cruz he took the vomito, and was saved by this treatment." (*AA* 14)

The text thus presents a treatment supposedly originating in Cuba as most successful. This is remarkable because the origin of the Shreveport yellow fever epidemic at the time was traced to Cuba as newspapers reported ("Yellow Fever at Shreveport"). Yet the question of origin or the by then accepted concept of transportability—which was most probably known to Bradshaw—never comes up in the novella that focuses on treatment and healing. With his promise that he shall not fail to try the yellow fever remedy and subsequently also recording her smallpox remedy, the physician, furthermore, remains the one to authorize Agnes's yellow fever treatment and actions. This is all the more remarkable since, as Nayan Shah has argued, the professionalization of medicine in the nineteenth century excluded alternative, and especially ethnic, medical practices (Shah 56; see also Starr). Bradshaw, on the other hand, entertains the possibility of the adoption of alternative medical practices. In his story the successful 'Spanish' therapy (of putting the patient's feet in hot and very strong mustard water and then applying salt mackerel to the fever patient's feet) is explained in much detail. Interestingly, the *Report of the Committee on the Yellow Fever Epidemic of 1873 at Shreveport* also states that the "most effective treatment included a mild cathartic (castor oil or magnesia), a hot mustard bath, crushed ice and lemonade, cool sponging, and mild diuretics" (qtd. in Carrigan, *Saffron Scourge* 327; Snell et al. 20–21). In the novella, the treatment is also conveyed to a black undertaker by Agnes. Like Agnes the black man is also fulfilling his part in fighting the epidemic, albeit on a lower social scale. By dictating the steps of her treatment to the black man, she assumes an authority that is not necessarily medical. The black man exclaims: "I knowed it was magic—somethin' like that, and not medicine at all!" (*AA* 13). The hierarchical social structure of African American undertaker—who believes in magic instead of science—and then female nurse and male doctor is solidified in the text. In providing a potential "Spanish" colonizer's recipe for the treatment, the narrative not only suggests a non-American remedy for the disease but also concedes a superiority to the "Spanish" disease treatment, and thus at least questions a WASP-ish identity construction that partly rests on a contrast to Catholic Spain. A critical stance toward the protestant clergy is also expressed in the narrative, when Agnes explains to her mother why she needs to go to Shreveport: "It is strange that we see no account of ministers or members of any denomination but the Roman Church volunteering to go to the stricken city.[95] All seem to stand aloof but them. How noble are those truly Christian and devoted women, the Sisters of Mercy!" (*AA* 7).[96]

Agnes, who constantly shows courage—"a girl of steady, powerful nerves, and cool temper" (*AA* 11)—and a seemingly never-ending devotion and selflessness, eventually dies of a broken spine and the severe internal injuries she sustains from a fall due to fatigue after caring too extensively for one of her many patients, a 12-month infant. Interestingly, only the full physical disintegration of her body—a broken spine—keeps her from standing upright and caring for her patients. Her sacrifice is complete. She wishes to be buried next to her former betrothed, George Harkness, who—despite their broken engagement—had followed her to the South and succumbed to the fever earlier in the story. Although diverging from satisfying readers with a traditional marriage plot, the two Northerners are reunited in death in the South. What makes Agnes so powerful in this scene is the fact that she is dying: it is she who dictates what is to be done in a "most composed manner" (*AA* 27).[97] This temporary reversal of power relations, a popular strategy of sentimental fiction, is also significant in terms of my argument of female emancipation, since Agnes is the one in control, not only in her dying hour,[98] but also when she is caring for her patients. At one point the male doctor endorses her superior quality as nurse and expresses his wish for her

95 Carrigan points out that despite reports of Protestant ministers fleeing in panic, clerical deserters were rather the exception than the rule (*Saffron Scourge* 341).

96 Interestingly the Sisters of Mercy—much like Agnes herself—have also given up the possibility of married life in a secular sense in order to care for their patients.

97 The description of Agnes's death is dripping with religious pieties and the sentimental language that is repeatedly found in deathbed scenes of Civil War nursing narratives. (cf. Laffrado 97). Louisa May Alcott's *Hospital Sketches* might be cited as an exception to the rule. Alcott with the description of John's death deliberately abstains from this approach.

98 "I have no fear of death, I am prepared for it"; "Come, Death, O come" (*AA* 27).

companionship and nursing care which he believes could only be possible if he were a woman: "Miss Arnold, you are worth all our nurses; and really I'm afraid all us physicians also put together. [...] I really begin to wish I was a woman myself so that if I should get the fever I might have you to nurse me well again." When Agnes tells him to "never mind about the being a woman" (*AA* 20) and promises to come should he fall sick with the fever, she points toward the possibility of a companionship across gender and professional divisions (physician-nurse). Since it was not uncommon anymore at the time that female nurses cared for male patients, the physician seems to refer to the professional divide.

In the short narrative form of *Angel Agnes*, yellow fever is not fully aestheticized into a language of disease that would represent the political and social crisis experience of the nation (as is the case in *Arthur Mervyn*). The Shreveport disaster serves as a formulaic setting to please a readership darkly fascinated by a fear of death and craving a tale of horror. For example, the novel opens with the exclamation of "Nothing but sickness! nothing but horror!" to be found in diseased Shreveport (*AA* 4). Later, when a nun who has fallen sick is described, we learn that the disease means the loss of one's natural self and the dethroning of reason (*AA* 18). *Angel Agnes* remains a sentimental tale of virtue, dedication, and generosity, featuring a strong female character. The narrative constructs Agnes as a social role model whose superior behavior is offered as remedy for the larger disease. A future female emancipation might be hinted at, but is not finally redeemed, as the strong Agnes has to die a martyr's death.

With *Angel Agnes* Bradshaw constructs a story with popular appeal which offers certain redeeming venues based on sentimental strategies of victimization and power reversal. The novella creates and relies on a narrative culture of fear and, at least temporarily, reverses patriarchal structures and questions a singularly WASP-ish identity construction. While the male doctor remains the authority by offering approval of Agnes's treatment, she also assumes that authority by lecturing others on the Spanish therapy. The novella thus at least temporarily reverses ingrained gender norms of the time as well as a prerogative of medical interpretation and treatment of diseases: by making the effective cure non-American—but Spanish colonialist—in origin and administered by a woman. *Angel Agnes* thus also puts forth a vision of female emancipation, a medical profession that acknowledges the role of women (nurses in this case) and an accepted co-existence of alternative cures and traditional (native) medicine as well as a critical stance against quarantine measures.

In 1873 yellow fever not only struck Shreveport on the Red River, but also traveled up the Mississippi as far as Memphis, Tennessee, a town with a population of about 50,000 at the time. Of the 15,000 persons who stayed in Memphis during the epidemic, approximately 7,000 fell ill, and 2,000 died (Carrigan, *Saffron Scourge* 111); the destructive force was thus comparable to that of the Shreveport disaster and was equally nationally publicized. It is probably through these channels that Bradshaw knew about young Martha Stephenson, in whose honor the citizens of Memphis planned to erect a monument at Elmwood Cemetery (see fig. 25). The documentation of these efforts as well as the preacher's remarks at Mattie's funeral service are part of Wesley Bradshaw's tale *Mattie Stephenson: The Sweet Young Martyr of Memphis* (1873) that fictionalizes the plight of the real person Martha Stephenson. With the death of its heroine announced on the first page, the text presents an account of Mattie's brave deeds and untimely death during the Memphis yellow fever epidemic. Owing to her extreme youth, the sanctification of this child martyr already sets in during her heroic nursing practices and is completed through her sickness and death. The narrative, however, is not only a fictionalized eulogy but a sequel to Bradshaw's earlier yellow fever novella *Angel Agnes*. In the first lines of *Mattie Stephenson* Agnes serves as a contrasting foil to characterize Mattie. Where Agnes is "exceedingly lovely" Mattie is merely "passably pretty," where Agnes is "very rich" Mattie is "poor," where Agnes is "engaged to be married" Mattie is "not yet entrammelled in love" (*MS* 19). Yet the text not only references Agnes to characterize the heroine of the Memphis epidemic (*MS* 18), it also features a prequel: the full story of the deceptive plot that ended the engagement of Agnes Arnold and George Harkness is revealed in the first chapter, entitled "The Unfortunate Courtship." Although the chapter is part of *Mattie Stephenson*, it has no direct connection to Mattie's tale other than to please the readers of Bradshaw's earlier novella before presenting them with another similar story.

Bradshaw promises to satisfy the curiosity "that has been excited in the public mind regarding to her [Agnes's] disappointment in marriage" ever since the publication of "the account of the heroic services and tragical death of Miss Agnes Arnold" (*MS* 3). He thus also elevates the importance of and demand for the marriage plot by his readers. In turn, Agnes's motivation to go to Shreveport is presented in a slightly different angle compared to the original piece. A note from George to Agnes was—according to Mrs. Arnold—"the final blow that parted George and Agnes forever in this world. It was immediately after this event that my daughter volunteered to go to Shreveport" (*MS* 13). We furthermore learn that Agnes's friend Sophia had succeeded in driving a wedge of jealousy between George and Agnes, but Sophia could not win George over for herself. And although George finds out about Sophia's deceit, he only arrives at the Arnold's place after Agnes is gone and is left to bemoan his and his fiancée's fate: "'Agnes! Yellow fever! I am her murderer!'" (*MS* 14). However, in terms of sentimental value, the revelation of Sophia's deceitful deed supposedly prompting Agnes's decision retrospectively elevates her sacrifice and death even further. Although the letter and its content are mentioned in the earlier narrative, the note's effect in hastening the protagonist's decision is not. To the contrary, as "Mrs. Arnold tried to rally Agnes about this, her first disappointment of the heart, [she] had the satisfaction of presently seeing her [daughter] quite merry" (*AA* 6). The newspaper's yellow fever reporting and Agnes's sense of Christian duty to help are given as motives (*AA* 6–7). The departure scene of Louisa May Alcott's *Hospital Sketches* (1863) may serve as an example for comparison: in the first-person account of Alcott, thinly fictionalized as Tribulation Periwinkle, the protagonist's mother wails as her daughter is leaving to become a volunteer nurse for the Union army. She "sees her off to war as though she were a son" writes Laura Laffrado (97). Laffrado reads the act of enlisting for (female) volunteer nursing as "a culturally sanctioned, asexual substitute for marriage" (97).[99] Furthermore, as Elizabeth Young points out, "Periwinkle is also more soldier than nurse in her experiences of military service" (Young 75) and can, in this respect, also be compared to Agnes Arnold. In fact, as a letter by her fiancé diminishes the prospect of marriage, Agnes chooses the substitution of volunteer nursing. The marriage plot is substituted by one of volunteer nursing. As George's letter has diminished the prospect of marriage, Agnes chooses to become a nurse. The narrative thus reverts to the commonly held assumption that the role of wife and the role of nurse (and by extension doctor) cannot be simultaneously fulfilled. This still holds true for Dr. Grace Breen in William Dean Howells' *Dr. Breen's Practice* (1882): Breen takes up "medicine because of a failed romance and ultimately leaves it because of a newfound one" (C. J. Davis 109–10).

After this introductory chapter that reframes the Angel Agnes story in even more conventional terms, Bradshaw follows his successful formula in structuring the course of action in *Mattie Stephenson*. We learn that both women were "actuated by the same motives" to volunteer to go to the fever districts and, in the words of the narrative, "help the afflicted" (*MS* 19). Mattie's volunteering is motivated "from pure childlike love and inborn bravery of heart" (*MS* 19). Refusing to be paid for her services despite her lack of money to buy clothes marks her as altruist and selfless. While these qualities echo those of Agnes, the reference to duty (also in relation and reference to a male military one) is more prominent in the earlier story. Agnes formulates it as a "duty to go and do what little [she] can toward alleviating

99 She has argued this in the context of Louisa May Alcott's *Hospital Sketches* (1863). On Alcott's *Hospital Sketches* see also Young 69–108.

the distress of those stricken sufferers" (*AA* 7). Despite the slight differences, the sentimental pattern readers know from *Angel Agnes* is applied again: this time with a marginalized poor protagonist as social role model and again with sick children and dead infants complementing the sentimental cast. Furthermore, the formal development from the unified tale in *Angel Agnes* to a more hybrid, yet also reductive, approach of a hagiography with documentary elements in *Mattie Stephenson* intensifies the focus on the sanctification already prevalent in *Angel Agnes.*

It is newspaper reporting that spreads news of the southern yellow fever disaster to the North and that attracts northern sympathy. This source of information serving as trigger to volunteer is the same in *Angel Agnes* and *Mattie Stephenson*. When Mattie Stephenson upon her visit in New England reads "about the dreadful disorder spreading from Shreveport along up the river, and the daily increasing lack of nurses," she decides to not return home but to go on to Memphis "to volunteer for the fearful work of nursing" (*MS* 19). Judging from the many references to her youth, Mattie is probably younger than twenty-two-year-old Agnes. Like Agnes, Mattie is briefly held up at the first quarantine station by reluctant officers who want to save her life, but who then let her pass as "they were too glad to accept the service of anyone willing to face the terrors of the pestilence" (*MS* 19). Mattie displays a fearlessness and bravery in light of the horrific scenes she encounters that is quite similar to Agnes. Mattie, however, does not actively promote her own cure or regimen or even discuss treatments with doctors as Agnes does. She offers a nursing care deeply craved by her patients, often simply staying with her patients while the doctors have to hasten on. At one instance, she merely postpones giving "the medicine left by the doctor" because her patient still slept and Mattie, we learn, "firmly believed in the common-sense rule that Nature heals the sick in slumber better than the physician" (*MS* 21).

Upon her arrival she experiences the literally contaminated atmosphere in the city of Memphis: "All over the place, wherever she turned her eyes, there arose clouds of smoke from burning tar and pitch, used as disinfectants. Men were engaged in scattering chloride of lime, phenol, carbolic acid &c., in all directions. The smell was positively frightful, and almost suffocating" (*MS* 20).[100] Seemingly unaffected by the spreading fear and suffocating atmosphere, Mattie promptly reports to the office of the Howard Association, a (secular) association that was founded in New Orleans.[101] In her first engagement Mattie is to care

100 These measures might have worked to some extent to keep the mosquitoes, who served as vectors, away from their next victims.

101 See Carrigan 346–50 on the association that was organized during the 1837 New Orleans yellow fever epidemic and incorporated in 1842; also see Carrigan for the

for a sick woman in childbirth. The contrast of the two females—the "shy young girl" (*MS* 20) and the agonized woman in labor—could not be greater and is openly noticed in the narrative by Dr. Williams, who is attending to the woman, as well as the messenger who takes Mattie to the "house of sickness and affliction" (*MS* 20). Mattie's "first care was to calm the patient's terror and excitement" (*MS* 21), and she succeeds as she "laid her cheek against the hot, saffron-hued forehead without the slightest fear" (*MS* 21). The symptoms clearly point towards yellow fever, yet Mattie's actions convey that she is neither afraid to contract the disease nor to face the woman's labor pains.

However, the feeling of solitude when she is with the sick woman weighs hard on Mattie. When her patient sleeps, the silence inside the sick room is contrasted with the street noises outside that conjure up images of war: "The silence, too was dreadful; but the noises now and then out in the street were still more awful; for the occasional vehicle that dashed along like a piece of artillery on the field of battle, Mattie knew to be a patient being taken to the hospital, or a corpse being hurried to the graveyard" (*MS* 22). Yet the war to be fought inside the room is the female one of childbirth. Despite the obvious differences between the two women, the "shy young girl" and the agonized pregnant woman, a bond between innocent Mattie and the sick woman is established by stressing their femaleness. Agnes's patient "began prematurely that sorrow which, for the sin of Eve, God adjudged all womankind should suffer" (*MS* 22); together they endure and accomplish the 'labor' of childbirth. When the woman delivers two babies, "one dead and the other dying [...], and both as yellow as gold" (*MS* 22–23), Mattie—probably due to her extreme youth and inexperience—fails to understand that the mother is also dying and is not able to respond to her encouraging words: "[T]he maternal ear was deaf, the mother's soul was summoned, and she heeded not the kind words and soothing voice" (*MS* 23) Mattie finds herself alone again, and she is facing death, "alone with three loathsome corpses" (*MS* 23). Yet although she was not able to save the mother or the children, she does not give up what she perceives to be her duty. She refuses to take a break after this initiation experience and "at once entered the sick room again" (*MS* 23). When her next patients, an old couple who fell sick after taking in four yellow fever orphans, quickly recover under her care, Mattie's maturation is completed. Patients and nurse resemble an ideal sentimental cast, and while the noble deed of the old gentleman and his wife does not immunize them against the fever but actually—as the narrative suggests—exposes them to it, they also do

role of the clergy during epidemics, 341–44. *Angel Agnes* exemplifies the role of the Catholic Sisters of Mercy in Shreveport.

not die and recover under Mattie's faithful care. At this point Mattie is textually elevated from "heroic girl" to "bright, ministering angel from heaven," "child saint," and "real handmaiden of God" (*MS* 23, 24): "[F]rom house to house, and from case to case, did young Mattie Stephenson flit, [...] nursing the sick, and, in her humble way, administering consolation to the dying, whispering the last word of piety and Christian hope into the many ears and hearts as the dark river flowed at their feet and engulfed them" (*MS* 23).

Providence is cited as the cause of and consolation for her early death. Mattie's last patient is a man whose physical size is in clear contrast to her delicacy. His corporeality provides a foil for Mattie's immateriality. Already more spirit than body, her transformation from heroic child to incorporeal saint is thus reinforced through focusing on the vulnerability of Mattie's body: "Mattie, through over-exertion with him, reduced her system so much, that she fell an easy victim to the contagion" (*MS* 24). Since direct transmission of yellow fever was already widely contested in the 1870s but also not entirely ruled out, it might safely be assumed that the word contagion takes on wider metaphorical meaning here, as a symbol for the inexplicability and violence of the disease. Mattie is diagnosed with yellow fever and taken to the hospital on the day her last patient dies. The "Sisters of Charity and Mercy, Howards, priests and clergymen of all denominations" assemble at the infirmary, vying "with each other in their kindness to the stricken girl" (*MS* 24). Mattie's passing away is described as "placid" and "peaceful" as "they had never seen before in a yellow fever patient," and her last words "God bless you all, I am going home" (*MS* 24) ring familiar in reference to the deathbed scene of Little Eva in Harriet Beecher Stowe's *Uncle Tom's Cabin*. The deathbed scene, circulating in the culture at large and employed here by Bradshaw, presents a "version of the ethic of sacrifice [...] that the highest human calling is to give one's life for another" (Tompkins 128).[102]

Known as Mattie Stephenson "from some town in the Northern States, but nothing more," a more complete identity including her home town is revealed only on the day of her death when a box with clothing and items suitable for the sick arrives from Towanda, Illinois (*MS* 27); it does not only reveal Mattie's place of origin but exemplifies Northern generosity to the South. The generosity is equaled by the people of Memphis: it is exemplified in the expensive casket and the enormous attendance at Mattie's funeral, including the mayor and several dignitaries serving as

102 Tompkins elaborates: "The power of the dead or the dying to redeem the unregenerate is a major theme of nineteenth-century popular fiction and religious literature. Mothers and children are thought to be uniquely capable of this work" (128).

pall-bearers of the "richest and most beautiful casket that money could procure" (*MS* 27). It could also be interpreted as desperate longing for redemption in light of the perceived power of the dead young Mattie Stephenson. The redemption of the unregenerate through the power of the dead or dying as a major trope of nineteenth-century popular literature has not only been pointed out by Tompkins (128). Mattie's sacrificial death provides a means for the Southern city's society to realign its values and norms and stabilize the group's coherence in light of the crisis of yellow fever which this Northern girl so boldly faced.

In the eulogy, reprinted as part of the narrative, a certain Reverend Boggs reminds the congregation of what Mattie did for the sick mother in childbirth, the first yellow fever patient whom she attended. She was a "slender, shy girl" and did the work others were not able to do because "[t]error had broken the tenderest ties of life; men had nerved themselves to face the danger by strong drink; women, otherwise ready with their sympathy and aid in that hour of agony, whose bitterness only a woman can know, stood aloof, with pale faces and parted lips" (*MS* 28). With this example, the reverend likens Mattie to the Good Samaritan, who—as an outsider—acted while most others shied away out of terror and fear. The quoted parable may also allude to the Howards, who refer to themselves as Samaritans. The reader also learns that the dead mother and Mattie now rest not very far from each other, which textually reunites the mother, an immigrant to the southern United States from Scotland, with the girl from Illinois and also stresses both women's sacrifice.

The tale ends with a supposedly authentic reprinted resolution of the Howard Association to not only lament the death of Mattie Stephenson and sympathize with her family, but also to erect a monument "in honor of her memory, and in justice to ourselves, and as an example to her race, [...] to mark the spot where she sleeps, and that her epitaph shall tell this sublime and beautiful story of her life" (*MS* 29). Not only this visual memorial marker, but also the short sentimental tale of Mattie's sacrifice narratively reunites North and South. It is not so much the image of marital reunion that realigns North and South in the visual memorial marker and the sentimental tale, but the sacrifice of this young Northern girl who will forever stay in the South, physically buried there and spiritually immortalized.

Another woman would have provided equally interesting material for a yellow fever tale. Although not fictionalized at the time, Cook's story has been documented in the *West Tennessee Historical Society Papers* (Wright, "Annie Cook") and in Jeanette Keith's book *Fever Season* (90–91, 158). Annie Cook of 34 Gayoso Street, Memphis, was the owner of an upscale brothel in that mansion where she and a woman named Lorena Meade, an 'employee' which she had not dismissed when the 1873 fever broke out, nursed yellow fever patients. Cook did the same during the devastating 1878 epidemic. Because she had turned her bordello into an infirmary, she was referred to as the Mary Magdalene of Memphis. When she again turned her brothel into a hospital during the devastating 1878 yellow fever epidemic, she caught the fever and died on September 11, 1878. She was buried at Elmwood Cemetery, where her grave remained unmarked until a monument was erected in 1979 (fig. 26). In January 1971 a Yellow Fever Memorial was dedicated in Tom Lee Park adjacent to the Mississippi river. It honors those who remained in Memphis during the frequent yellow fever epidemics in the 1870s (fig. 27).

Fig. 25. Mattie Stephenson Memorial. Photo by Vivian Taylor Arendall. Find a Grave. *27 Mar. 2004. Web.*

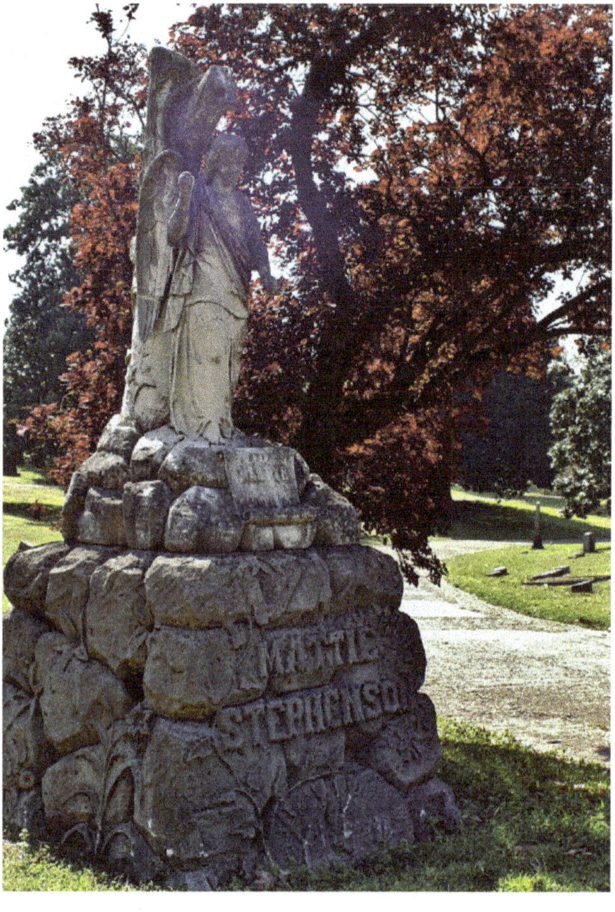

Fig. 26. Annie Cook Memorial. Photo by Melissa Bridgman. 26 Feb. 2007. Web.

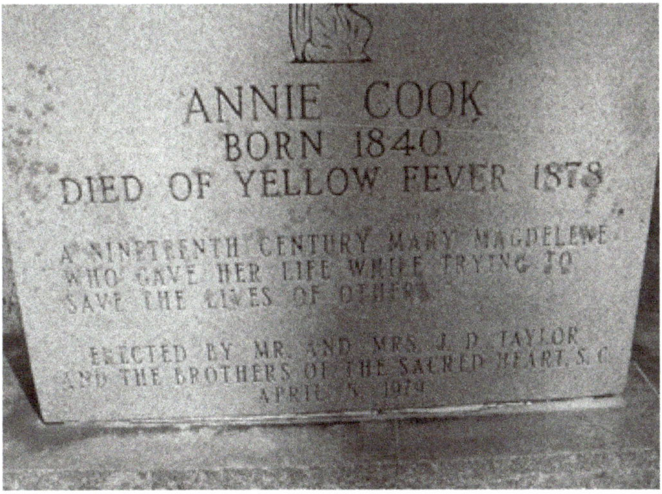

Fig. 27. Yellow Fever Memorial, Memphis. Design by Harris Sorrelle, 1971. Memphis Art Project. *Web.*

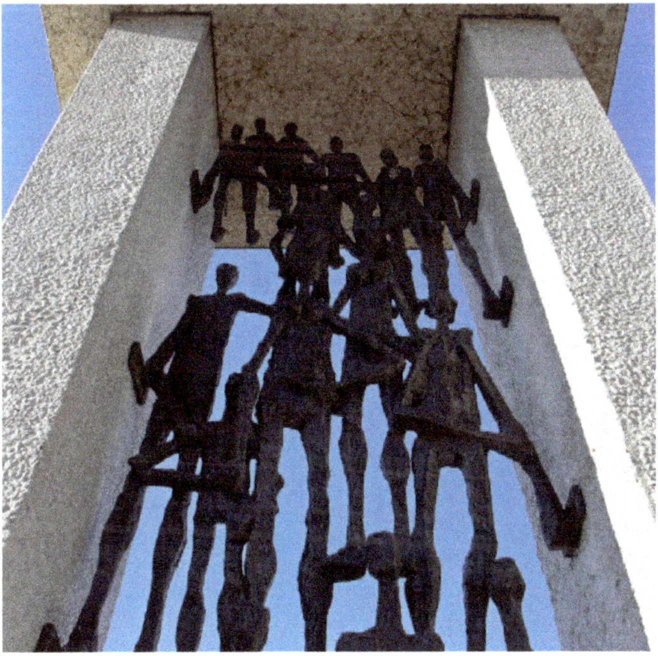

4.4 "Volunteers to the fever district": Reversing Gender Roles in Elizabeth Stuart Phelps's "Zerviah Hope" (1880)

After the 1873 fever more outbreaks in the South culminated in the devastating 1878 epidemic during which, by one estimate, twenty thousand people died in the lower Mississippi Valley, with a death rate of 10 percent of the population in some cities such as Memphis (Patterson 857–58; "Major U.S. Epidemics"). Elizabeth Stuart Phelps's short story "Zerviah Hope" that was first published in *Scribner's Monthly* in 1880 features a yellow fever epidemic on the South Carolina seaboard as well as Phelps's first actively practicing woman doctor—other such characters were to follow—with the telling name of Dr. Marian Dare. It focuses on the self-sacrifice of the title character, a male nurse with the gender-ambiguous name of Zerviah Hope (Morris 141; Wegener 12).[103] The story is set in the small South Carolina town of Calhoun ("ZH" 78) during a particularly devastating yellow fever epidemic.[104] It begins with a steamship departing from its course to permit a group of "[p]hysicians from New York" to disembark as "[v]olunteers to the fever district" ("ZH" 78). A "short passenger," who has made no acquaintances on board the ship and is only later identified as the story's title character, inquires about the lady whom he presumes to be a nurse. He learns that "[s]he's a she-doctor. Doctors, the whole of 'em. There ain't a nurse aboard." When Zerviah Hope further speculates that many nurses are probably to be found in Calhoun, it is the woman doctor who is the first of the three doctors to reply and thus speak in the story. Exhibiting "a quick and clear-cut, but not ungentle voice" and speaking "in a business-like tone" she informs him that there are no nurses and that the place is perishing; she thus indirectly invites Zerviah to join them. Larger towns, such as Savannah, are in the focus of the authorities which Dr. Dare deems "natural and right" ("ZH" 78). In fact, while more people died in the cities due to higher population numbers, smaller inland towns were often hit much harder by yellow fever and displayed significantly higher mortality rates since the inhabitants often had

103 Zerviah was King David's older sister. While she is hardly described in 2 Samuel 17:25, her three sons are mentioned as David's soldiers; they are referred to with the matronymic connotation of "Zerviah's sons." David relies on his sister's sons' protection and advice, yet also recognizes them to be motivated by evil. David's false trust in them leads him to conspire with one of them in evil-doing.

104 Savannah, which is mentioned in Phelps's story, had been hit by a particularly devastating epidemic in 1876 (with a mortality rate of 3 percent, according to Patterson 858). The 1878 epidemic hit the entire lower Mississippi region with national reverberations. The succession of epidemics in the 1870s probably informed Phelps's writing.

not built up immunity during earlier outbreaks. As a result, the virus found more susceptible victims and could spread faster. Although the causation could not yet be explained, observations of mortality rates were made at the time.

The medical field found itself in a major period of transition in the 1870s: not only did the germ theory of transmission (also with respect to yellow fever) slowly take hold, but the increasing number of women doctors also influenced the outlook of the profession. In 1849, Elizabeth Blackwell had become the first woman to receive a medical diploma in the United States; others, like Dr. Marie Zakrezweska, had followed. As the Civil War ended, several hundred women had begun practicing medicine,[105] and Phelps accompanied their rise in several of her writings and "culturally, socially, and professionally" helped legitimate the "figure of the American medical woman" (Wegener 2). Two of Phelps's short stories, "Our Little Women" (1872)[106] and "Hannah Colby's Chance" (1873), show the transformation of two young women into professional physicians. Her novel *Doctor Zay* (1882) represents Phelps's best-known treatment of the character of a woman doctor.[107] Like "Zerviah Hope" the novel is an example of role reversal drawing attention to the gendered patterns and power struggles in doctor-patient relations. Yet Phelps's interest in the topic was already apparent in the 1860s and 1870s when she engaged the topic in several essays. In an 1867 essay in *Harper's New Monthly Magazine* Phelps commented on the still difficult but increasingly trodden path of women doctors "What Shall They Do?": "Be a doctor? and be sure that you could be few things more womanly or more noble. The brave pioneers? God bless them for it!? have broken the way for you. It is an easier way now than the path of the idle or the ill-paid" ("What Shall They Do?" 523). As Frederick Wegener has shown, Phelps in her essays argued against the skeptics and in favor of more women receiving a medical degree based on

105 By 1880 approximately six percent of practicing physicians were women. The first female delegate to the American Medical Association was admitted in 1876 (C. J. Davis 107).

106 See Jean Carwile Masteller for an analysis of "Our Little Women" as a story of empowerment for young girls as readers (esp. 138). The protagonist Lois is determined to leave her working-girl past behind and become a professional physician.

107 Two novels that had a woman doctor as central character were issued in short sequence of Phelps's short story and her novel *Doctor Zay* (1882), William Dean Howells's *Dr. Breen's Practice* (1881) and Sarah Orne Jewett's *A Country Doctor* (1884). While Howells' *Dr. Breen's Practice* is a "negative portrayal of a female physician," Jewett's *A Country Doctor* "tells the story of a woman who declines marriage to become a physician" (G. R. Thompson 164–65).

their skill and professionalism and on the economic success of already practicing medical women—she explicitly mentions their "pecuniary value" ("What They Are Doing" 1; see also Wegener 4). Phelps furthermore identified the need for medical women assisting women patients who were often reluctant to "disclose symptoms to male practitioners" and thus welcomed the possibility to consult doctors of the same sex (Morantz-Sanchez 52).

In her journalistic prose, Phelps did not only foster the education of women doctors but also argued for their coeducation, which would provide for the training of men and women "under identical disciplinary conditions" (Phelps, "Experiment" 1), much in the vein that separate is indeed not equal.[108] Since Phelps's close acquaintance Dr. Mary Briggs Harris attended the Boston University School of Medicine and enabled her to personally observe the class and its training, the school often serves as a model in her articles. Phelps's conviction of what Cynthia Davis calls the "viable principle of commensurability" (106) is equally reflected in her imaginative writings. In "Zerviah Hope" the two male doctors accompanying Dr. Dare stand for opposing views regarding female physicians. One of them, Dr. Frank, has attended a course of lectures with the female doctor and—true to his telling name—"spoke to her with an air of *camaraderie*, at once frank and deferential" ("ZH" 78; emphasis in original). Despite his skeptical views regarding the medical education of women, the proven excellence of this particular woman doctor influences his conviction: he respects Dr. Dare as someone who has "outranked him at graduation" ("ZH" 78) and also recognizes her as a "lady" whose family he knows. Thus Dr. Dare's professional distinction as well as her status as a woman of higher social rank is confirmed. The other physician, Dr. Remane, more clearly represents the prevalent view of the time: he "never consulted with doctresses" ("ZH" 79). Dr. Dare, as "a single, highly educated, economically autonomous New Woman" (Smith-Rosenberg, *Disorderly Conduct* 245) poses a threat to white masculinity. While the text clearly problematizes the changing gender roles, it also points toward equality and partnership between the sexes. A male/female fellowship between the three physicians is confirmed early in the story and in light of the unifying effect of the impending disaster: they lean against each other and even Remane moves closer to the others in a gesture of wishing each other well before separating and individually

108 Phelps was an adamant proponent of women's rights and wrote "The Experiment Tried" for *The Independent*, which had started as an antislavery paper and now advocated women's suffrage.

confronting the crisis and the patients it brought forward ("ZH" 79).[109] The signs of human fellowship are equally represented in the marriage plot-induced relationship between North and South, or more precisely in Northern dispatches of "food, physician, purse, medicine—that spoke from the heart of the North to the heart of the South, and upheld her in those well-remembered days" ("ZH" 81)

In the short story, yellow fever and its destructive force is referenced with an allusion to Psalm 91 as "[t]he pestilence [that] walked in darkness, and the destruction wasted at midday. Men died, in that little town of a few thousand souls, at the rate of a score a day—black and white, poor and rich" ("ZH" 80). Furthermore, the disease functions as a leveler disregarding race and class, but not explicitly gender in this enumeration. This does not mean that Phelps disregards the effect of the disease in literal and metaphorical terms on gender. It is the yellow fever crisis that seems, as one critic puts it, to submerge "[a]ll sex-based hierarchies of the day" (Wegener 11). Phelps moves the question to the foreground with her radical choice of characters and the characterization of her main figures with respect to gender roles. As in her novel *Doctor Zay* that features a woman doctor and a male patient, Phelps makes the nurse male and the doctor female, calling into "question the association of femininity and frailty" (C. J. Davis 115).

The male and female physicians who are entering "the afflicted region of Calhoun," that seems almost completely shut off and shunned from the rest of the world:

> The quarantine laws tightened. Vessels fled by the harbor mouth under full sail, and melted like helpless compassion upon the fiery horizon. Trains upon the Shore Line shot through and thundered past the station; they crowded on steam; the fireman and his stoker averted their faces as they whirled by. The world turned her back upon Calhoun, and the dying town was shut in with her dead. ("ZH" 80)

When a "glum passenger"—later identified as Zerviah Hope—asks to be landed as well, no one notices him at first, until Dr. Dare invites him into the space of their boat: "There's room for you" ("ZH" 79). Tellingly, the woman doctor provides another example of her attentiveness. She seems to intuitively grasp the desperate situation they are about to face, noticing the effect isolation and constant fear of infection has on the people. When observing their "negro boatman" Scip, she detects "a kind of terror for which we find that animals, as well as men, instinctively refrain from seeking expression," and wonders whether "all the people in Calhoun

109 When they land in silence, "[t]he four passengers stood for a moment upon the hot, white sands, moved toward one another, before they separated, by a blind sense of human fellowship. Even Remane found himself touching his hat" ("ZH" 79).

would have that look" ("ZH" 78). When Dr. Frank offers his help, picking up an idle pair of oars, Dr. Remane reprimands him for he should not exhaust himself. The exchange exemplifies the social and hierarchical structure within the story. Later it is the boatman who finds a "corner to spend the night" for nurse volunteer Hope ("ZH" 80), which might also foreshadow their reliance on each other.

All three physicians master the trek from the landing dock to the afflicted city alone, a fact that seems most important to the woman doctor. When Dr. Frank asks Dr. Dare whether he can serve her in any way, she thanks him but confirms her self-reliance, offering her hand in a gesture of farewell. For Dr. Marian Dare this incident represents "the first moment when the consciousness of her sex had made itself oppressive to her since she ventured upon this undertaking. She would have minded presenting herself to the Relief Committee of Calhoun, accompanied by gentlemen upon whom she had no claim. She walked on alone, in her gray dress and white straw hat, with her luggage in her own sufficient hand" ("ZH" 79). When the "reticent passenger" approaches her to inquire about "the best way of going to work to offer myself as a fever nurse in this place," she commends him for not going to Savannah. And after assessing for herself that "[p]lainly, this poor fellow was not a gentleman," she even allows the volunteer nurse what she could not allow her professional colleague earlier, to carry her heavy bag ("ZH" 79). After being told that she will need him as a nurse the next morning, he introduces himself as Zerviah Hope, and Dr. Dare takes down his name in her note-book ("ZH" 79). Apart from confirming the woman doctor's independence from her male peers, the exchange also shows her acceptance of Zerviah as her inferior aide. It thus promotes a reversal of conventional gender roles, the subordination of the male nurse under the female doctor.

The first part of the story, entitled "Prelude," ends with a direct address to the reader that assures the truthfulness and authenticity of the tale ("ZH" 80).[110] The first-person intervention also clarifies that readers are not to expect a romantic tale or a marriage plot, as the "story does not deal with love or ladies" nor include "tender passages between the fever-physicians." The passage also establishes the figure of the woman doctor as a brave human being and as a scientist, but it mainly reveals her function as key to an understanding of the short story's male title character, namely "that certain missing fragments in the history of the person known as Zerviah Hope we owe to her. She hovers over the tale with a distant and beautiful influence, pervading as womanly compassion and alert as

---

110 "I have nothing further to say about the story before I tell it, except that it is true" ("ZH" 80).

a woman's eye" ("ZH" 80). Vision on a literal (observing Zerviah as well as her patients empathetically) and a metaphorical level (seeing Zerviah's potential as nurse) plays an important role in the story. In this sense, the woman doctor's vision is not reduced to the medical gaze that separates the patient's body from the patient's person (theorized by Foucault in a French cultural context), but she 'sees' both body and identity (in Zerviah's case); Phelps thus qualifies and genders the gaze.[111] What Antje Dallmann asserts in regard to the character of Dr. Zay in Phelps's novel of the same title, can also be applied to the woman doctor in the short story: "biomedicine as a discourse is instrumental, since it naturalizes the social, and, through the character of a woman doctor, gives scientific, moral, and emotional authority to women. Thereby, the text also appropriates and genders the medical gaze, rendering it less universal and at the same time more comprehensive" ("Doctors" 131).

In the course of the story Zerviah takes care of the worst yellow fever cases, and those most discarded by society that might qualify as Other: "[h]e sought the neglected, and the negroes. He braved the unclean, and the unburied" ("ZH" 81), and Dr. Dare watches him with a slight touch of emotion. Asked by Dr. Frank about her "fancy to the fellow," she insists on her professionalism and curtly replies that she's "been in practice too long to take sudden fancies. There is no profession like ours, Doctor, for putting the sympathies under double picket guard" ("ZH" 80). If there is a nod to the marriage plot it is one that is not carried out but muted. For Zerviah, the bond between Dr. Dare and himself remains the only one that counts for him. She is the only uninfected person he speaks to: "He was always pliable to the influence of a woman's voice or to womanly manner. He had, in the presence of women, the quick responsiveness and sudden change of color and sensitiveness of intonation which bespeak the man whose highest graces and lowest faults are likely to be owing to feminine power" ("ZH" 81). His feminized position and his possession of or at least responsiveness to female gender characteristics is what secures Zerviah's "remarkable success as a nurse. He was found to be infinitely tender, and of fine, brave patience" ("ZH" 81). Yet it is only the combination of male and female traits that characterizes Zerviah as the ideal nurse. Phelps, as in her later novel *Doctor Zay*, thus fictionally comments on the arbitrariness of stereotypical gender roles (cf. Donaldson 103). Similar to a reference in *Angel Agnes*, soldierly qualities are accredited to the volunteer

111 Lawrence Rothfield has theorized the "medical gaze" in a British context for the nineteenth century (*Vital Signs*).

nurse and almost super-human or angelic qualities are conferred upon him, complete with halo and an incorporeal, but radiant presence:

> He went to his task as the soldier goes to the front under raking fire, with gleaming eyes and iron muscles. The fever of the fight was on him. He seemed to wrestle with disease for his patients, and to trample death beneath his feet. He glowed over his cures with a positive physical dilation, and writhed over his dead as if he had killed them. He seemed built of endurance more than mortal. It was not known when he slept, scarcely if he ate. His weariness sat upon him like a halo. He grew thin, refined, radiant. In short, he presented an example of that rare spectacle which never fails to command spectators—a common man possessed by an uncommon enthusiasm. ("ZH" 81)

Again at this point in the story, the narrator confirms the credibility of the story by pointing to the people who knew Zerviah Hope, even without being personally known by him: "I have been told that, to this day, many people personally unknown to him [...] were unable to speak it because of choking voices. I have often wished that he knew this" ("ZH" 81). Communication as another means of transmitting information seems to break down in light of the crisis. While on a literal level the inability to speak refers to people's reverence, the possibility of communicating or transmitting the disease is referenced as well. It is curtailed by an absence of communication. Furthermore, the foreboding character of these lines of knowing or rather not knowing, of not being able to profess his good reputation, is confirmed when Zerviah not much later finds out that his secret has leaked. As it turns out, Zerviah has taken the job as nurse to atone for a murder he has committed and was convicted for. His secret has finally followed him south on board the *Mercy* and through the words of Scip, the black boatman, to Jupiter, Dr. Remane's assistant, the whole town knew. Zerviah's first impulse is to put a spatial distance between him and those who know. When he reenters town in desperation, it is Dr. Dare who confronts him about what she refers to as "a hateful rumor" ("ZH" 83).

Due to the reversal of conventional gender roles as a result of the inverted pattern of male dominance, communication in this situation again fails. Zerviah, who has committed the murder out of love for a woman, respects Dr. Dare as his professional superior and although he craves her compassion, he does not want to take advantage of what he perceives as a female quality and cannot utter his remorse:

> He wanted to go on speaking to this woman [Dr. Dare], not to defend or excuse himself, not to say anything weak or wrong, only to make her understand that he did not want to excuse himself; in some way, just because she *was* a woman, to make her feel that he was man enough to bear the burden of his deed. He wanted to cry out to her, "You are a woman! Oh, be gentle, and understand how sorry a man can be for a deadly sin!" but his lips were parched. He moved them dryly; he could not talk. ("ZH" 83)

Dr. Dare, in return, expresses her faith in him and sends him back to his patients. The muted or at least one-sided communication between the two can also be read as a symbolic means to control the spread (or communication) of the disease. Frederick Wegener has pointed out that "Dr. Dare's reaffirmation of his human worth deepens the kinship [Zerviah] senses between them" (Wegener 12). The exchange equally affects Dr. Dare and her understanding of and reliance on their relationship, yet she instinctively hides the physical and physiological female side of herself: "She drew her veil; there was unprofessional moisture on her long, feminine lashes" ("ZH" 84). The people of Calhoun take somewhat longer than Dr. Dare to re-align the image they had pieced together in their heads and are only able to recognize Zerviah again for what he did when they find out that he has put all of his nurse's wages into the relief-contribution boxes of the local charities. Relief committee members are subsequently searching for him and require Dr. Dare's help in locating him; they learn that she has contracted the fever and Dr. Frank is taking her cases. Her illness is not defined as a failure of strength due to her femaleness but is explicitly not gendered.[112]

While Dr. Dare is sick with the fever, Zerviah, who does not know about her plight, is called to Scip's hut. The atmosphere clearly emanates death and loneliness with the solitary palmetto tree that "looked like a corpse, though there was life in it yet" ("ZH" 85), and the urgency and desolation of the situation is conveyed in a matter-of-fact medical telegram style: "Scip was very sick. Hope had sent for Dr. Dare. She had not come. Scip was too sick to be left. The nurse found his duty with the negro. Scip was growing worse" ("ZH" 85). When in a brief interlude Zerviah is able to leave the hut, the place of death and sickness, he has a vision of people tending their sick loved ones in the town. The passage that is saturated with biblical allusions ends with Zerviah's promise, spoken in prayer, to "not leave the creetur [sic]" and stay in the swamp (86). According to the resolution, a changed set of metaphors of war characterizes the following description: "The nurse and the plague, like two living combatants, met in the miserable place and battled for the negro" ("ZH" 86), who is too sick to be left alone. The spatial distance between female doctor and male nurse is amplified in the mode of narration. Zerviah finds himself physically outside of town, unreachable and alone in "a hard place for a man to die" ("ZH" 85), and this

112 The non-pathologization of female illness is reminiscent of Louisa May Alcott's representation of nurse Tribulation Periwinkle's fever in *Hospital Sketches*. Her illness is implicitly equated with the male soldier suffering from his war injuries (see also Young 75). In Phelps's story the suffering of female doctor and male nurse from yellow fever is similarly equated.

is also reflected in the self-reflexive figural narrative style, as well as the reference to each single day that conveys time's slow passing among the sick: "It was Monday, but no one came. It was Tuesday, but the nurse and the plague still battled alone together over the negro. Zerviah's stock of remedies was as ample as his skill. He had thought he should save Scip. He worked without sleep, and the food was not clean. He lavished himself like a lover over this black boatman; he leaned like a mother over this man who had betrayed him" ("ZH" 86). The intimate connection and absolute dedication conveyed in the description of the patient-nurse relationship stands out as we, for example, never witness anything similar between the three doctors and their patients. However, it seems too far to interpret a homosocial bond into their relationship as Holly Furneaux has done in nineteenth-century Britain regarding male nursing and gentleness.

Zerviah fervently battles for the black man's life ("ZH" 85) but loses him, only to realize that he now has "*got it*" too ("ZH" 86). The black boatman Scip and the male nurse Zerviah Hope remain the only yellow fever victims of the story whose suffering and death the reader witnesses, and although the narrow-minded Dr. Remane also dies, his passing is not further elaborated on.[113] So while, in fact, as Phelps writes "black and white, poor and rich, clean and foul, saint and sinner" ("ZH" 80) died alongside each other, the focus of the story remains on the suffering outsiders or Others. The emphasis of the passage of disease realization is solely on Zerviah:

> His professional experience gave him an excruciating foresight of his symptoms, and their result presented itself to him with horrible distinctness. As one by one he passed through the familiar conditions whose phases he had watched in other men a hundred times, he would have given his life for a temporary ignorance. His trained imagination had little mercy on him. He weighed his chances, and watched his fate with the sad exactness of knowledge. [...] "They would have come if they had known. They would not have let me *die* alone. I don't think *she* would have done that. I wonder where she is?" ("ZH" 87; emphasis in original)

Only subsequently, his self-pitying thoughts wander to what they and later *she*, Dr. Dare, would have done, had *she* only known. He does not believe, in other words, in a deliberate abandonment. The fact that Dr. Dare does not know where Zerviah is in the week when they are both ill, and of Zerviah knowing that she would have saved him had she only known, strengthens the bond between them.

---

113 "The young Northerner, Dr. Remane, was gone,—a reticent, brave young man" ("ZH" 88).

Zerviah is trapped inside the hut and inside his diseased body, and his vision is restricted: "Through the wooden shutter, Zerviah could see the lights, and the lonely palmetto, and the grave" ("ZH" 87). His dying wish is for "a great, white, holy frost […] for these poor devils that have borne so much!" ("ZH" 87). Yet before Zerviah's death "a little party from the city rode up, […] Dr. Frank was with them, and the lady, Marian Dare." Her first name is given, and—in an equally intimate manner—her name is not connected to her being a doctor but with a female noble character. She seems fragile, "pale, and still weak," after recovering from the fever ("ZH" 88). The narrative suggests that Zerviah sees her before his eyes close: "She knelt beside the bed, and put her hand upon his eyes. […]. Let us hope that they knew her before they closed" ("ZH" 88). The importance of vision and of seeing is stressed again here, but the factuality of the recognition is only revealed later. In the postscript to the story we learn that "he rested, after her hand had fallen on his eyes" ("ZH" 88). Zerviah is, as Wegener suggests, thus "redemptively linked to her once again at the end." Their association "as fellow healers from the North" has a "restorative function" (Wegener 13). Wegener argues that the story manifests what historian Paul H. Buck in the 1930s has called the "'bond of sympathy underlying the hostility of the divided sections'" and thus aligns itself "with the work of those who 'wrote of the sections at last united and truly reconciled by the generosity of deed and attitude of the North'" (13).

It is in fact the released convict, the Other in many respects, whose generosity the people of Calhoun most openly appreciate and remember in the end. He had killed the new lover of the woman he loved because Zerviah believed that this act would save her. In turn, he has lost everything and suffers for what he did, wishing to repent for his sins by becoming a nurse. As a trope this also alludes to the plight and story of the South and Southerners who have fought and lost for the cause of the Confederacy and who are now primarily but not singularly suffering from the yellow fever epidemic. So the immediate connection and bond between the suffering people of Calhoun and their Northern beneficiaries is established through the male nurse. In a second step it is extended through Zerviah's personal bond to Dr. Dare, the trained Northern physician. Her (female) emotionality, mostly professionally restrained or actively hidden in the course of the story, comes to the fore at the moment of his confession and at the crucial instance of his death, to (re)establish the special bond (between physician and nurse, man and woman, North and South). After witnessing Zerviah's death "[s]he came out, and tried to tell about it, but broke down, and sobbed before them all" ("ZH" 88). Explicitly referred to as "a martyr's death," ("ZH" 88), the sanctification of Zerviah even conjures up a possible connection to Abraham Lincoln. The redemptive act is complete as the frost puts an end to the disease and the story.

> In the morning, when they all awoke, these of the sorrowing city here, and those of the happy city yonder; when they took up life again with its returning sunrise—the sick and the well, the free and the fettered, the living and the dead—the frost lay, cool, white, blessed, on his grave. ("ZH" 88)

4.5 "The fever creeping into her veins": Yellow Fever as Liminal Experience in Mollie E. M. Davis's *The Queen's Garden* (1900)

Mollie Davis's novel *The Queen's Garden* (1900)[114] is set during one of the last great yellow fever epidemics in New Orleans in the late 1890s. Like many yellow fever narratives, it employs the trope of an orphan, yet with a twist. The protagonist Noel Lepeyre has already lost her mother and father at the beginning of the novel and thus before her confrontation with yellow fever.

Orphaned at age seven, she has no concept of family and her solitude defines her character: Noel was "used to being alone" (*QG* 3) having lived with three distant old relatives and experienced the presence of death as a well-known companion: "aunt Hester, mama's sister" (*QG* 4), and then aunt Harlowe who, on her deathbed, confided Noel to step-aunt Mitchell. The latter died six months before the story is taken up. Noel is left to care for herself and becomes a teacher at a small country school. Early on in the story—and after the deaths of her three aunts—Noel at the age of nineteen travels to New Orleans to meet a fourth aunt: Margaret Chrétien, called "Tante Marguerite" (*QG* 8). She finds her aunt ill with yellow fever and herself caught in a terrifying atmosphere and confined to a house emanating death and decay. She longs for the motherly guidance of her long-lost aunt, the adoption by whom is posthumously confirmed by Dr. Andrew Grafton, the doctor who attends to Madame Chrétien (in front of him she calls Noel "my beloved niece and adopted daughter, Noel Lepeyre," *QG* 129). The adoption is never actively pursued as aunt and niece never meet to become mother and daughter, and Noel is left an orphan again at the end of the novel. The plot has Noel undergoing a rite of passage: she is not only faced with other people's deaths but her own death as well. Her yellow fever-infected aunt remains an absent presence paired with the disturbing presence of the mulatto servant, clearly marked as Other by use of language (she speaks broken English) and appearance (a "meagre, weazened, yellow old creature" [*QG* 26] that to the protagonist conjures up the image of a voodoo witch who seduces young women in order to destroy them). The only other characters Noel speaks to and

114 In the following I will use *QG* for *The Queen's Garden*.

interacts with in the novel are male: a veteran she meets on the way to her aunt; the physician Dr. Grafton, the former lover of her aunt and now her doctor; and a newspaper reporter, reassuringly named Richard Strong, whom Noel falls in love with.

The rational elements in the novel (represented by the doctor and the newspaper reporter) clearly promote a belief in the effectiveness of a rigidly followed quarantine in light of a yellow fever epidemic. On a structural level the quarantine, the strict separation of sick and healthy (in order to prevent the spread of the epidemic), is mirrored in the narrative's representation of spatial dichotomies and of inside versus outside. The logic follows the relationship between medicine and morals (dating back to antiquity) that suggests countering illnesses by sustaining or restoring social order.[115] Although the *Queen's Garden*'s use of binary oppositions to restore a supposedly lost order is most obvious on the spatial level of within and without, it is also transferred to the levels of self and other, male and female, old and young, sick and healthy, city and country and thus transcends a separate spheres ideology on various levels. The politically-motivated quarantine tactics described in the novel ultimately fail and the boundaries are blurred by a transgression of borders (spatial and bodily). Noel and the man she falls in love with transgress the borders assigned to them, fall sick, and survive the fever. And although physically and psychologically scarred, they are enabled to build their own tangible paradise on the property Noel has inherited. Read in a fiction-as-symbolic-action approach, it is only through the transgression of boundaries as well as the transgressive disease experience that this transformation is made possible. In the following I will trace the spatial and other dialectic oppositions in the novel whose strict separation is offered as a means to control yellow fever but ultimately fails, thus offering a critique of those same measures.

Mollie Moore Davis, was born in 1844 in Benton County (later Calhoun County), Alabama and grew up in west Texas. Her father was a physician and her husband a newspaper editor. Davis thus knew the two professions that not only influence the subject matter of her writing but also her observational realist mode in describing the psychological state of her characters, such as the effect of the house quarantine on *The Queen's Garden*'s protagonist. Already at age sixteen Mollie Moore was identified as a poetess in the 1860 census. With the outbreak of

---

115 See Mary Douglas who argues that "ideas about separating, purifying, demarcating, and punishing transgressions have their main function to impose system on an inherently untidy experience. It is only by exaggerating the difference between within and without, above and below, male and female, with and against, that a semblance of order is created" (4).

the Civil War she shifted her focus to patriotic poetry supporting the Confederate cause (Francis 61). In 1874 she married Major Thomas E. Davis and wrote mostly short fiction for an emergent market of juvenile magazines. In 1879 they were forced to leave Texas for financial reasons and settled in New Orleans, where her husband was offered a position as an editorial writer and later became an editor for *The Picayune* until his death in 1914. New Orleans, once booming with economic opportunity during the antebellum era, had become a poor city in the Gilded Age.

> [T]he city was dirty and poorly lit, few streets outside the downtown area were paved, and the water supply was unsafe. Disease infested the place. Not only endemic illnesses such as typhoid, smallpox, malaria, and diphtheria, but also recurrent epidemics—a devastating attack by yellow fever had killed four thousand the previous summer—gave New Orleans a frightful reputation. (Brady 103)

Yet, Davis did the best she could with the little money the family had left after her husband's business went bankrupt in Texas (Brady 102). Although it was not considered the place of residence for Anglo-Americans, she moved her family to the French Quarter that, after its golden days in the 1830s had seen a gradual deterioration with only a few respectable Creole families remaining (after several financial crises, the Civil War, and postwar depression) (Brady 104). From 1885 Mollie Moore Davis held Friday reception days that became gradually known as salon readings, which, for example, were attended by Kate Chopin, when visiting from St. Louis (Brady 110, 113; Toth 326). An illustrious circle of writers also frequented the Davises' household: "among them George Washington Cable, Lafcadio Hearn, Grace King, Ruth McEnery Stuart, Booth Tarkington, Hamlin Garland, and Julia Ward Howe" (Francis 62; see also Brady 109). It was the literary scene and a community of writers that helped New Orleans to garner new recognition.[116] While still writing for the juvenile market, Davis's poems and stories also appeared in *Harper's* and *The Atlantic Monthly*. In the 1880s and 1890s Davis published several works of fiction, many of which draw upon the local color (for plots and characters) of her adopted home.

The Queen's Garden also begins in a classical local color fashion and emanates an impressionistic quality. Another popular trope of yellow fever fiction

116 Women writers such as Grace King, Mollie E. Moore Davis, and Ruth McEnery Stuart, Elizabeth Jane Poitevant Nicholson (pseudonym Pearl Rivers), the editor and publisher of *The Picayune* (1876–96), and the journalist Elizabeth Gilmer (Dorothy Dix), a newspaper associate, influenced public opionion on questions of race relations, women's rights and social reform in the New Orleans of the last two decades of the nineteenth century (Bryan 8, 77).

is equally employed, that of foreign or unacclimatized—in the terminology of the day—persons travelling to a region not only unknown to them in custom and manner, but—more importantly—infested with yellow fever. The concrete location, New Orleans, for example, is the same in George Washington Cable's *The Grandissimes* which has Joseph Frowenfeld together with his family moving to the South, only to fall victim to the then-raging epidemic (see ch. 5.3). Agnes Arnold, the protagonist of Wesley Bradshaw's novella *Angel Agnes* is actually admitted to the region by the quarantine officers because of her earlier presence and acclimatization during a New Orleans epidemic. On her way from Texas to Louisiana, nineteen-year-old Noel Lepeyre is similarly travelling through a landscape that is foreign to her.

> There were sugar plantations on either side, where the cane waved and glistened under the yellow rays of the setting sun; and occasional groves of orange-trees, whose stiff, round-bunched green threw into bright relief the silvery shining banana-clumps beyond. Long stretches of half-cleared swamp-land, where bearded moss hung motionless from the bare limbs of girdled trees, alternated with fields of artichoke, dust-gray in the hot September haze. (*QG* 1)

Noel Lepeyre's foreigness to the surroundings is enhanced by her looks. Yet, while her light and almost transparent outward appearance—her "white neck," "blue-gray" eyes and her "ashen-blonde" hair (*QG* 2–3)—signifies her as Other, the connection to the unfamiliar and exotic Creole culture is established through Noel's invisible biological heritage, her blood:

> The landscape, poetic, semi-tropical, unfamiliar, harmonized, to Noel's dreaming fancy, with the foreign speech of a group of girls over against her. [...] She did not understand the musical tongue, but something within her—her father's blood—responded to its soft accents, its caressing tones and slurring syllables. [...] Apparently there was nothing foreign about herself except her name. Her fluttering neighbors were dark-haired, velvet-eyed, plump, bewitching. Noel was tall and slim—much too meagre, indeed, for beauty. (*QG* 2)

Noel had, by what is described as a "special decree of Providence" (*QG* 9), chanced upon the address of her father's sister, French Creole "Tante Marguerite," while leafing through her father's papers (*QG* 6). Aunt Marguerite had replied and invited her to New Orleans. Yet there is also something uncanny about the invitation, and Noel is left wondering whether her aunt will be able to communicate with her. While on a literal level this refers to speaking English, the possibility of disease transmission is referenced in the communicability metaphor as well. While reading her aunt's letter "she shivered; the phraseology of the letter was so remote, so strange, so unreal" (*QG* 6). There is a reference in the letter of fairy-tale like quality that Noel cannot decipher: "Claude, thy father, was used to call me La Reine Margot, in the old days before we quarreled and he went away" (*QG* 7). This riddle sets Noel on a quest.

On the train she meets an "old gentleman" (*QG* 3) who introduces himself as "John Henry Steele, a late major in the Confederate States Army" (*QG* 13); his name and the military affiliation, which make him a companion to Noel's late father, emanate reassurance. Steele, in mentor-like fashion of the typical coming-of-age plot, joins her on the ferry-boat that is—rite of passage-like—crossing the Mississippi River (*QG* 11). When landing, Noel's insecurity is reflected in the instability of the dock—also functioning as threshold—where "the treacherous undercurrent at that moment [was] gnawing away the very point upon which the ferry-landing was constructed" (*QG* 12). Yet Noel's coming-of-age journey only begins there and her first view of the city foreshadows the horrifying experiences she is about to face, "[a] girl of nineteen—a girl like that! alone at night in a strange, wicked, devouring city!" (*QG* 14). Yet when no one meets Noel at the station as promised, Steele gallantly stays at her side and delivers/accompanies her to the door of her aunt's house. The streetcar, only recently introduced to the city of New Orleans, serves as their means of transport; it attains the quality of a "swift flight […] through the dim streets" and "the loud, insistent clang of its bell, its amazing curves and dangerous doublings, disquieted Major Steele almost as much as they did his companion" (*QG* 16). New Orleans is depicted as a city between "the mundane and the exotic, the mysterious and the fantastic" (Francis 62). Neither Noel nor the major, who would "prefer a buggy and pair of mules" over the street-car (*QG* 16), are apparently 'acclimatized' to the city as they enter the French Quarter where neither of them has been before. Noel is "appalled by the forbidding strangeness of the narrow side street, whose peaked roofs seemed almost to meet in the strip of sky above. The standing water in the open gutters nauseated her, the unintelligible chatter of the children swarming the pavements confused her wearied senses" (*QG* 17). Without a direct indication of the infestation of yellow fever in the city at this point the narrative in a naturalist fashion confronts reader and protagonist with the type of environment that throughout the nineteenth century served as description of the ideal miasmatic 'breeding ground' for yellow fever. The encroaching and unfriendly atmosphere is underlined by an aural reference: "a barrel-organ, ground by a ragged negro lad, was wheezing forth a melancholy tune" (*QG* 18). It is at this point that Noel cries out her wish to "go back" (*QG* 17).

When approaching a group of men stationed in a sentinel-fashion, they learn that the parti-colored red and yellow flag identifies a yellow fever house, and Major Steele, now defined in terms of age as the "old Confederate officer" (*QG* 18), "uttered a horrified ejaculation" (*QG* 19) and hurries his warden forward. The house they finally locate "had the air of a prison" (*QG* 19), and the description foreshadows the mansion's function for Noel. She refuses Steele's offer to accompany him and instead enters the house of her aunt, sending him away with a promise to never forget him. The Major perceives her "light figure [as] poised, butterfly-like, on the threshold of the wide door. She was gazing with eager eyes before her, and into her own new life. 'Even now she has forgotten me! [...] it is the way of youth.'" Noel's posture and outlook is contrasted to the veteran's aged body who "trudged away, limping, bent, and travel-worn" (*QG* 21) boarding the electric car again, this time "too weary to be apprehensive of its rocket-like vagaries" (*QG* 22).

The first person Noel encounters in Madame Chrétien's house is Marcelle, the mulatto house servant who had been mentioned in her aunt's letter: "Marcelle thrust her face through the opening; a wrinkled yellow face, framed in a lofty tignon, with deep-set yellow-brown eyes and overhanging brows" (*QG* 21). The yellow complexion of the mulattress may or may not be a reference to the impeding fever threat. As Noel passes the threshold she exits her old and enters "her own new life" (*QG* 22). The following chapter's title, "Within" spatially situates her inside her aunt's house and her new life, a life that begins without the presence of her aunt and instead of that of Marcelle and her unfamiliar Creole diction: "'Madame Chrétien ees een hair baid'—'Her'—'Hair baid, mamselle. Since today she ees a leetle seeck'" (*QG* 25). Noel cannot hide her dismay and alarm and wants to be taken to her aunt immediately, but Marcelle tells her that her aunt will not be able to receive her before the next day, although she refers to Madame Chrétien's illness as a "bagatelle of a migraine" (*QG* 27). Imagining Marcelle as a practitioner of voodoo who attracts young girls only to destroy them, Noel's vague fears increase: "What if this meagre, weazened, yellow old creature were one of those wicked enchantresses of whom she had read? One of those voodoo witches who tole young girls to destruction" (*QG* 26). Only the visual recognition of her father's portrait calms Noel again: "On the threshold, where she halted trembling, Noel's fears instantly vanished. The first object which met her roving glance was a portrait of her own father" (*QG* 27). It also strengthens Noel's connection to New Orleans through her family ties. The importance of vision and imagination continues as a connecting thread throughout the story and also serves to signify the onset of the disease.

To Noel, aunt Marguerite is merely present as the "mysterious unseen [aunt] Number Four," visually existing to her niece only in a portrait in the dining hall. Upon entering the garden, a fairy story of her childhood returns to her memory and she deciphers the reference in her aunt's letter: The "*Young Queen* [...] *La Reine Margot*" (*QG* 30), in the diction of Noel's father refers to her father's sister she has not yet met. The 'Queen's Garden' (the novel's title) is the very space she finds herself enclosed in now. The scenario is comparable to that coined by Sandra Gilbert and Susan Gubar as "The Madwoman in the Attic." The heiress finds herself in the attic—or, in Noel's case—in a house and enclosed garden.

The next morning, Noel awakens to the sound of "a smothered wail, half pain, half anger, like the cry of a wounded animal" (*QG* 34). She is further confused by the mosquito net with its misty folds that adds to her feeling of confinement. In this chapter—forebodingly called "Apparitions"—Noel's fears intensify. She sneaks out of her room and hides on the upper hallway. From her vantage point she watches Marcelle's distorted movements and animalistic outcries when three nuns apparently inform her about the fate of her mistress. To Noel, the three visitors "had the appearance of spectres, or ghouls! in their long yellowish robes; and their strange head-coverings, which were drawn across the lower part of their faces, leaving visible only their angry and threatening eyes" (*QG* 36). Noel's limited point of view prevents her (and the reader likewise) from witnessing the effects of the ravaging yellow fever outside (such as, for example, piles of shrouded corpses being carted through the cities' streets). However, what Noel does see seems to register more horribly in her mind: she "continued to stand, paralyzed by terror" (*QG* 36). *The Queen's Garden* does not boldly exploit the horrors of yellow fever epidemics, such as describing the gruesome symptoms of the many suffering victims, but the feeling of calamity is transferred to a description of the psychological state of the novel's protagonist. When Noel's hiding place is discovered, she is only briefly able to discern the figure of a man, "the thin, dark, benignant face with its white beard and gray hair" (*QG* 36–37). Recognizing what seems to be a physician "as a human being like herself, the blood flowed once more to her face, her feet were loosened and without even hearing his stern order, [...] she fled precipitately to her chamber, where she fell half fainting upon her bed" (*QG* 37).

What has loomed over the story as an imminent but not yet pronounced threat is now, for the first time, recognized and described as yellow fever by Marcelle: "'Madame Chrétien has that fiev'—la fievre jaune. She was souffrante yesterday, pauvre enfant; an' she has been afraid eet was that yellow fiev'" (*QG* 38). Marcelle is most skeptical (if not outright hostile) about the doctor and the nurses and the practice of quarantine now enforced upon the house: "They have nail a flag on the door; they have place' some guard there, so that nobody may enter in that door, or go out in that street" (*QG* 37). Although Marcelle wishes to re-establish her own authority as nurse which she has acquired during the illness of Madame Chrétien's husband, her role—with all other servants gone after the first sign of the fever—is confined to that of chamber maid and cook, while "[a] trained nurse was in attendance of the patient" (*QG* 40).

The novel fictionalizes the Louisiana Board of Health's house quarantine policy of 1897 that had never been enforced in New Orleans and required the placing of parti-colored red and yellow flags at the doors of yellow-fever infected houses to prevent persons from entering or leaving without board permission. The policy provoked "violent public opposition" in a city that was "notoriously casual" about yellow fever epidemics, having defined 'strangers' as scapegoats for epidemics so that "'acclimated' New Orleanians could view the problem as something other than their own" (Francis 62–63; Carrigan, *Saffron Scourge* 10). According to Carrigan, "New Orleans newspaper editors often insisted that 'our' city was the healthiest in the Union—*except* for the strangers."[117] Disregarding xenophobic tendencies, Mollie Davis's husband urged New Orleans citizens to cooperate with the house quarantine in his *Picayune* editorials (Francis 62). The Davises had arrived in New Orleans in 1879, one year after the most devastating epidemic in the South, but they had first-hand knowledge of several milder epidemics in the late 1890s. They were aware of the fact that "[p]eople often refused to report yellow fever cases" and escaped "their 'enforced imprisonment' through the back doors of flagged houses (Francis 62–63; Carrigan, *Saffron Scourge* 10).[118]

In Davis's novel, Doctor Grafton with regard to young Noel refines the yellow fever quarantine policy within the Chrétien household in even stricter terms: "But le docteur Grafton had ordered that Mamselle Lepeyre, being totally unacclimated, should come in contact with no one, not even Marcelle, who had had the fever—oh, but yaas, in '57, when the fievre jaune was the fiev'!" (*QG* 41). The belief of yellow fever as a stranger's disease and a belief in the immunity of acclimatized people as the leading paradigm is also conveyed and underlined in the representation of this measure. The arrangement Noel is to follow has apparently also been endorsed "by madame herself [...] though burning with fever" (*QG* 42). Noel is not ready to accept nor fully understand what is referred to as "the strangeness of her situation" (*QG* 44); she wants to nurse her aunt herself, arguing that she has nursed sick people before (and even witnessed the death of a young child):

> Then she felt a pang of remote, intangible pity for the woman lying sick in another part of the house; then a procession filed swiftly through her brain, and vanished, leaving her heartsick—a ghostly procession of guardians and warders, which began with the shadowy figure of her father, and ended with step-aunt Mitchell lying in her coffin-bed, white and placid, and—at last—still. (*QG* 44)

117 While the argument is valid to the extent that strangers often were yellow fever's principal and first victims, natives were not immune.

118 See also Carrigan, ch. "The Yellow Fever Panic of 1897," 141–66.

This realization of her aloneness is followed by a seemingly never-ending nightmarish week mirrored in a succession of chapters entitled by the days of the week and attaining the quality of a prisoner's diary, Monday through Friday (chs. 6–10), Saturday and Sunday (chs. 12–13). The novel ends with chapters 14 and 15: "Claude's Way" and "Love's Way," already in those titles offering another 'way' or solution to live with and through yellow fever.

The space of her aunt and herself (of sickness and health respectively) in the house are now clearly separated, and Noel sets out to explore her new surroundings, dreaming of the "White Days" (*QG* 49) ahead, and not knowing that in "the region beyond the wide dividing hall, where Madame Chrétien lay" she is "already battling for her life" (*QG* 49). Noel finds the courtyard a sanctuary (and a temporary escape) and experiences "an ecstasy of amazement and delight at sight of it" (*QG* 50). The dense foliage brought about by the September sun, the butterflies and birds are contrasted to the life not present within the walls of the house. Noel is caught in a daydream of "La Reine Margot […] '*the most beautiful young Queen that ever was*'" who walks through the garden followed by Noel's father (*QG* 53). Noel is now certain that she has found the Queen's Garden of the fairy tale which Claude Lepeyre, her father, had always told her. She identifies the Spanish dagger tree as the one on which "the Prince from Beyond the Wall wrote his name," and she deciphers the initials A.G., by now distorted from the growth of the tree. In the garden Noel, having shed her old life of poverty, no longer wears the clothing she has arrived in, but she sees the reflection of her "own white-robed image" (*QG* 56) in the glass, dressed in the garments her aunt has had specially made for her. A brief glimpse to one of the upper windows and the recognition of a nurse's cap reminds her of the disease's presence again, but she immediately reinterprets the scene and her presence in what she refers to as "the enchanted Palace" to the "Beauty and the Beast" (*QG* 56).

Still elated from her fairy-tale phantasy, Noel is full of hope when she finds a note on her breakfast table the next morning saying that "Madame Chrétien finds herself better" (*QG* 57). In order to prevent the transmission of disease, the communication between aunt and niece remains restricted to a written exchange. Her aunt's earlier letter of invitation to her house and the note are the only signs of her existence for Noel. When Noel explores spaces in the house she has not been to, she finds the door to Madame Chrétien's apartment locked, and a room she enters from the dining room that had been locked so far greets her with a "funereal atmosphere" that "pervaded the dim vastness. The antique furniture, cumbrous, obsolete, and handsome, which would have made the mouth of a collector water with longing desire, repelled the country-bred young girl" (*QG* 60). The dichotomy of the separated spaces, emanating life and death, quickly sends her back to the space originally assigned to her. The dichotomy of the *country*-bred girl now living in the *city* is alluded to with a reference to the "rumble of street noises" outside. Noel is curious to explore the city as she remembers it from only two days ago, yet it is the garden whose "call" she follows instead, picking up a dust-covered book from the library on her way out of the house. The book, a copy of Moore's 'Melodies,' bears Madame Chrétien's maiden name, Marguerite Lepeyre as well as the initials A.G. Ruminating about the two letters reminds Noel again of the tale her father told her when she was a young girl. She already knows that the young queen in her father's story is her aunt, la reine Margot, and she now suspects her father of having been her aunt's follower and helper (henchman). Still speculating about who the prince in the story might have been, she locates stairs leading out of the garden, when she is taken aback by a sigh, "a longing, passionate, murmourous vital breath" (*QG* 65). This vital sign (of love) is immediately put in contrast to the (deathly) space "on the farther side of the garden; where the sick woman lay, and her nurses and doctors came and went, incessantly, noiselessly, anxiously" (*QG* 65). Back on the bench in the garden a longing for companionship grows in Noel.

When Noel receives the same message from her aunt the next day, she realizes that the notes are prefabricated. Noel believes that her aunt must have "written these messages herself when she felt the fever creeping into her veins" (*QG* 68). The expression represents the disease as clandestinely transgressing bodily boundaries and taking hold of a space within. And the scheme her aunt has devised relies on anticipating preparations to save her niece by deceiving her with the production of false textual evidence to be laid in front of her by Marcelle daily. It is a one-sided way of communicating with Noel in order not to communicate the disease to her. To Noel, yellow fever seems too abstract a phenomenon to be afraid of: "The yellow fever? But why should she be afraid? She, who had never known an ache or a pain in her life!" (*QG* 69). It is interesting to note that pain seems to refer to her physical pain only, as Noel has certainly experienced the pain of loss before in her life. The realization of her own fearlessness however, intensifies her wish to see Tante Marguerite, and when she again fails to convince Marcelle, she lapses deeper into the "present isolation […] all at once oppressed by the loneliness, the solitude and silence" (*QG* 70) and again clings to the hope that the notes of her aunt were no deception.

The omniscient narrative voice informs us that Noel only later learned about the "side court with a separate entrance from the street to the other part of the house; a small stairway by which the physicians came and went. Old Marcelle slipped in and out of the infected apartment like a shadow; choosing the hours when Noel was sleeping, or sitting in the garden." Noel, while not being able to "look[] into a human face," is herself being watched from the sick-room by Doctor Grafton and her aunt who "had followed her movements from time to time about the sunny close below—'Claude's daughter! Claude's daughter.' The cry was ever upon the sick woman's lips" (*QG* 71). Noel is kept from this knowledge, and an allegorical description of the Garden of Eden with Noel, aka Eve, picking a sour orange symbolically underlines her ignorant state: she does not know "that the city itself, girdled by a fast narrowing cordon of quarantine, was scorching in the breath of the pestilence; she felt only the unbroken solitude; she heard only—a sigh!" (*QG* 72). Her fantasies of "far-off islands of citron and spice, of [...] the land of the pomegranate and the nightingale, the land of the Thousand and One Nights, the land of the wonderful Fairy Story" (*QG* 73) make her isolation bearable. The discovery of a marble Cupid guarding the garden's fountain momentarily breaks her solitude as—after cleaning Cupid's face—not only the statue returns her look, but also a young man who "looked—and laughed! down into his neighbor's [Noel's] garden" (*QG* 77). Noel immediately leaves the garden, promising herself never to return. The next morning presents her with yet another note from her aunt, and, abstaining from the garden, she discovers a new space within the house, "the boudoir of Madame Chrétien" adorned with "a bit of embroidery. [...] The femininity of the place appealed to Noel" (*QG* 80). The private room inside the house functions as much as a gendered space as the—since recently—male-dominated, and thus (in Noel's phantasy) forbidden, space outside. Noel reconstructs her aunt's life in the portraits she sees of her only son and her husband, and connects what she sees to the words she remembers from Marcelle, recognizing aunt Marguerite "[a]t the cradle, at the schoolroom, at the marriage, at the death of M'sieu, her husband, at the tomb of her only son!" (*QG* 81). By identifying "Anatole Thierry Chrétien de la Vigne" as her aunt's husband, Noel is again left to ponder the identity of the Prince. She abandons her resolution not to enter the garden again and discovers the signed book by Moore "now swollen out of all proportions" (*QG* 82) which she discerns not as her fault but as the fault of "the Man who Laughed" (*QG* 82). She has barely reached the fountain "when some object came flying through the air with a whizzing sound and lighted plump on Cupid's head" (*QG* 83): a "wreath of red roses" (*QG* 83). Noel's isolation is broken when the wreath thrower identifies himself by the reassuring name of Richard Strong and already knows her name from having picked up the handkerchief with which she had cleaned Cupid the other day. Noel is enchanted by the voice, "it was so *heavenly* to hear the sound of a human voice once more; any voice!" (*QG* 86), She learns that the courtyard on Richard's side (a male-dominated space) is "mostly a dumping-ground for dirt and rubbish," and she gets to know the "hoarse, abrupt voice" of a redheaded parrot who chases her away "frightened and mystified" (*QG* 87). Later in the story, it is the parrot who has access to the other side (outside) and who—by mimicking the undertaker's cries passing by with their carts—brings to Noel's realization not only what is happening outside but that her aunt has died: "'La morte! La morte!'" (*QG* 111). When the parrot announces the death of her aunt, Noel is linguistically excluded: "No sound disturbed the silence of house or court except an occasional croak from the parrot in his window up among the purple roofs, [...] Noel did not understand the words, but their sinister echoes vaguely disturbed her peace" (*QG* 111).

When the next day, a Friday—and possibly in allusion to the day of Christ's suffering—brings no flowers but Madame Chrétien's—her name also underlining a Christian connotation—usual note to her breakfast table, as well as "hurried tramplings and uneasy whispering beyond the inexorable partition wall" (*QG* 88), death assumes a very real presence and "[s]he reproached herself for having talked lightly, and with a stranger! while her aunt was lying yonder ill—perhaps, even unto death" (*QG* 88–89). Although resolved never to enter the garden again, the temptation of the forbidden and also of the unknown disease lures her into the garden and Noel descends the stairs at nightfall. She purposely seats herself "whence she could not see the reproachful window of the sickroom" (*QG* 89–90) nor the gallery from which Richard Strong had descended once. Shielding herself purposely from being faced with the imminent disease threat, Noel undergoes the first step of her rite of passage as her garden prison transforms into a garden of love. Joined by Richard, Noel is able to reconstruct what lies behind her father's story, namely a true account of her father's life in that same house and garden. The passage Richard uses to enter the garden is her father's, i.e. "Claude's Way" (*QG* 93). Andrew Grafton, who moved on to become a famous physician, was Marguerite (then) Lepeyre's lover. But her parents had chosen a different husband for her. Marguerite's brother Claude quarreled with his sister for the sake of his friend Andrew and then left. Yet years later a sign of Claude Lepeyre arrives in the form of Noel's letter. It is Richard who is able to add this twist to the story: "Lately, she [Marguerite Lepeyre] has held a letter in her hand which she has kissed many times and read over and over to her old servant" (*QG* 97).

The importance of seeing and of vision is again stressed in this scene. Richard has fallen in love with Noel although he could "not see [her] face at first" and has just "heard [her] voice" (*QG* 99). He has been watching her from behind that grille ever since" (*QG* 99). Noel is barred from having that same visual knowledge of her aunt. From her limited perspective, she is spared a visual confrontation with the disease's horrifying symptoms. The narrative refrains from sensationalist renderings of the epidemic and instead focuses on its unseen psychological effects (through isolation and fear). Noel explains to Richard:

> "But I have not even *seen* my aunt Marguerite. She is ill, very ill, I fear. She has the yellow fever"—"What!" the interruption was a hoarse cry of alarm; he threw out an arm as if to shield her from some tangible danger. "Madame Chrétien has the fever! Oh, you must go away. You must not approach her room. Promise me, promise me!" "But, indeed, I would *see* her! I would nurse her if they would allow me. I long to go to her!" (*QG* 100; emphasis mine)

Being a newspaper reporter, who in his self-understanding helps "to turn the world over every night" (*QG* 104), Richard Strong represents and endorses the official view of quarantine and urges Noel to comply with the measures prescribed for her. He furthermore operates as her relay station to the world outside, also providing the knowledge that is kept from her:

> "Is it then so terrible, the yellow fever?" she asked, incredulous. "It is very terrible," he replied. "There is a great deal of it in the city. There are flags everywhere, marking the infected houses, and guards are placed at the doors to prevent people from entering or coming out. The entrance to my own quarters is from an alley, so I have not seen the flags on this house-door. I did not know there was fever here. Many people are dying. The dead are buried almost before—Oh, promise me that you will not enter Madame Chrétien's room, no matter what may happen. Promise!" (*QG* 101)

Strong has lived in New Orleans a "long time" (*QG* 101) and has never had the fever which might point to his fearlessness being grounded in his belief in the paradigm of acclimatization. Although not a New Orleans native, Noel is seemingly not afraid either and refuses to grant his wish to promise her compliance (*QG* 102).

With regard to the representation of New Orleans in literature, Violet Harrington Bryan has pointed to southern "writers [who] have used the seductive lushness of the beautiful tropical landscape and the eminence of death through natural or human-caused violence to epitomize the romantic myth of New Orleans" (Bryan 22). The strategy of presenting the flora and fauna as exotic and seductive (in the form of a night-blooming cereus) but also as terrifying and destructive (in the form of invading yellow fever beetles) becomes apparent in an interposed chapter that does not mark another weekday of Noel's imprisonment. It details the intimate encounter of Noel and Richard with a cactus flower coming into bloom. Yet, what might symbolize the awakening sexuality of Noel is immediately counteracted by images of impending doom with so-called yellow fever beetles invading the garden. These beetles—far from being connected to existing speculations about an insect vector for the transmission of yellow fever—were called yellow fever beetles by "superstitious folk" who believed they come into being "by the first fetid breath of the pestilence" (*QG* 113).

At first, however, the description of the beautiful flower suggests that the (tragic) love story of Noel's aunt and Dr. Grafton is about to repeat itself. Noel and Richard watch hand-in-hand under the full moon and declare their love for each other. "Snow-white and lovely, like a bride awaiting her bridegroom," the flower is an allegory for Noel and her longing and possibly consumption of marriage: "the exquisite blossom, wide open,—a radiant wheel,—swayed as if to spirit music on the up-curved bracket-like stem; the slender petals whispered to some invisible Presence; the golden heart quivered as if under the caress of an unseen lover" (*QG* 103). The passage invokes female sexuality for a nineteenth-century readership. While implicitly performed, the official confirmation of Noel and Richard's marriage is forestalled. It is not so much the fact that Richard admits to being poor, that is echoed by Noel's confession of poverty and their mutual resolution to address the problem with hard work, but the presence of the yellow fever epidemic and the quarantine measures that foreclose their happy union. Once the quarantine policies are lifted from the house, Richard promises to come and "claim [her] for [his] wife" (*QG* 105). At this point, however, Noel not only remains trapped within the house and adjacent garden, but the remaining communication channels are shut down as well. Returning to the house that night, "[a]ll was silent there; silent as sleep" (*QG* 107), with sleep as the sister of death darkly foreboding the latter. Noel's attempt to communicate the happiness she has just experienced is furthermore curtailed when she finds a note she has written to her aunt torn and no flowers from Marcelle or note from Madame Chrétien as usual on her breakfast table the next morning.

More alarmingly, the yellow fever that had been kept outside of Noel's realm has entered the same, the space of the Queen's or Noel's garden as well as her own body: "It struck her, too, as she crossed the garden, that the sunshine was too bright; it gave her a slight sensation of pain about the temples; the vivid yellow of the nasturtiums in their round bed, the scarlet of the geraniums against the house-wall irritated her nerves" (*QG* 109). The colors of yellow and red point to the fever patient's skin coloring or the quarantine flags, and the "sensation of pain" irritating Noel's nerves alludes to the transgressive power of the disease in the same sense as when her aunt had felt it "creeping into her veins" (*QG* 68) earlier. The beautiful flower, the bride of the night before is withering away; its decay forebodes Madame Chrétien's death and Noel's illness: "A few limp, yellowish white petals straggled from the inclosing sheath; a sickly odor exhaled from them. It was like a corpse from which even the still beauty of death had departed. Noel touched it caressingly, pityingly, but shrank away, repelled by the cold, damp lifelessness of the thing but yesternight resplendent with vitality" (109–10). Noel interprets the flower's symbolism in the same way, leaving however the sentence unfinished: "'Perhaps it is an emblem of'—" (*QG* 110). Death assumes a very real presence for Noel who experiences "yellow-fever-induced nightmares in which the images of rich gardens are replaced by ones of ghosts, ghouls, menacing men in yellow-white robes, sickly odors of contagion, a rat lumbering across the garden path, and yellow fever beetles descending by the thousands and literally possessing her." She has contracted the fever and in turn, "her mind inverts, exaggerates, and invents" (Francis 65) a horrible vision that is taking place in the gothic enclosure of the prison-like garden:

> She stifled a cry of terror! Her white gown was alive with crawling beetles, black, heavy-winged, and tenacious. She tried to brush them off; but they were creeping up her sleeves, clinging to her throat, caught in the meshes of her hair, alighting with whirring wings on her bosom, falling upon her face. She fought them with frantic hands, running about the court [...]. They were everywhere, loathsome, horrible; crawling along the walks, dashing themselves clumsily against lattices, swinging to flower-buds, dropping heavily upon benches and into jardinieres—darkening the very air and filling it with a ghastly, corpse-like odor. (*QG* 112–13)

The horrifying description of Noel's infestation with the crawling beetles that represents her frantic state of fear induced by the fever offers a realistic insight into the horrors of the disease. The representation of this fever-induced vision is complemented by a description of Noel's yellow-tinted and bloodshot eyes, symptoms widely accepted as pointing to her infection with the fever: "She looked around with bloodshot eyes, whose luminous gray was faded to a wan yellow" (*QG* 116). The Cupid fountain has turned from a symbol of love to a symbol of death, "[t]he unkempt walks were thick with dead beetles; the fountain, choked with them, had stopped playing" (*QG* 116). In line with the foreboding symbolism, love—personified in Richard—does not return to the garden that night. Noel "moved like a ghost" to the threshold of her aunt's apartment only to be greeted by silence, "like the silence of death" (*QG* 114). She longs to be comforted by a woman who has also experienced male rejection, as the Prince also had once ceased to come to her aunt.

Noel's ordeal continues, and "[t]he Sunday stillness was the most terrifying yet" (*QG* 115). While her sense of hearing remains overtly intact, Noel suppresses her sense of vision. Barely noticing that "Madame Chrétien's window blinds were flung wide open" (*QG* 116), she shuts her eyes and sinks into a fever dream, calling for her father and Richard, dreaming of judgment day. When she is roused by a clanging on the street door (*QG* 117), she perceives the coffin bearers entering:

Noel closes her eyes again in order to not see the "the Black Thing," the coffin that bears her aunt's corpse (*QG* 119). An auditory event, Marcelle's wailing, breaks the Sunday stillness (*QG* 119) and restores Noel's sense of vision and recognition, yet also intensifies her frantic and ill state: "'She is dead! She is dead! And I shall never see her!' whispered the half-crazed girl, staring through the lattice with dry eyes" (*QG* 119–20). After her aunt's "hasty burial" (*QG* 121) the "sun sank in a sea of sulphur-colored cloud" (120): a circumstance not only reflecting the fever patient's skin color but referencing the fact that sulphur was used to disinfect the sickrooms of the city. When night falls, the beetles return, and the air of the infected mansion enters the garden:

> The beetles, which had seemed dead, lifted their shell-like wings and flew aimlessly hither and thither, thickening the air; and a poisonous smell stole down on the vapory air from the infected mansion, and mingled shamelessly with the pure scent of the night-blooming jessamine, and the rank breath of the triple-horned datura. (*QG* 120)

The description seems to reverberate a miasmatic theory of disease transmission, whereas the fact that Richard Strong has also been lying afflicted with the fever for two days points to an infectious transgression of boundaries. When Noel perceives the muffled groan (*QG* 121) of Richard calling her "He is sick, my Richard. He is calling me" (*QG* 122), she hurries to him taking the reverse route of Claude's Way, climbing up the wisteria tree like her father and young Andrew Grafton. Richard tries to send her away when she is about to enter the private space of his apartment: "'Do not come in, Noel! You shall not touch me, I tell you! Go away, Noel, I command you! Do you not see that I have the fever—the *yellow fever*,' he shrieked frantically. 'Go away, Noel'" (*QG* 123). In line with the quarantine policies Noel should neither enter the room nor touch him and thus perform the fusion of their bodies' boundaries enabling the transgression of the disease. Noel disregards his wish, and the narrative leaves the two seriously ill lovers reunited on and beside Richard's bed.

The point of view shifts to an hitherto unknown medical student named Max, whom Richard in his agony calls for. The same Sunday night Max Warren enters Dr. Grafton's office, asking him to check on his friend Richard Strong. Dr. Grafton promises to see after the news reporter as he is about to depart to visit Madame Chrétien's niece, who is now the sole heir of the estate under his guardianship. He finds Noel at Richard's side, "a bright spot burned scarlet in either cheek; her eyes rolled wildly; she moistened her parched lips incessantly with a red tongue. The lamp gave out a stifling smell. The heavy atmosphere reeked with contagion" (*QG* 132). Noel, who consciously meets Dr. Grafton the first time, focuses on the fates of Richard and her aunt, whom she will never see, when she tells him: "'He is very sick. He has the yellow fever. And La Reine Margot is dead, and I will never see her'" (*QG* 132). She conjures up feelings of Grafton's boyhood by referring to "Claude's Way," the name her father and Grafton had invented for the secret garden path which Grafton, sometimes called the Prince, used to enter the garden: "the garden of La Reine Margot! The way so long untrodden by a dispossessed Prince. 'Claude's Way.' Love's way!" (*QG* 134). At this point, Richard is unconscious and Grafton believes it is too late for him. He lifts up Noel, "her hot head fell against his neck; her fevered breath burned his cheek" (*QG* 134). The parrot croaks "*La Morte! La Morte!*" (*QG* 135).

The last chapter picks up the narrative after some time has passed ("she had arrived weeks ago at the gate of the Queen's Garden", *QG* 137), and is entitled "Love's Way." Noel has survived the fever and enjoys the "late October sunshine" in the garden: "It was as if a new summer had entered the close, treading out with beneficent feet all vestiges of that brief and awful moment when decay and death had dwelt there" (*QG* 136). Dr. Grafton has "piec[ed] out for her the old Fairy Story, making it whole, and more lovely" for Noel, who has become "his young ward" (*QG* 137). We encounter her again in the

> rusty black frock in which, in company with Major John Steele, she had arrived weeks ago at the gate of the Queen's Garden. Her illness had left her frightfully emaciated and pale almost to deathliness. Her gray blue eyes were heavy; her lips had lost their rosy bloom; the corners of her mouth drooped pitifully. "Yes, she is ugly, Claude's daughter. And yet she reminds me, somehow, of Marguerite!" (*QG* 137–38)

Noel has aged physically and spiritually, having undergone a rite of passage that has led her to inherit her aunt's house and thus freed her from a status of dependency on men as well as her status of the locked-away '(mad)woman in the attic.' The doctor reminds Noel of the life ahead of her and that it is only the old people in her life that have died, relying on a dichotomy of age and youth: "'Old, all of them! And quite ready to creep out of life. Or else careworn, and disappointed, and miserable. Or too pure and lovely to linger in a world like this'" (*QG* 140). And indirectly referencing Richard Strong he adds: "'But when one is young and strong and passionately in love with love and life! That you will admit, Noel, that is different'" (*QG* 140). At this moment, in a deus ex machina move, Dr. Grafton presents Noel with Richard and reunites the two young lovers: "He was as colorless and wraith-like as herself. They might have been, in their pale ethereal beauty, two disembodied spirits, meeting, after their release from earthly life, in some divinely sheltered bower of Paradise!" (*QG* 141–42). The lovers' reunion is rendered in realist terms, their suffering from the epidemic has left both of them scarred, but the force of their youth has also conquered the disease. Whereas the yellow fever infection may be read as punishment for Noel's blossoming and transgressive female sexuality, she also survives the epidemic and inherits a new life. Noel and Richard have the opportunity to finish the story of La Reine Margot and her Prince. At least, this is what Doctor Grafton hints at or hopes for: "'She's like Margot.' Like Margot! Like Youth! Like Love!" (*QG* 142).

In contrast to other yellow fever narratives the focus of the story is neither on physicians or nurses, nor on their actions or heroic deeds. The nurses and doctors in *The Queen's Garden* just come and go to the sick patient's room "incessantly, noiselessly, anxiously" (*QG* 65), using a small hidden stairwell. The patient they attend to eventually dies. The novel's protagonist Noel Lepeyre is a young 'unacclimated' woman who desperately wants to nurse her aunt as she has previous experience in caring for the sick, but she is not permitted to see or communicate with her due to the enforced policy of quarantine that the family doctor adapts to the Chrétien household in even stricter terms. The novel also points to a professionalization of medical practice as not only Noel, also to prevent her infection, is kept from nursing her aunt, but also the long-time mulatto servant "who had had the fever [...] in '57, when the fievre jaune *was* the fiev'!" (*QG* 41; emphasis in original) is replaced by an experienced nurse: "A trained nurse was in attendance upon the patient," and Marcelle would be permitted into the sick room to prepare Noel's food and that of "that tr-r-enn nurse" (*QG* 39) the linguistic difficulty in pronouncing the qualification ('trained') also pointing to Marcelle's indignation with the circumstance. Marcelle similarly despises the doctor and cannot understand that her previous yellow fever experience, tending to Madame Chrétien's husband, and her knowledge of herbal tea cures is so utterly rejected: "'Me, I did not desire those doctor. Have I not nurse that yellow fiev'? Ees eet that I do not know the tisanes for that fiev'? But no'" (*QG* 39).

The doctor does not emerge as a full-fledged character in the novel until the last chapter when the narrative focus shifts to him, introducing him as "the famous physician [...] a tall, spare man, with a look of great strength and vigor about his person, despite his sixty-odd years" (*QG* 125). Doctor Andrew Grafton is immersed in grief over the death of the woman he has always loved but was prohibited from marrying. He has failed to save her and feels "farther away from [her] than ever!" (*QG* 126) as she now lies reunited with her legal husband and only son in her tomb. The absence of any represented action in Madame Chrétien's chamber while she is sick with the yellow fever underlines the focus of the novel on the physical and psychological effects of yellow fever in realist terms rather than a sensationalist account of suffering in the sickrooms, or the endless succession of funeral carts on New Orleans streets, or shrouded and tarred corpses awaiting burial in the cemeteries by purposely blocking out those spaces. The only two other infected characters in the novel are Noel Lepeyre and Richard Strong. While especially the effect of the fever on their minds and their bodies is conveyed, their recovery as well as any possible contribution of Dr. Grafton remains untold. The doctor hints at their youth, and one might take the virility of Richard's last name as another sign for his survival. Noel, as one critic has pointed out—detecting "a pun on Lepeyre and *the payer*" (Francis 67)—has to pay the price for her rite of passage into a new life in New Orleans. The liminal experience of her confinement and her illness has not crushed Noel, whose first name refers to the birth of Christ and thus the possibility of her own re-birth.[119] A more pronounced and incidentally ironic commentary on the novel is, in fact, that no matter how strictly a quarantine policy is enforced on a political level and reflected in a separation of spaces on the narrative level (of non-communication and visual restriction), a transgression of boundaries is inevitable as love, sexuality, and death (here also in the form of the epidemic disease) will transcend them—and with it a simple separate spheres ideology—and unite what cannot even be artificially kept apart. The consequence of the transgression, the disease experience, is in itself a transgressive phenomenon and, largely kept off-stage in the narrative, remains unpunished.

4.6 The Transformative Potential of Yellow Fever Narratives

According to Nina Silber "the language of romantic and sentimental reunion reached a crescendo" in the aftermath of the "profound misery and devastation of the 1878 yellow-fever outbreak" (Silber 65). This language is visible in Bradshaw's writing, yet also, in a more refined way, in Phelps's story. While Phelps makes use of sentimentality, she does not pursue sentimental outcomes like the adherence to a marriage plot or love story between doctor and nurse. In contrast to Phelps, Mary Floyd's novel *The Nereid* still relies upon a conventional marriage plot between the heroine, who serves as a nurse during the yellow fever epidemic, and her second husband who realizes and accepts Leda as a woman with a profession (be it as a teacher or nurse). Furthermore, a sense of community among the women of *The Nereid* and especially of those women surviving the epidemic is retained and strengthened.

With *Angel Agnes* Bradshaw constructs a popular story which offers certain redeeming venues based on sentimental strategies of victimization and power

---

119 Giving birth can also be read as liminal experience.

reversal and with a female heroine who takes control of her life when her engagement is severed by her fiancé in the North. She helps the afflicted in the South where she dies a martyr's death to redeem the latter. In terms of gender dynamics in the story, the male doctor remains the authority by offering approval of Agnes's treatment, yet she also partially assumes that authority by lecturing inferiors on the Spanish therapy. The novella thus at least temporarily reverses ingrained gender norms of the time as well as a prerogative of medical interpretation and treatment of diseases: by making the effective cure non-American—but Spanish colonialist—in origin and administered by a woman. *Angel Agnes* thus also puts forth a vision of female emancipation and a medical profession that acknowledges the role of women (nurses in this case).

Mattie Stephenson repeats the pattern of *Angel Agnes* and similarly remains a sentimental tale of virtue, dedication, and selflessness. Mattie's sacrificial deeds as well as her final sacrifice are offered as remedy and means of redemption for the larger disease. The visual marker put up in her memory as well as Bradshaw's fictionalization of her story imaginatively serves to reunite North and South. Nina Silber's image of 'marital reunion' is translated into one of spiritual adoption and veneration of this girl from the North by citizens of the South.

The possibility of a companionship across gender and social divisions that is only hinted at in *Angel Agnes* is carried through in Phelps's realist short story. Although the relationship between Zerviah Hope and Dr. Marian Dare is never presented as one carried out on equal terms, its representation serves to establish the special bond between physician and nurse, man and woman, North and South. During the yellow fever crisis, North and South are doubly reunited by the help and assistance received from the North provided by the characters of Zerviah Hope and, by extension, Dr. Marian Dare, yet also by the bond of kinship established between the two unequal partners in the course of the narrative. The conventional marriage plot is replaced by a no less sentimental plot of healing. In this sense, the fictionalization of the catastrophic experience of yellow fever in the three texts serves to destabilize conventional patterns of dominance and thus—at least from a Northern literary perspective—enables national healing.

Richard and Noel are both scarred from the yellow fever epidemic: she is no beauty, and neither is he after the illness. Their marriage is built on a partnership on equal terms. Different from the generation before them, they accept each other freely and enter into a marriage in a way Susan Donaldson has called "the spirit of New Woman, New Man, and New Marriage" (106).

5 Race and Racial Relations in Yellow Fever Writing

5.1 Theorizing Yellow Fever and Race

Three facts in particular point to the importance of looking at race and racial relations with regard to yellow fever. First, many of the most popular novels in the nineteenth-century United States focus on the consequences of racial oppression and on religion (Samuels, *Reading the Novel* 19). Adding to this, Samuel Otter ascertains that "[f]ever and race are yoked across nineteenth- and twentieth-century American fiction" (Otter 31–32), from *Arthur Mervyn* (1799/1800), and William Faulkner's *Absalom, Absalom!* (1936), to John Edgar Wideman's "Fever" (1989) and *The Cattle Killing* (1996). The enduring association may have to do with the resonant events of 1793 and also with the figurative links between fever, color, and exposure (Otter 31–32). Secondly, after 1820 yellow fever was largely a Southern disease, and the American South was defined by its race relations. Thirdly, the contagionist school of the origin of the disease argued early on that yellow fever did not originate in America but was imported by ships, people and cargo arriving from the West Indies. Many abolitionists, while not necessarily following the particular theory of a West Indies or African origin, believed that the practice of slavery and the slave trade resulted in divine punishment in the form of yellow fever (see also Bell 18). While neither school of thought was entirely correct (none of them suspected the mosquito to be the pivotal figure in the process), the particular explanations became part of the cultural and political debates.

Ever since the first major yellow fever epidemic that hit the young nation's capital in 1793, the history and experience of yellow fever was intricately linked to the history of racism in the United States. During the nineteenth century, blacks were often considered to have a low risk of infection with yellow fever. At the same time they were also often characterized as dangerous carriers of the disease (Humphreys, "Appendix II" 193). Pathological research had a decisive influence on the perception of race and the belief in a rather low susceptibility of Africans to the disease. Medical writing of the eighteenth and early nineteenth century furthered this view by arguing that persons of African origin and French Creoles were less prone to the fever due to their longer residence in the climate. The theory of so-called seasoning and acclimatization was clearly favored over immunity due to an innate disposition (Jackson, *A Treatise* 249–51). The Scottish surgeon Colin Chisholm—so fervently attacked by American physicians for his contagionist stance—wrote in 1822: "The influence of colour, or more properly speaking of idiosyncrasy in the negro constitution was so great at Grenada, that, in my practice, at least, only 4 had the fever, of those exposed to it, and only 1 in 83 died of it" (*A Manual* 174). He continues: "In negroes the manner in which this disease came on was, in some respects, different from that in whites" (183). It is statements like these—although its author might have been criticized for his general contagionist stance—that stuck in people's minds.

African Americans suffered equally from yellow fever and probably even more than whites from its economic effects that stirred xenophobic tendencies. An illustration from August 16, 1879 in *Harper's Weekly* (fig. 28) shows poor African Americans in ragged clothing walking barefoot through a city street while carrying their few possessions. Two young children are each seated on a mule and a cow respectively, and an emaciated old man is crouching on a small wagon drawn by the mule. A woman is carrying an infant and dragging another young child behind her. The caption of the illustration reads: "En route for Kansas: poor Negroes fleeing from the yellow fever in Memphis." The 1879 epidemic affected Memphis and the whole lower Mississippi Valley at a time when more than 20,000 African Americans migrated from Nashville to Kansas. The so-called Exoduster Movement of 1879 was led by Benjamin 'Pap' Singleton (1809–1892), a former slave born in Nashville, Tennessee, who was later accorded the title of "Father of the Exodus" (Painter 100). Since whites would not sell their farmland to the free African Americans in Tennessee, they trekked to Kansas by steamboat, train, or horseback via river towns in Missouri, Mississippi, and Louisiana. Many of the migrants were poverty-stricken and looked unwashed and sick. Stigmatizing the migrating African Americans as potential disease carriers, city officials in St. Louis in particular imposed unnecessary quarantine measures to discourage future migrants ("Western Migration"). Already during the Civil War period freed slaves had consistently been marked as "carriers of smallpox, dysentery, and yellow fever when in fact just as many were dying from exposure and starvation. [...] African-Americans mostly, if not exclusively, entered the medical records as suffering from contagious diseases and illnesses, while other medical problems remained unreported" (Downs 36; see also Humphreys, *Intensely Human*). In *Sick from Freedom* Jim Downs convincingly argues that the lack of adequate food, shelter, and clothing were the actual culprits of a debilitating African American health during the war and reconstruction. Poverty and unemployment more than anything else paved the way "for the spread of epidemic diseases such as smallpox, cholera, and yellow fever" (Gretchen Long 102). Yet the high mortality and morbidity rates among African Americans were widely interpreted a sign of racial inferiority and looming extinction, implicating the so-called innate inferiority of the black body (cf. Downs 103).

Although countertexts to the dominant nineteenth-century narratives and racial theories of inferiority exist, they are rare. For example, Frederick Douglass made a point in linking black skin color, racism, and fever in "Colorphobia in New York" (1849):

> Equating fever and racism, Douglass identified a new population of sufferers. He expressed his sympathy for the unfortunate white victims of 'colorphobia,' a perceptual disease which he described as 'malignant,' an 'epidemic,' and a 'strange plague.' Outlining the physical and mental symptoms of this fever, Douglass advised that the infected be treated with ridicule and indignation. (qtd. in Otter 32)

Fig. 28. "Negro Exodusters en route to Kansas, fleeing from the yellow fever." Photomural from engraving. Harper's Weekly *16 Aug. 1879: 652. Images from the History of Medicine. National Library of Medicine (NLM).*

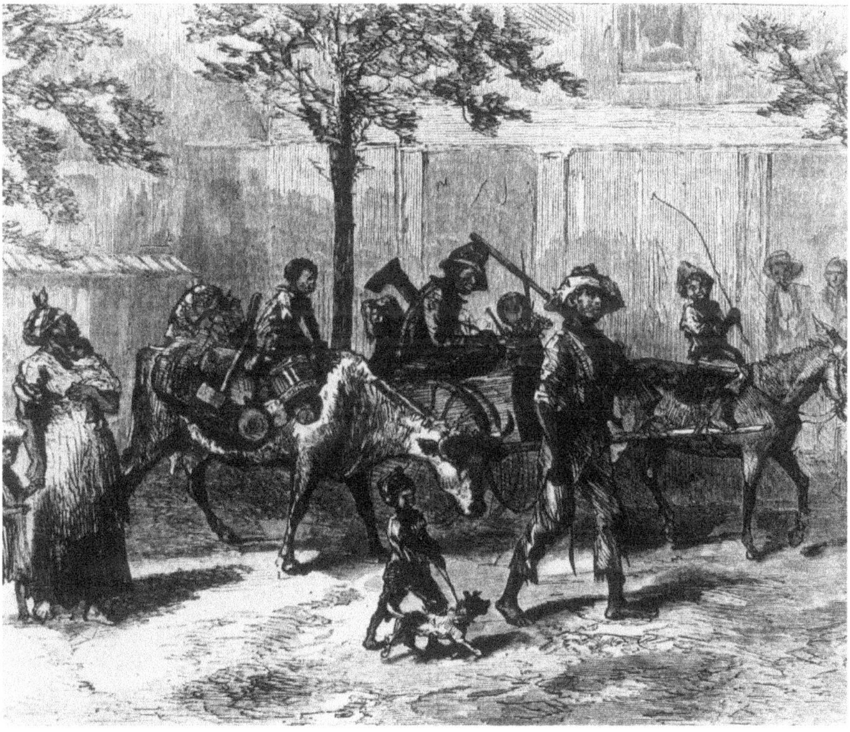

Humphreys calls for more attention to be given to "the delicate question of variations of racial susceptibility to the disease" ("Appendix II" 193). While the historiographic research on black immunities begun by Kiple and King in the 1970s and continued by Sheldon Watts in the 2000s is certainly important (Kiple and Kiple; Kiple; Watts), this chapter focuses on the representation of the Other and the intersectionality of race, gender and ethnicity in relation to the experience of yellow fever. The crisis situations that are often symbolically paired with yellow fever in the narratives of this chapter are connected to race relations, slavery, and abolitionism, or they feature African American, Irish American, German American, Creole, and European encounters with the real and the metaphoric disease. This thematic complex is not geographically bound to the American mainland or the American South in particular but is also located within a complicated realm of social, political, and economic exchange between the United States and the Atlantic, Carribbean, and Pacific seas, thus the transnational dimension of the disease is foregrounded.

5.2 Yellow Fever at Sea

In much of nineteenth-century fiction "[w]ater rushes up on the shores of the sea novel in ways that are difficult to reproduce since we have lessened our dependence on the sea as a means of transportation" (Samuels, *Reading the Novel* 160–61). Both canonized and lesser known fiction of the nineteenth century that critically address expansion, border crossing, and racism in seafaring narratives or adventurous explorations of the far West also includes a yellow fever theme.[120] This section explores the yellow fever experience at sea in its relation to racism and in light of a growing racial hybridization. It reads the sailing ship as "a living, microcultural, micro-political system in motion" (Gilroy 4). Altough Paul Gilroy's ship allegory proves useful in this chapter, the majority of the works under discussion fall into the rubric of classical sea novels written by white males in the vein of Herman Melville. Additionally I look at an American translation and publication of a French novella having the sea as a setting that allegorizes yellow fever from a Northern European perspective.

---

120 Yellow fever references, for example, are present in the following adventure novels of the frontier or the West: James Fenimore Cooper's *Wept of Wish Ton-Wish* (1829); James Hall's *Legends of the West* (1832); Baynard Rush Hall's *The New Purchase, or, Seven and a Half Years in the Far West* (1843).

Published in the mid-1830s, Edgar Allan Poe's novel *The Narrative of Arthur Gordon Pym* (1837) lays bare the results, contradictions, and anxieties of a "racist and pro-slavery mind" (126), Gesa Mackenthun writes:

> As probably no other writer at his time, Poe articulates the fear ravaging the American South after the black rebellions of Haiti and Nat Turner, as well as the anxiety, among pro-slavery and antislavery circles alike, about the growing racial hybridization that the peculiar institution produced. (126)

The young Arthur Gordon Pym is hiding as a stowaway on the slave deck aboard the *Grampus* when a mutiny erupts on the ship and many of the crew are either killed or put to sea in a small boat. Together with the captain's son Augustus and a mutineer who regrets his participation in the uprising, they hatch a plan to regain control of the *Grampus*. Pym emerges from the lower deck disguised as the ghost of a dead soldier; he startles the superstitious mutineers, and takes over control of the ship with the other survivors of the small counter-rebellion. After a storm hits, they drift on the Atlantic on the wreck of the *Grampus*. When they encounter a horrifying ghost ship, they are first exposed to a smell, described as "hellish—utterly suffocating—insufferable" (Poe 517) before they see twenty-five or thirty human bodies scattered on the deck "in the last and most loathsome state of putrefaction" (Poe 518). "From the saffron-like hue of such of the corpses," Pym concludes that the ship's company

> had perished by the yellow fever, or some other virulent disease of the same fearful kind. If such were the case (and I know not what else to imagine), death, to judge from the positions of the bodies, must have come upon them in a manner awfully sudden and overwhelming, in a way totally distinct from that which generally characterizes even the most deadly pestilences with which mankind are acquainted. (Poe 519)

Far from providing the rescue so desperately sought by Pym and the few surviving crew members of the *Grampus*, the gruesome sight weakens their spirits and continues to haunt them. They realize that the plight of the passengers on the ghost ship could be their own destiny. The scene is also reminiscent of slave ship horrors, of bodies bound together in the narrowest of spaces during the Middle Passage, and exposes the guilt of those beholding the scene. It furthermore exposes deeper fears of the violent consequences of the slavery system, such as the successful slave revolt in Haiti (1791–1804) or possible future "slave rebellions in the South" (Rowe 53). Racial fears are thus symbolically paired with shocking yellow fever scenarios. Both can only be cured in an acceptance of the "racial hybridization" (Mackenthun 126) brought about by the slavery system.

Herman Melville's novella "Benito Cereno" (1855) chronicles a slave rebellion on board a Spanish merchant ship, the *San Dominick*, in 1799. Since essential information is withheld from readers, the story—at first—seems to simply present the fate of a badly damaged ship after rounding Cape Horn. Tossing supplies and fresh water over board due to heavy winds, the ship's crew, including every officer with the exception of the captain, become sick with scurvy and some develop fever and die. The slaves survive. This is the version told to Captain Amasa Delano, who encounters the *San Dominick*. The fever story seems plausible to Delano because two beliefs—although disputed at the time—were still held by him: that slaves were immune to the fever and even that they were its potential carriers. The story critically exposes these racist yellow fever myths as false, when the fictitiousness of this version of the ship's fate is revealed. Namely, that during a slave rebellion on the *San Dominick* every crew member except for the captain, Benito Cereno, was killed by the slaves. As a punishment for the deception and the cruel treatment of Cereno, Babo, the intelligent leader of the rebellion, is violently struck down by the supposedly civilized sea captain Delano. The question of moral righteousness of using violence against violence remains open in Melville's text and has been answered in favor of the slaves' leader Babo by postcolonial and postmodern critics who have read the novella as an anti-racist and abolitionist text.

Before writing "Benito Cereno," Melville published three other works with yellow fever references: *Omoo: A Narrative of Adventures in the South Seas* (1847), *White Jacket, or, The World in a Man-of-War* (1850), and *Redburn: His First Voyage* (1849). *Omoo* is an episodic novel based on Melville's own experience in the South Pacific. Shortly after being rescued from the island of Typee and boarding the British whaler *Julia*, an ill-managed ship, the narrator befriends the ship's physician. When he is relieved from active duty because of a lame leg, he spends his time playing chess with Doctor Long Ghost and reads his books, of which "a learned treatise on the yellow fever" (*Omoo* 35) is specifically interesting to him. When two men fall sick and die, yellow fever is suspected as the cause but is never confirmed. All crew members live under terrible conditions. The disease changes the fate of the whaler when the captain also falls ill and the vessel changes its course to reach the nearest island, Tahiti. For the soldiers suffering under the dismal conditions, the island presents an opportunity to free themselves from the cruel military rule. Their mutiny fails and the soldiers are shackled, and in a reversal of the white gaze they are exposed to the eyes of a native audience: "During this period, we were the lions of the neighborhood; and, no doubt, strangers from the distant villages were taken to see the 'Karhowrees' (white men), in the same way that countrymen, in a city, are gallanted to the Zoological Gardens" (*Omoo* 129). The novel offers an imperialist critique by fashioning the observers of Polynesian culture themselves into objects subjected to the gaze of the Other. This, of course, also extends to the narrator, who is aware of his gaze returned when he describes himself as observing Polynesian culture: "All this gave us a fine opportunity of making observations." (*Omoo* 129; see also Banerjee, "Civilizational Critique" 219). Melville's civilizational critique functions through an exposure of the imperialist gaze. It is worth noting that the situation which serves as a catalyst is brought about through a health crisis experienced within the confinement of the whaler. The fever presents an existential threat, from which there is no escape on board the ship. Only the arrival on the island, a much more variegated space, casts away the disease. The perception of the Other and an acceptance of a more diversified society is presented as cure for the larger disease that plagues society.

White Jacket is based on Melville's service aboard the Navy frigate *USS United States*. The novel is one of Melville's most politically critical works presenting practices of abuse (flogging) common in the United States Navy. In *White Jacket*, the *USS United States* becomes the frigate *Neversink* that is rounding Cape Horn. The novel's title refers to the narrator's clothing and introduces the symbolism of the color white (later expanded with the white whale Moby-Dick). The frigate's surgeon's steward, called "Pills," is described as having "a yellow-fever tinge upon his pallid face" (*White Jacket* 695). In fact "so many of those who would fain minister to our own health [...] look so much like invalids themselves" (*White Jacket* 694). The ship's authorities are represented and thus criticized as part of the diseased U.S. system. In *White Jacket*, Melville uses the microcosm of the ship as symbol of the U.S. American nation to expose the ill practices of class distinction, segregation, and slavery.

The idea of the ship as allegory for the United States can also be found in Melville's semi-autobiographical novel *Redburn*. Here, it is an emigrant ship named *Highlander*, en route from Liverpool to New York City, that becomes a "plague-ship driving through a stormy sea" (*Redburn* 378).[121] Harold McCarthy has described the ship as "a familiar Melville metaphor, a social microcosm, with a rigid division of its spaces as determined by money and without regard to human need or even to human life" (409). Yet before the actual return journey of the ship, the novel describes young Wellingborough Redburn's first voyage as a sailor working before the mast, not being allowed in the area of the officers who command the ship. The strict hierarchical structure of captain, other officers, crew,

---

121 Regarding the analysis of *Redburn*, I am indebted to Carmen Birkle's manuscript "Infecting the City upon a Hill: American Plague Narratives."

cabin passengers, and later—on the return journey—emigrants, taints Redburn's view of the people on the ship as one family and the captain as father figure. The journey from New York City to Liverpool represents the young merchant boy's rite of passage, and—once in Liverpool and given liberty ashore—he observers extreme poverty: wandering down a street called Launcelott's Hey, he witnesses the death of a poor mother and her children with no one willing to help him save them. Thus, ironically, Redburn utterly fails in emulating the knight Lancelot's noble deeds on the street named after him.

Liverpool is a city of commerce, based on the riches it had gained as Europe's center of slavery. The legacy is still very present to Redburn, who critically comments not only on the heroic statue of Admiral Nelson, who famously demonstrated British naval power in the Battle of Trafalgar, but focuses on the statue's harsh contrast to the "four naked figures in chains" at the base of the pedestal (fig. 29).[122] They

> are seated in various attitudes of humiliation and despair. One has his leg recklessly thrown over his knee, and his head bowed over, as if he had given up all hope of ever feeling better. Another has his head buried in despondency, and no doubt looks mournfully out of his eyes, but as his face was averted at the time, I could not catch the expression. These woe-begone figures of captives are emblematic of Nelson's principal victories; but I never could look at their swarthy limbs and manacles, without being involuntarily reminded of four African slaves in the market-place. (*Redburn* 198)

In fact, Nelson and the Navy relied on black sailors, many of whom were ex-slaves from the West Indies and America. Their service paved the way to liberty. In this vein, the black steward from the *Highlander* is able to walk around with a white woman in Liverpool, something that would be impossible in New York City, where the "couple would have been mobbed in three minutes; and the steward would have been lucky to escape with whole limbs" (*Redburn* 259–60). A critical stance toward slavery is clearly expressed in Redburn's recognition of the man's right to "humanity and normal equality" and his cynical comment that "we Americans leave to other countries the carrying out of the principle that stands at the head of our Declaration of Independence" (*Redburn* 260).

---

122 Interestingly Lisa Lowe also chooses a visual confrontation of Nelson's column in London as a fitting illustration of her book *Intimacies of Four Continents*. It shows artist Yinko Shonibare's ship in a bottle, which was installed on the fourth plinth in Travalgar Square 2010–2012, to critically confront Britain's colonial and imperial past and expose its continued presence. The point is echoed in Lowe's book which illuminates the "intimacies" of freedom and subjugation, privilege and degradation, and possession and expropriation.

Fig. 29. Nelson Monument in Liverpool, England. 27 Aug. 2008. Photo by Man vyi. Wikimedia Commons. Web.

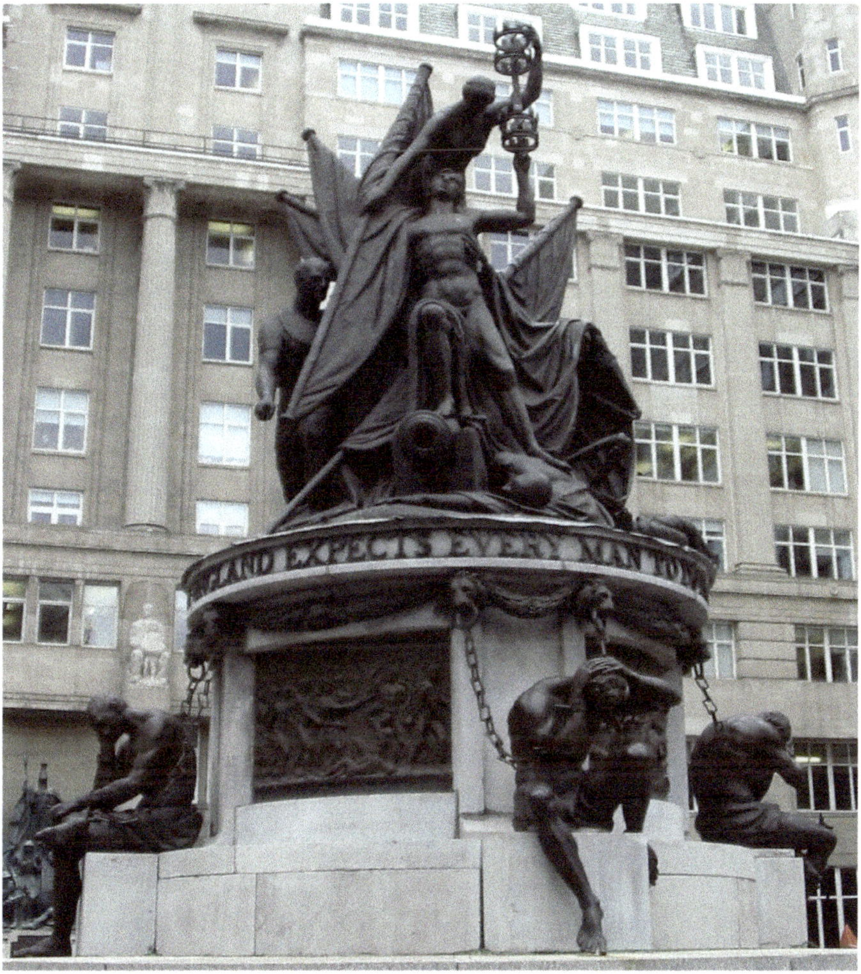

That the city is furthermore a main port of European emigration becomes clear when Redburn watches Irish, Germans, French, Danes, and Scots prepare for their voyages at the docks. He contemplates in a rather pathetical fashion:

> There is something in the contemplation of the mode in which America has been settled, that, in a noble breast, should forever extinguish the prejudices of national dislikes. [...] You cannot spill a drop of American blood without spilling the blood of the whole

> world. […] No: our blood is as the flood of the Amazon, made up of a thousand noble currents all pouring into one. We are not a nation, so much as a world. (*Redburn* 216)

Reasonably matured once he boards the *Highlander*, now bound for New York City, Redburn criticizes racism and the treatment of immigrants to America by describing the conditions on board. Most of the emigrants are recent survivors of the Irish Potato Famine; they are "stowed away like bales of cotton, and packed like slaves in a slave-ship; confined in a place that […] must be closed against both light and air" (*Redburn* 313). Their situation easily conjures up the Middle Passage of Africans to the New World. It seems unsurprising to Redburn that "fevers and plagues are the result" (*Redburn* 313) and notably a "malignant fever" breaks out in the emigrant quarters, which he attributes to the confinement and lack of food, but also to "their personal uncleanliness" (*Redburn* 369). The "fear of contagion" (*Redburn* 370) takes hold among all people on board and the emigrants start introducing zones of quarantine that prove useless on a ship as Redburn explains: "On land, a pestilence is fearful enough; but there, many can flee from an infected city; whereas, in a ship, you are locked and bolted in the very hospital itself. Nor is there any possibility of escape from it; and in so small and crowded a place, no precaution can effectually guard against contagion" (*Redburn* 372). The dehumanization of the fever patients works on two levels. Firstly, they suspect only the worst from each other and "all looked upon each other like lepers" (*Redburn* 373). Secondly, when the fever deaths subside, and the weather conditions allow for it, the emigrant quarters are disinfected, which Redburn compares to "cleaning out a stable, [rather] than a retreat for men and women" (*Redburn* 375). Although the *Highlander* eventually reaches New York harbor and, quite ironically, sails past the "pale yellow flag" that symbolizes the residence of the quarantine officer and to Redburn seems to "symbolize the yellow fever itself, and strike a panic and premonition of the black vomit into every beholder, all quarantines all over the world" (*Redburn* 386–87), the ship passes uninterrupted. Yet, for the emigrants their vision of a better future has already been weighed against the loss of loved ones and the racism endured on board. Using the fever-stricken ship as "social microcosm" (McCarthy 409), a "microcultural, micro-political system" (Gilroy 4), Melville criticizes American nativism directed against the Catholic Irish as well as an inherent racism and disregard for humanity and equality as principles of the Declaration of Independence. With *Redburn*—and in this sense similar to Charles Brockden Brown's *Arthur Mervyn*—he argues for an acceptance of a more heterogeneous makeup of U.S. society, which begins on board the emigrant ships. He only asks us to "consider, how best the emigrants can come hither, since come they do, and come they must and will" (*Redburn* 379).

James Fenimore Cooper was the first major American writer to include full-fledged characters of Africans, African Americans, and Native Americans in his works. He also wrote several sea novels, of which at least two represent an experience of yellow fever. In the life story of *Ned Myers; or, A Life before the Mast* (1843), Cooper recounts the story of his shipmate whom he met while serving on the merchant ship *Sterling*. Ned Myers rejected his status as a British subject and became a U.S. citizen, only to be captured by a ship of the Royal Navy during the War of 1812. He survived and in 1843 met Cooper again, who authored his biography. In one of the episodes Myers briefly encounters yellow fever, prevalent in New York City at the time he gets there. Having previously been in Charleston overseeing the discharging of sugar casks, Myers is unfairly blamed for a fatal accident to one of the slaves there (*Ned Myers* 79). He is forced to pay a sum for the athletic African American, which he cannot afford, and for which he has to hand over the fore-topsail instead. In order to pay for it, he signs up for a ship bound for the fever-stricken New York. Cooper represents a critique of the absurd system of slavery, in which human beings are denigrated as mere commodities, where the loss of life means nothing more than the loss of money. His subsequent lack of money forces Myers to risk his own life, not only at sea—which seems a calculable risk—but also in the fever-infested city of New York. Yellow fever and slavery both represent liminal experiences of closeness to death. An existential threat is inherent in both the disease and the peculiar institution. In this sense, an allegorical reading of *Ned Myers* suggests a critical assessment of the practice of slavery whose continued presence, like a yellow fever epidemic, threatens the United States' social cohesion.

Cooper's second novel with a yellow fever theme—*Jack Tier, or, The Florida Reef* (1848)—is set at the time of the Mexican-American War and focuses on the relationship of the sailor Jack Tier and the captain Stephen Spike on board the *Molly Swash*. Unknown to everyone but Spike the brig is bound for the Florida Keys to traitorously sell ammunition to the Mexican government, with which the United States is at war. The plan fails and Spike is fatally wounded. He is taken to a small naval hospital at Key West where Jack Tier nurses him. Here Jack Tier's identity is revealed: s/he is the captain's abandoned wife Mary Swash, whom Spike marooned on an island twenty years earlier when he had become interested in another woman. On the island she nursed a seaman named Jack Tier dying of yellow fever who had also been left on the island: "The poor fellow caught the yellow fever the very next day, and did not live eight-and-forty hours" (*Jack Tier* 485). She decides to take over Tier's identity, assuming the role of a man, and has been sailing ships ever since, knowing that she would find her husband again. Jack

Tier has actually only been taken on board the boat back in New York City harbor by Spike because his African American steward and cabin 'boy' of many years, Josh, remembered Tier as a handy steward's assistant and original crew member of the *Molly Swash*. The combination of female nursing, yellow fever, gender identity, and African American knowledge—and possibly bonding between the races—makes this novel an interesting proposal for a more equal makeup of the American society in successfully facing health and military crises.

While the canonized authors mostly use yellow fever as a metaphor in their critical assessments of race, the hybrid racial makeup of U.S. society, and the practice of slavery, a much lesser known author follows in their footsteps as far as the setting and form of his novel is concerned. John Sherburne Sleeper's *Jack in the Forecastle, or, Incidents in the Early Life of Hawser Martingale* (1860) is most interesting for its continuous recurrence and political functionalization of the yellow fever theme. The novel is the semi-autobiographical story of Hawser Martingale, who is determined to go to sea. His wish is ridiculed by his kinsman, Captain Tilton, who also threatens him with the presence of yellow fever in the Dutch (later British) colony of Demarara. Tilton nevertheless signs Martingale up for his first voyage on board the *Dolphin*. At the beginning of the novel, the risk of yellow fever is thus introduced as an imminent threat connected to seafaring, especially between the United States and the West Indies. Luck is with Martingale when he finds that the province "had not been so free from yellow fever at that season for several years" (Sleeper 51). Yet the unpredictability and suddenness of the disease is also a factor that adds to its seriousness and ever-present threat.

When, some time after, Martingale is about to embark on a voyage in the service of the Dutch Creole Captain Lordick of St. Bartholomew and Saba, he is not able to prove his American citizenship. The fact of his identity is existential since the Royal Navy during the War of 1812 continued its practice of taking seamen from American ships by force. In order to avoid being impressed by the British, Martingale is provided with the papers of the captain's younger brother, who recently died of yellow fever. Although hesitant to abandon his American identity, Martingale is eventually convinced by Lordick's argument and accepts the citizenship of St. Bartholomew. Due to his exposure to the sun, he has apparently already assumed the Other's identity, since he "looked as much like a creole as any person on board" the ship (Sleeper 281). His false identity—in appearance and on paper—saves him in the course of the voyage from being shanghaied when he is interviewed by a British officer who came on board. Yet, Martingale is eager to resume his "native citizen[ship] of the United States" (Sleeper 300) once they reach Grenada.

The fact of Martingale's assumed identity and quick shedding of the same is remarkable with regard to his decision to stay in Grenada. It is almost as if Martingale has not only taken over and later shed the Other's name but—more importantly—has acquired immunity to yellow fever. While in the West Indies, Martingale "enjoyed excellent health, with the exception of an occasional attack of intermittent fever" (Sleeper 340). 'Intermittent fever,' most likely malaria, was already treated at the time rather successfully with quininc. Two events eventually provoke his departure from Grenada: firstly, his impending appointment as civil officer of the district and connected need for an oath of allegiance to the British government. Secondly, the reporting of several sudden deaths due to yellow fever on the island, even among those who consider themselves acclimated. In September 1816, Martingale leaves Grenada for St. Lucia and Martinico and sums up his experiences during his four-year residence:

> I was brought into communication with people of different nations, different characters, and different modes of thinking; of different politics, philosophy, and religion; all of which has a tendency to eradicate or weaken early prejudices, liberalize opinions, and inculcate charitable views of human nature. While such a relation with people of other countries can never diminish the feeling of patriotism in a well-balanced mind, it will lead a person to discover, acknowledge, and respect, in other communities and other nations, much that is good and worthy of commendation. (Sleeper 351)

His assessment and vision of a beneficial difference of people, nations, and communities testifies to his personal and political maturation.

At Martinico the disease Martingale has managed to evade for so long comes back with a vengeance and is referred to as the "King of Terrors" that is taking the strong men, as well as the young, and the beautiful (Sleeper 353). Martingale feels protected from "this West India pestilence" by his acclimatization and "had no fear of yellow fever" (Sleeper 354). Yet the acclimatization has also turned him into an Other, including a dark-complexioned skin: "I had been so long in the West Indies that I had lost the distinguishing marks of a Yankee. And my broad accent, my swarthy complexion, my unseamanlike costume, adapted to the climate, all seemed to contradict my statement that I was an American sailor" (Sleeper 354). He boards a vessel, the *Betsey*, that is bound for the United States. The ship—like Redburn's *Highlander*—is an allegory of America. Reminiscent of Edgar Allan Poe's disguised guests who seem to be oblivious to the Red Death in the short story of the same name, the people on board the *Betsey* celebrate the fact that "they had left the yellow fever far behind, and congratulated each other on their good fortune" (Sleeper 357), only to realize that the disease is among them, with a seaman named Smith in a feverish state. A crewman named Gaskell represents those who rejoice in times of crisis and use it for their own benefit:

> He loved to talk of the yellow fever; he set that fearful disease at defiance, and said he never enjoyed himself so gloriously as he had done the year previously at Savannah, when the yellow fever was sweeping off the crews of the shipping in that port by hundreds, and he found employment as a carpenter, and cleared ten dollars a day by making coffins for the "Yankee" sailors. (Sleeper 358–59)

Shortly after Smith, the captain is also diagnosed with yellow fever and Martingale takes over the navigation of the *Betsey* while also tending to the sick. Eventually everybody on board except for Martingale and an officer named Mr. Ricker are infected. Martingale describes the inevitability of escape on board a ship as opposed to yellow fever raging in a city, where retreat is possible: "And no one, not familiar with such scenes, can form an idea of the distress which a mortal sickness produces on board a ship at sea" (Sleeper 363). With many more sick and Gaskell plundering the wine casks, the brotherhood Martingale forms is with the black cook, who assists him in taking care of the sick. When the cook also falls ill, Martingale nurses him and—despite the advanced state of the disease—the black man recovers. What Martingale achieves with the African American, he is not able to manage with Gaskell, who eventually also falls sick. Martingale attributes this to Gaskell's proneness to fear: "He urged me to bleed him, which I undertook, and opened a vein in each arm, but the blood would not flow; the vital current seemed to be congealed by fear" (Sleeper 364). The novel thus promotes anxiety and panic as the most powerful factors in affecting the disease's mortality rate and contagiousness.

Beyond the metaphorical use of yellow fever that signifies the constant existential threat seafarers face, Sleeper fictionalizes the occurrence, origin, and constant risk of yellow fever in the West Indies. However, the character Martingale never catches the fever while living in the West Indies because he blends in and fully accepts the hybrid makeup of the many island societies. His attitude is thus promoted as a cure for the disease that could be applied to the United States. Sleeper makes this quite clear by presenting the yellow fever ship as a microcosm of the diseased U.S. society on Martingale's voyage back to his homeland. Martingale does not differentiate between treating the rebellious Gaskell and the black cook.

The last example in this section, Émile Souvestre's novella "Mathieu Ropars" (1868), uses the experience of the sea and seafaring on the Atlantic as background to functionalize yellow fever allegorically. The disease itself becomes the Other that is invisible and highly contagious; it causes existential fear which leads to death. Both the European-American publication history and the novella's view on yellow fever from the European side of the Atlantic add a transnational angle.[123] Yellow fever is connected to "Havannah or Brazil" (28) in the novella but is able to reach the Western tip of France as an unseen passenger on ships.

Similar to the isolated spaces of ships represented in the novels discussed earlier, Souvestre builds his tale upon the frigate *Thetis* and two small islands, or rather "two large rocks" near Brest, France, in the Bay of Roscanvel. On the first island called Treberon a lazaretto is located. It is only in use when sick passengers or crew from an incoming ship need to be hospitalized. The second island, the Ile des Morts or Isle of the Dead, contains the principal magazine belonging to the naval arsenal. Each island is only permanently inhabited by one man and his family. Dorot is already stationed at the Ile des Morts when his old ship-mate Mathieu Ropars accepts the post as quartermaster on the neighboring island Treberon. Ropars becomes related to Dorot by marrying Dorot's cousin Geneviève. They have two daughters, Josèphe and Francine; while Dorot and his wife, who soon dies, have a son named Michael. The death of his wife brings Dorot closer to his friend Ropars and the mutual visits are greatly enjoyed by all. The novella begins with such a visit by Dorot and his son Michael to the cousins' island home. They behold a frigate anchoring far out, which is quite unusual for a returning ship. They suspect that it might be a quarantine measure and are able to discern the ship as the *Thetis*. The frigate is Monsieur Gabriel's ship, an old friend of the Ropars and especially of their oldest daughter Josèphe, who had spent a week at the lazaretto three years earlier. Due to the otherwise extreme solitude on the island, the hospital patients provide a welcome diversion as they bring news from abroad or from the mainland—yet, they may also bring disease. Dorot cautions Ropars not to tell his daughter that Monsieur Gabriel is about to return, as the ship arrives "from the Havannah [sic]" ("MR" 18). Ropars answers his friend's remark with a prayer. The fact that he points out their island's freedom from crime or sin speaks for an understanding of disease as God's punishment.

---

123 The novella first appeared as *Le garde du lazaret* (Brussels: A. Lebègue, 1852) and was published as *The Isle of the Dead, or, The Keeper of the Lazaretto: A Tale of the Yellow Fever* in London (1863) and as "The Lazaretto-Keeper in the *New York Illustrated News* (1863). The story thus first appeared in the United States at the height of the Civil War and shortly after the Emancipation Declaration (January 1, 1863). It was republished as "Mathieu Ropars" in May 1868 by editor William Young. The translations of Souvestre's original French narrative differ in the three English versions. The title character who is referred to as Matthew in the two 1863 English versions becomes the French 'Mathieu' in the 1868 collection. In my discussion of the novella I will cite from the 1868 American version, abbreviated as "MR."

Dorot and Michael have hardly left when a longboat appears and approaches the Isle of Treberon bearing a yellow flag. Ropars opens the hospital for the boat passengers, and when he returns to his family he asks for his daughters, silently wishing he had sent them to the Ile des Morts with his friend. Geneviève is horrified when her husband tells her that the longboat of the *Thetis* has landed nurses and physicians as well as eight men sick with yellow fever. It seems clear to the two of them that none of them will leave his bed alive. Concurrently, the second part of the novella opens with an explanation of the terrible and deadly effects of yellow fever. Ropars has witnessed the disease in his military years at sea and has related "that butchery" ("MR" 27), as he calls it, to his wife. He believes that he has escaped the disease only by a miracle. Ropars and his wife do not fear for themselves but mostly for their daughters. The island has become their prison since violating quarantine would result in Ropars's discharge. He tries to divert the fears of his wife by speaking lightly of the danger:

> [H]e set himself seriously to soothing the terror of Geneviève by underrating the danger that they incurred. After all, they were not here in a state of things that favoured the disease; they had not to contend against the enervating sun of the Havannah or Brazil; this was not one of those awful contagions that spread from house to house like a fire, leaving behind it the dead alone—it was a disorder partly spent, and from which, with certain precautions, escape was easy. The chief and the most indispensable of these precautions was to avoid going near the apartments occupied by those who had been brought into quarantine, and never to stay to leeward of the lazaretto. ("MR" 28)

The girls are forbidden to approach the quarantine grounds and to expose themselves to the wind blowing from the hospital. They promise obedience to their mother who explains in tears that neglect of the measure would result in "the disease, or even death itself" ("MR" 28). Even Ropars, who usually enjoyed the exchange with the patients, ceases all intercourse with the hospital, and is only informed every evening by the tolling of the bell that more graves are being prepared to receive the dead. Vacant places in the hospital are soon filled by new arrivals from the frigate, indicating an increase of fever patients, while no convalescents ever appear on the hospital's terrace. The daily boat with provisions and medicines never touches the shore, and "sailed away in an apparent hurry, that bespoke the fear of contagion" ("MR" 29).

To Ropars and his wife the actual deaths remain 'unseen,' the disease reigns beyond their vision, and the invisibility leads to a temporary feeling of security: "[s]eeing that it was possible to live in contact with the formidable malady, they half forgot, both of them, that is was also possible to die" ("MR" 30). When the first sick arrived, Ropars had inquired about his friend Monsieur Gabriel who was then found to be in good health. Yet not before long, he receives a note "steeped in vinegar" ("MR" 30) telling him that M. Gabriel is on the island, the writing resembling that of a man tremulous with sickness. Ropars discards all previous caution and hurries to the hospital. He is not admitted and learns that chances for the recovery of his friend are nil.

Unremarked by their parents the two girls Josèphe and Francine experience their rite of passage: watching from beyond a thicket, they see four men from the hospital descending to a ravine carrying a corpse. While the younger girl, Francine, hides her face in her sister's bosom, Josèphe boldly looks at the scene before her. When she beholds the face of the dead man and recognizes it as Monsieur Gabriel, she cries out. Her outburst of "inexpressible horror," her "grief and terror" ("MR" 36) is not heard as the noise of the falling body covers it. Vision is functionalized as a means of contagion. Josèphe is diagnosed with yellow fever shortly after the encounter and dies. For the parents, "grief had preceded their loss" ("MR" 42), and they turn their attention to Francine because the "[b]reath of the contagion, like the sea-blast, spares nothing, and at any moment may send the living to rejoin the dead" ("MR" 45). The couple determines the sea to be their only hope, and Ropars breaks the quarantine laws to carry Francine to the Ile des Morts, which is no longer symbolically the island of the dead but that of the living. His night journey attains a biblical quality as Ropars is walking through the water at low tide without clear vision. He leaves his wife almost senseless with terror ("MR" 51), and—when he returns from his trip—finds Geneviève unconscious, lying next to their dead daughter. Although a physician momentarily restores her spirits, she falls into spasms and then into a stupor, very similar to the fate of her daughter. Terror has induced her sickness. Although the symptoms were not those of the contagion which was raging at the hospital, she dies of the fever ("MR" 64); yet not before she has seen her healthy daughter in the distance over on the Ile des Morts for a last time. Geneviève's death is the last one on Treberon.

Souvestre's approach to yellow fever is an allegorical one which equates the disease with existential fear, i.e. death brought about by an unknown Other. Although the disease is specifically identified as yellow fever and Ropars's experience of it at sea is cited as evidence, the symptoms are not portrayed in a realistic manner but are reduced to those of a high fever and a loss of vision, with the characteristic black vomit absent from the description. Those suffering from yellow fever are hidden from view in the hospital, a space that is never narratively explored, except for Ropars 'opening' it for the arriving patients, doctors, and nurses. When he seeks to gain information on his friend Gabriel he is not admitted. This invisibility and lack of knowledge feeds into the fear of contagion. Panic and terror are presented as an actual cause of the disease. In the narrative, only those who grieve and suffer from the loss of a loved person contract the disease: Josèphe mourns Monsieur Gabriel, and Geneviève greatly suffers from the loss of her daughter. Thus the patients in the lazaretto must also have experienced grief and suffering before being struck by illness. Furthermore the absoluteness of death—everyone who contracts the disease is bound to die—adds to the horror the yellow fever in *The Isle of the Dead* emanates. The fact that yellow fever did reach Northern European shores, but was never experienced there in any way close to an epidemic event, possibly added to its perception as a horrific but invisible and unknown threat known to be generally located in the West Indies and the Americas, the realms of other, hybrid and dangerous societies.

5.3 New Orleans: Race Capital, Disease Capital

The city most intricately and tragically linked to yellow fever after 1820 in the United States is New Orleans. The geographical location of the city, which was built on an area below sea level and just below Lake Pontchartrain and its connected swamps, furthered a seasonally changing occurrence of floods, often followed by diseases (Ryan 26). New Orleans was also a major city of the Atlantic slave trade until the Civil War. The following section will explore these two dimensions of the city—as capital of the slave trade and as disease capital—and how both formations are represented and interfaced as imaginative spaces in literature and culture. Yet far from branding New Orleans in the nineteenth century as being the one or the other or both, the city was, of course, also characterized by its polyglot culture and linguistic diversity, as well as its cultural diversity founded in Native American, Spanish, French, and African roots.[124] New Orleans had only become a part of the United States with the Louisiana Purchase in 1803. Thus, English was not the dominant language and Catholicism rather than the Protestantism of the English colonies the prevailing religion. The French-speaking or 'Creole' population consisted primarily of descendants of the French colonial

---

124 In mid-century, Charles Gayarré promoted the ethnic reconciliation of New Orleans cultures in his four-volume *History of Louisiana* (1854). He relied on an ideology of 'whiteness,' which only included Spanish, French, and Americans. He believed that Native Americans would peacefully disappear and Africans would continue to provide the labor force. In the 1840s Alexis de Tocqueville also commented on the racial situation. He spoke of a "third race" that existed in Louisiana and saw two solutions: a strict partition as promoted by Gayarré or a continued racial hybridization, of which the latter seemed more viable to him (Tocqueville 388–89).

period and of French colonial refugees from the Haitian Revolution.[125] This group dominated New Orleans during the first two decades of the nineteenth century, when little more than 20,000 people lived in the city. The introduction of the steamboat in 1812 and the expansion and commercial prospects of the cotton and sugar economies attracted English-speaking migrants. The large mixed-race free population, called free people of color or *gens de couleur libres*, numbered almost twenty thousand at its peak in 1840.[126] A tradition of inter-racial liaisons was supported by informal institutions, such as the quadroon ball (social occasions for white men and free women of color), or *plaçage*, a practice by which a white man literally 'placed' a woman of color under his protection; in many such cases the man would provide a home for the woman and their children. Two developments can be seen as consequences of New Orleans racial relations: on the one hand, racial 'sciences' that denigrated the mixing of races flourished in New Orleans.[127] On the other hand, spaces of black resistance formed in the swamps around New Orleans. The so-called maroon communities allowed former slaves and their Native American allies to operate relatively autonomously.[128]

By 1850 New Orleans had become the second-busiest port and financial center after New York and had a population of 116,000, making it the largest city in the American South and the fourth largest city in the United States. Waves of immigration from the Caribbean and Europe and a steady stream of English speakers from other states had ensured the steady growth of the city. Between 1847 and 1857, 350,000 immigrants entered the United States through New Orleans and many of them remained in the city (S. E. Thompson 34). They were fleeing from the Great Famine in Ireland and from political repression following the 1848

---

125 Following Arnold R. Hirsch, Joseph Logsdon, and Gwendolyn Midlo Hall, I use the designation 'Creole' in its eighteenth- and early nineteenth-century sense, meaning people of European descent born in Louisiana or New Orleans (Hirsch and Logsdon xi; Hall 60).

126 The rather large mixed-race free population has its roots in the eighteenth-century French and Spanish practice to manumit the children they fathered with slave women. After the Haitian Revolution many free people of color also entered the city (cf. Manganelli 40).

127 For example, Josiah Nott and George Gliddon, authors of the 'ethnology' *Types of Mankind* (1854); proslavery physician Samuel Cartwright, all of them frequently lectured in the city, on mulatto degeneracy and polygenesis (a theory of the separate origins of the various human races) and on so-called 'slave diseases' that caused mischievous behavior.

128 The swamps around New Orleans as spaces of resistance were fictionalized by Victor Séjour "Le Mulâtre (The Mulatto)" in 1837.

revolutions in Germany and France (February Revolution).[129] Between 1852 and 1853 alone, over twenty thousand Irish and German immigrants arrived in New Orleans. Never exposed to yellow fever before, their immunological defenselessness enhanced the devastating progression of the disease in the summer and fall of 1853. From the eight to nine thousand yellow fever victims more than seven thousand came from recent immigrant groups. Even before the devastating epidemic of 1853, "[f]or New Orleanians, yellow fever was much more than a disease; it was a measure and a test of cultural belonging, [...] and the response to an epidemic distinguished in the public's mind the city's cultural 'insiders' from its 'outsiders'" (S. E. Thompson 27). In this line of argument, however, white Creoles and people of African descent were put into the same category of 'insiders' and seen as immune or less prone to the disease. For the Creoles it was thus pertinent to base the 'insiderness' on 'acclimatization' rather than on a shared biology with the black or mixed-race population. The explanation also signaled to recent immigrants the opportunity to get 'acclimatized' to the city and its diseases. "Americans" new to the city, and immigrants could adapt to the culture of the place and acquire immunity. That differences existed can also be seen in the yellow fever mortality rates, which for white residents is given at 7.4 percent and at 0.2 percent for the black population (Pierce and Writer 48–49). To assume an immunity of large parts of the black population dating from earlier exposure in the Caribbean or Africa seems unlikely, since the importation of slaves had been banned in 1808 and only an internal American slave trade continued. Through the numbers it can be asserted that while blacks were as likely to fall ill, they had a lower mortality rate. It is not surprising that debates like this sharpened rather than soothed "racial and cultural tensions" (S. E. Thompson 27). Because of this unique status, New Orleans served writers as a prism shedding light onto questions of national, cultural, and racial identity; noteworthy examples follow.

In her anti-slavery novel *Uncle Tom's Cabin; or, Life Among the Lowly* (1852) Harriet Beecher Stowe depicts slavery's aberrations exemplified in a symbolic New Orleans setting. The Northerner Ophelia, who comes probably closest to Stowe's intended readership, deems New Orleans "old and heathenish" (216). The most brutal excesses of slavery are depicted on the Louisiana plantation of evil Simon Legree. In *Romance of the Republic* (1867) Lydia Maria Child uses two New Orleans mixed-race women to imagine a racial, cultural, and sectional

129 The cultural impact of French and German speakers is reflected in the increase of newspapers catering to these constituencies. The publications thrived especially during the antebellum period.

reconciliation after the Civil War. In order to achieve this, she uses a pre-war New Orleans setting and a cast of characters available in the city. Picking up the controversial issue of interracial attraction or "cross-racial desire" (Samuels, *Reading the Novel* 126), Child proposes the acceptance of interracial marriages as important steps on the way to a national solution. In short, Child speculated about the ways in which a stronger United States could emerge from the ashes of the Civil War. That she intended the national rather than the personal importance of her text can also be seen in her choice of title: instead of sticking to the originally longer version "Lovers and Memories: A Romance of the Republic" she decides not to emphasize the sentimental but the national potential and to go with the simple form (cf. Samuels, *Reading the Novel* 126). However, a heavily didactic purpose indebted to sentimental fiction is apparent in *A Romance of the Republic*. Child could be classified as a 'romantic racialist' who presents an alternative narrative of national identity in her counter-romance that is also heavily indebted to sentimental fiction: the stock elements from orphans, tragic partings and reunions, to switched infants are all represented.

Furthermore, the tragic mixed-race character was an important figure in sentimental antislavery literature, which is also often referred to as the tragic mulatto genre (e.g. Gillman): the characters appear to be white but have black ancestry and thus suffer under slavery and other race-based social ills. They command increased sympathy from a primarily white reading audience who could see their own features in their white visages. Rosa and Flora Royal, the protagonists in Child's *Romance* are two beautiful young sisters growing up not knowing that they could be claimed as slaves because their father never freed their (previously purchased) quadroon mother. When their father dies without having manumitted his daughters, they are endangered to be sold as slaves and smuggled out of the city by Rosa's suitor Gerald Fitzgerald who knows their secret. However, Fitzgerald never actually planned to marry Rosa and hides her and Flora on his Georgia plantation. When he sexually harasses Flora, she manages to escape to Boston. Rosa gives birth to the son of Gerald Fitzgerald and names him after his father. At the same time Gerald and his Northern wife Lily Bell also have a son whom they unknowingly also name Gerald Fitzgerald. Rosa switches her mixed-race child with the child of Gerald and Lily Bell and then escapes to New Orleans with their child. From New Orleans Rosa sails to Europe and leaves the baby with a Mr. Duroy, the cousin of her former music teacher Madame Papanti.

Besides the aberrations of slavery the cruelest disease taking away the lives of loved ones—and also intricately linked to New Orleans—is yellow fever. While family members were often forcibly separated because of slavery or disappeared after attempts to escape it, there still existed a hope to locate, find, and identify those lost family members. The same was not the case with those perishing from yellow fever. Once in Europe, Rosa learns from a letter that the whole Duroy household has died of yellow fever. When Flora later tries to locate her lost sister in New Orleans, she finds everyone she used to know either dead or gone. She is told that her sister boarded a ship bound for Europe, which was reported to be lost at sea. Flora "drove to Mr. Duroy's, and found strangers there, who said the former occupants had all died of yellow-fever,—the lady and gentleman, a negro woman, and a white baby. Flora was bewildered to find every link with her past broken and gone" (Child 263). Yet both Rosa and Flora never learn the true identities of those supposedly dead from yellow fever. The child survives and later calls himself George Falkner, is sold into slavery and escapes from it. Rosa's actual son, who is called Gerald Fitzgerald like his father, is raised as a white gentleman in the Fitzgerald household. Nineteen years pass since the events in New Orleans, when the Civil War begins and Gerald Fitzgerald meets his half-brother George Falkner. They become close friends before Gerald Fitzgerald, Rosa's son, is killed in the war. After his true identity is revealed to him, the white George Falkner goes off to Europe with his slave wife and their daughter and takes on the name of his father again, Gerald Fitzgerald. "Neither of the two stays at home or in the republic," Shirley Samuels points out ("The Identity of Slavery" 171). In the end, it seems as if Child did not fully trust her own vision of a cross-racial American future. It is true that the two Royal sisters Rosa and Flora both marry white husbands and decide to live in Boston after Rosa's return from Europe; yet they have always passed as white (the premise on which the narrative is built) and thus make it easy for the white reading audience to accept the cross-racial marriage.

Although yellow fever only takes a minor role in *A Romance*, it needs to be asserted that it manages to sever the ties between loved ones without regard to their racial affiliation. Slavery, of course, also cruelly separated families, but it only affected those who were defined as slaves (disregarding their outward appearance). Child's audience did not need to be educated about the devastating and horrifying effects of yellow fever, which—I would like to argue—serves as an allegory for the aberrations of slavery to those looking in upon it from the outside.

Yellow fever is also employed as an allegory of a more mystical apocalyptic kind and comes upon the people as a retribution for the practice of slavery in Baron Ludwig von Reizenstein's serial novel *The Mysteries of New Orleans (Die Geheimnisse von New Orleans)*. Reizenstein was a German aristocrat born in Marktsteft at the Main river, who emigrated to the United States in 1848 and eventually wound up in New Orleans, where he worked as an editor and journalist.[130] In *Die Geheimnisse von New Orleans* he fictionalized the horrors and traumatic experience of the 1853 yellow fever epidemic for many recent voluntary immigrants and paired it with the African American trauma of slavery. The text was published serially in the German-language newspaper *Louisiana Staats-Zeitung* in 1854 and 1855. *Geheimnisse* aims to imitate the tradition of gothic urban mysteries popular both in Europe and in the United States, which put the respective city at the center of the narrative to expose violence, corruption, and exploitation, and which often did not refrain from describing deviant sexualities.[131] Steven Rowan, who rediscovered the novel and translated it into English in the 1990s, refers to *Geheimnisse* as "one of the first trash novels in America" (Rowan, "Baron von Reizenstein's"). Yet the novel was not banned shortly after its publication for its sexual explicitness and depiction of a lesbian relationship or for accusing thinly veiled real citizens of misdemeanors, but for its antislavery, pro-black stance (Rowan, "Baron von Reizenstein's").

In the course of the novel Captain Marcy of the United States Army sets out for an expedition to find the source of the Red River, which supposedly marks "the region of *yellow fever*" (Reizenstein 3; emphasis in original). Upon his return to New Orleans, he attends a social function. In a conversation with Prince Paul of Württemberg the military man states: "[I]f I were an abolitionist, I would like to believe that slavery was to blame for yellow fever" (Reizenstein 443). Marcy refers to the argument of abolitionists, who see the presence of yellow fever as a result of the aberrations of slavery:

> [Captain Marcy] spoke of the first appearance of the yellow fever in New Orleans in 1769 and he rejected the assumption that this disease had been introduced by a British ship that had arrived with a cargo of slaves from the west coast of Africa. "You do not appear to be an abolitionist, Captain," the prince of Württemberg remarked at this point.
>
> "How did you come to this perilous question, Prince?" the captain asked tensely.
>
> "Because you oppose the notion that we have the importation of slaves to thank for this," the prince of Württemberg asserted.
>
> "Now I understand you, Prince—you are of the opinion that, if I were an abolitionist, I would like to believe that slavery was to blame for yellow fever."

---

130 Despite his involvement with his own newspaper *Alligator* and with the *Louisiana Staats-Zeitung* Reizenstein usually identified himself as "draftsman, architect, engineer, suveyor, or civil engineer" (Rowan, "Introduction" xix).

131 Examples of this genre are *The Mysteries of Paris* (1842) by Eugène Sue; *The Mysteries of London* (1844) by George W. M. Reynolds; and *Quaker City, or the Monks of Monk Hall* (1845) by George Lippard.

> "To be sure," the prince responded. "But since you so boldly cast doubt on the correctness of the common opinion that yellow fever came with a slave ship, I would not harbor the least suspicion that you are an abolitionist." (Reizenstein 442–43)

In their conversation the Prince recounts the belief in slaves as carriers of the disease. The men's discussion results in the uneasiness of the misogynistically portrayed female guests who do not know what to make of the term 'abolitionist.' Instead, they speak among themselves about the ungallant ways of the gentlemen "to talk about such incomprehensible things in the presence of [...] ladies" (Reizenstein 443). Noticing their discomfort, the captain apologizes, also on behalf of the prince, and promises to make good for his rudeness by telling a story. The story that unfolds is the one that has been told from a different angle earlier in the novel. The Captain reports from his expedition in search for the source of the Red River where he hoped to find the *Mantis religiosa.* His avid listeners immediately connect the Latin term to "a *wandelndes Blatt* [stick insect] or a *Gottesanbeterin* [praying mantis] in German, since this creature looks like a leaf on one side, while from the other side it always raises its front legs in the air, folded together, as if it were trying to pray" (Reizenstein 445). Captain Marcy's *Mantis religiosa,* however, is not an insect—as he continues to explain—but a plant "that contains the germ of destruction" (Reizenstcin 66) with "the dreadful capacity to cause the plague of yellow fever" (Reizenstein 445). Marcy also speaks of a mystical black man called Hiram, who is a Freemason, supposedly 200 hundred years old, and has come to take revenge upon the South for slavery. Hiram has supposedly thrown the seeds of the poisonous plant, which is known only to him, into the cisterns of New Orleans. The trope of well poisoning by an unpopular Other is established throughout literature and has also been conjured up in relation to the 1793 yellow fever in Philadelphia (see footnote 41).

The devastating 1853 yellow fever epidemic in New Orleans was still fresh in Reizenstein's mind when he wrote his novel. The outbreak precipitated intense controversy in terms of future control of the fever. The importation theory—that yellow fever is imported through the city's ports from where it then spreads—was widely established at the time. Reizenstein's fictional theory of local origin and deceitful conduct of an apocalyptic black figure is thus all the more interesting from a cultural studies perspective for its vision of race. It suggests that the disease can be contained by exploring and destroying its source, the *Mantis religiosa* plant and its distributor, the mystical Hiram bringing the yellow fever with him to prepare the way for a black messiah. The apocalyptic vision of race is carried through, with Hiram dying at the end and leaving a black emperor to rule in Haiti (reminiscent of Toussaint Louverture's role during the Haitian Revolution, 1791–1804).

The ending with a partly successful black rebellion mirrors white fears of a similar revolution spreading to or erupting in the United States. It can only be controlled by the abolition of slavery. Yet the city has forgotten all about the fever—and the threat of slavery—and the author leaves readers with the warning "Ruin awaits him who does not take heed!"

Reizenstein became friends with novelist George Washington Cable in the early 1880s (Rowan, Introduction xiii, xxiv). The latter was inspired by Reizenstein to create a character modeled after the German in his novella "The Entomologist" (published 1899, fourteen years after Reizenstein's death). Reizenstein—a hobby lepidopterist—had named a new species of moths he discovered after his friend Cable, *Smerinthus cablei* (Rowan, Introduction xxiv). Yet the title character of Cable's novella was a not very flattering version of Reizenstein; he is depicted as "a dried-up, obsessive pursuer of bugs and butterflies," who "becomes involved with the sexually aggressive wife of a neighbor, and [...] dies of yellow fever" (Rowan xxiv–xxv). Yellow fever here is employed in a moral sense of divine retribution ("The Entomologist"). While Cable does not specifically focus on racial relations in "The Entomologist," he problematizes race and represents the disease in the novel *The Grandissimes* (1880), in the short story "Tite Poulette" (1879, 1883), and in *Dr. Sevier* (1884). Cable's history *The Creoles of Louisiana* (1884), which also includes descriptions of yellow fever, goes back to a United States Census Bureau commission to provide a historical sketch of antebellum New Orleans for a special section of the Tenth United States Census (1880). A revised version of the text became *The Creoles of Louisiana*. Far from presenting a nostalgic version of pre-Civil War New Orleans, Cable's history is a critical and realistic account of life, including descriptions of the city's frequent epidemics: "Between 1810 and 1837 there were fifteen epidemics of yellow fever" (Cable, *The Creoles of Louisiana* 219). He continues by giving the numbers of the many subsequent epidemics. The gruesome account of the devastating 1853 epidemic covers several pages and ends with the staggering numbers "of nearly thirty thousand residents [...] ill of the yellow fever, and [...], nearly sixteen thousand" dead (Cable, *The Creoles of Louisiana* 302). Yet, Cable also recalls that

> [i]n the very midst of these visitations, it was the confident conviction and constant assertion of the average New Orleans citizen, Creole or American, on his levee, in the St. Charles rotunda, at his counting-room desk, in the columns of his newspaper, and in his family circle, that his town was one of the healthiest in the world. (*The Creoles of Louisiana* 292)

In his report Cable exposes this false security, usually referred to by acclimated citizens, as "an absurd belief in his entire immunity from attack" (Cable, *The*

Creoles of Louisiana 292). Since Cable's work was not altogether favorable to Creole society, it encountered heavy criticism in New Orleans. His fictional works received a similar reception.

Cable published his first stories and novels when New Orleans was faced with a waning of Reconstruction and the acceleration of racial hostilities. He fictionalized what came to be regarded as the picturesque life of Creoles, their dark secrets, and their entanglement in old family feuds. He introduced the peculiar cultural geography of New Orleans to a national audience. With the representation in Cable's *Old Creole Days* (1879) and *The Grandissimes: A Story of Creole Life* (1880) New Orleans not only came to be regarded as the capital of Louisiana's plantation life but was also dreadfully linked to the brutal treatment of black slaves. The dichotomy of the city's attractive diversity of African, Creole, and Anglo-Saxon cultures on the one hand and its connection to natural disasters (floods), diseases (yellow fever), and the brutalization of blacks on the other is typically represented in much of later nineteenth century literature (cf. Skaggs 156).

In *The Grandissimes: A Story of Creole Life* (1880)[132], Cable provides a realistic portrait of race and class relations in New Orleans at the start of the nineteenth century, immediately following the Louisiana Purchase in 1803. The central political and historical episode of the novel is the transfer of the Louisiana territory to the United States. Cable implicitly parallels the Purchase and the ensuing cultural conflicts with those of the Southern Reconstruction between 1865 and 1877 (cf. Bryan 22). Both political decisions led to the establishment of new power relationships that needed to be negotiated on cultural terms. Cable's novel achieves this by representing New Orleans Creole society through the lives of the extended Grandissime family, including its members from different races and classes. The dichotomy between the romanticized description of Louisiana plantation life and the aberration of the system of slavery on which it is built, provides the foil for the two protagonists of the novel to develop their arguments. Honoré Grandissime, a descendant of the white Creole branch of the Grandissime clan, becomes the mentor of the young Joseph Frowenfeld who has recently arrived in New Orleans from Philadelphia. Their conversations revolve around the peculiar situation of racial mixture in Louisiana, of white and black Creoles and of Anglo-Saxons. While the idealistic Frowenfeld advocates abolitionism and social reforms as the only possible future of an interracial society, Honoré Grandissime is caught in his family's racist past that relies on the system of slavery.

---

132 In the following, for simplicity's sake, I will use *G* for George Washington Cable's *The Grandissimes: A Story of Creole Life* and "TP" for his short story "Tite Poulette."

A recurrent theme of the novel that is intertwined with the idea of acculturation and acclimatization to the region—specifically also to its diseases and yellow fever—is taken up early in the novel. When the Frowenfeld family approaches New Orleans, the metaphors connected to the city suggest violence and death. Observing from their vantage point on board a ship, they are disappointed by "a land hung in mourning, darkened by gigantic cypresses, submerged; a land of reptiles, silence, shadow, decay" (*G* 11). Ironically, and not known as vectors in the transmission of yellow fever, "jubilant mosquitoes [are] spinning about each head" at this morning of first disappointment of the Frowenfelds (*G* 10). Although some believe that the air is actually kept pure by the mosquitoes, as the captain tells them, he also advises them: "keep out of the sun and stay in after dark; you're not 'acclimated,' as they call it, you know, and the city is full of the fever" (*G* 14). The Frowenfelds are eventually assured "that to live in those swamps was not entirely impossible to man" (*G* 12). Already on the third day after their arrival, Joseph Frowenfeld falls ill of yellow fever, the symptoms of which are described in a realistic manner. He is helped through his illness by a "blue-turbaned black nurse" (*G* 16) and by Doctor Charlie Keene, and he eventually recovers. Yet while he has mastered this part of the acclimatization process, his whole family, father, mother, and sisters, have not.

The concept of acculturation is also featured in the conversations between the newcomer Frowenfeld and Honoré Grandissime, who furthermore stresses that Southern society requires submission to its customs: "You cannot afford to be entirely different to the community in which you live; is that not so? […] You must get acclimated […] not in body only […] but in mind—in taste—in conversation—and in convictions too" (*G* 46). Honoré predicts that Frowenfeld will be molded into society's shape and not the other way around: "My—de'-seh, the water must expect to take the shape of the bucket." "They all do it—all who come. They hold it for a little while—a very little; then they open their stores on Sunday, they import cargoes of Africans, they bribe the officials, they smuggle goods, they have colored housekeepers" (*G* 46). To which Frowenfeld replies: "One need not be water!"—but he also changes and adapts his behavior and speech to society's demands. Honoré is actually more changed by Frowenfeld in the course of the narrative than the other way around. He attempts to right the wrongs done in the name of his family to the Nancanou family, who have their land returned to them. Honoré also acknowledges his octoroon half-brother who shares the name with him and brings him into the family business as a partner. The money that his darker brother brings into the business is, of course, one key motivation, a fact that the white brother also acknowledges, at least to himself.

In the beginning yellow fever serves to acclimatize Joseph Frowenfeld—"an American by birth, rearing and sentiment, yet German enough through his parents" (*G* 10)—and molds him into a member of New Orleans society. He even gains enough influence on Honoré to change some of his beliefs. Towards the end of the novel the narrative function of the fever changes from being a rite of passage for newcomers to New Orleans to now also affecting the Creoles. Although the Louisianans will not be granted suffrage to participate in the Presidential elections in the fall of 1804, "the people are feverish" (*G* 389) from the excitement. Joseph Frowenfeld tells his friend Doctor Keene: "[T]hey have voted Honoré Grandissime a traitor; they have voted me an encumbrance; I hear one of them casting that vote now" (*G* 389). The times are about to change, which holds true for Louisiana in 1804 as it does for the South after Reconstruction, when the novel was written. Honoré has taken the first steps in repaying old debts and embracing his mixed-race brother but is—at this point—punished for it. The conversation of Frowenfeld and the doctor ends with the latter resuming his practice as physician because "the yellow fever was bad again" (*G* 391). Yellow fever is paralleled with the disease of slavery and its inheritances. Both are not yet healed—racial tensions, in fact, seem to be accelerating in 1804 as well as after the end of Reconstruction when *The Grandissimes* was published.[133]

Cable's short story "Tite Poulette" (1883) focuses on the tragic situation of mixed-race individuals and also presents a post-Reconstruction rendition of the tragic quadroon/octoroon motif discussed earlier in connection with Lydia Maria Child. It also critically approaches the racially discriminatory practice of the quadroon ball and the system of *plaçage* arrangements, in which a Creole man would 'place' a free woman of color under his protection, providing a home for the woman and the children resulting from the relationship. The melodramatic story is built around the contrast between 'Tite Poulette (little Poulette), the innocent "daughter" of Madame John and "the wicked city" ("TP" 222) as Kristian Koppig, the newly arrived Dutch accountant calls New Orleans. Koppig—in a quite voyeuristic way—watches the activities in the *plaçage*-supported house of Madame John from his window across the street. As in her youth going out to the quadroon ball, the widow is now paid for her "dance of the shawl" ("TP" 220), which serves as a metaphor for "the beautiful exterior and the decadent, morally corrupt interior of New Orleans" (Bryan 16). Madame John tells

133 From Cable's manuscript notebook we know that he "meant to make *The Grandissimes* as truly a politcal work as it ever has been called—not a *party* thing, but a *principle* thing" (qtd. in Tregle, Jr. 177; emphasis in original).

Poulette about the fate of being mixed-race, that Poulette will be lonely "all [her] poor life long. There is no place in this world for us poor women. I wish that we were either white or black" ("TP" 221). The short story draws attention to the intersectionality of race, gender, and class within this system of oppression. Koppig describes Poulette as "one of those whom the taint of caste has cursed. She lives a lonely innocent life in the midst of corruption, like the lilies [...] in the marshes" ("TP" 222). Sensing that he is attracted to the young mixed-race woman, he finds himself in a moral dilemma as he imagines the "horror of mixed blood" ("TP" 222–23). When he falls sick with a fever, he is nursed by Madame John "who was the best yellow-fever nurse in a thousand yards round" ("TP" 215). Madame John tells Koppig that tending to him is nothing compared to caring for yellow fever patients; she nursed "a lady and gentleman once—a Spanish lady and gentleman, just off the ship; both sick at once with the fever—delirious—could not tell their names. Nobody to help me but sometimes Monsieur John! I never had such a time,—never before, never since,—as that time" ("TP" 240). Despite his reluctance to break the law and his moral principles, Koppig proposes to Poulette. It is only at this divisive moment that Madame John produces the papers to prove that her 'daughter' is actually the daughter of the Spanish couple who died of yellow fever in her boardinghouse. Freeing Poulette from her mixed-race status by making her a yellow fever orphan might have sounded reasonable to (mostly Northern) readers, to whom yellow fever figured as the cruel disease of the South. Yet, the deus-ex-machina trick must also have seemed a lie to many of those who suffered under the discriminatory system (cf. Bryan 17).

In *Dr. Sevier* Cable almost completely blocks out the question of race to focus on class instead. Besides Dr. Sevier, the second protagonist of the novel is John Richling, a disinherited and thus impoverished member of the aristocracy. His equally poor wife Mary is a descendant of the Northern working class. The quadroon landlady of the first apartment John and Mary Richling rent is the only black character in the novel. Cable knew that it would be much easier to make his case for social change with the agrarian Richling than with poor blacks or poor immigrant whites. Cable argues for the moral responsibility of wealthy people, such as Dr. Sevier, to help those poor (i.e. John and Mary Richling) with whom his readers could relate and who had the chance to overcome poverty.

The novel is set during the 1850s, the decade that saw several horrifying yellow fever epidemics and that mostly affected the many immunologically naïve immigrants that came to New Orleans since the late 1840s. Various immigrant groups are at the center of the novel and at the center of attention of Dr. Sevier, who at least tries to act charitably—and according to his name—as their 'savior.' Yet a naturalistic tone is already prevalent in this 1884 novel of Cable:

> So the July sun rose up and moved across the beautiful blue sky [...], and as the last night passed into the first twinkling hour of morning the month chronicled one hundred and thirty-one deaths from yellow fever. The city shuddered because it knew, and because it did not know, what was in store. People began to fly [sic] by hundreds, and then by thousands. Many were overtaken and stricken down as they fled. Still men plied their vocations, children played in the streets, and the days came and went, fair, blue tremulous with sunshine, or cool and gray and sweet with summer rain. How strange it was for nature to be so beautiful and so unmoved! (*Dr. Sevier* 282)

Here we see a development in the functionalization of the fever away from a metaphoric toward a realistic description of its course, uninterrupted and unchangeable by natural or human efforts.

The development is continued in Lafcadio Hearn's novella *Chita: A Memory of Last Island* (1889)[134]. The story is based on the 1856 Last Island hurricane that hit Isle Dernière (or Last Island), a barrier island and pleasure resort southwest of New Orleans. The novella was first published in *Harper's Monthly* in 1888 and bears Ralph Waldo Emerson's dictum as a motto: "But Nature whistled with all her winds, / Did as she pleased, and went her way" (*Ch* n.pag.). I read the novella in terms of its critical approach to racial appropriation, as well as the text's framing within a natural and a yellow fever disaster.

Part one of the narrative begins with the "cataclysm" and the "fury of a storm-flood" (*Ch* 14), in which Dr. Julien La Brierre of New Orleans is separated from his wife Adèle and their daughter Eulalie during a shipwreck caused by the hurricane. Later, the body of a child is found as well as the corpse of a fair-haired woman who is identified by her wedding band as Julien's wife. The physician is rescued by a ship and returns to New Orleans half a year later in February 1857, certain that both his wife and daughter are dead.

Part two introduces the Spanish fisherman Feliu Viosca and his wife Carmen, who is described as "a little brown woman" (*Ch* 68). The couple has buried their firstborn Concha/Conchita at Barcelona before coming from Europe to a little Gulf island off the coast of New Orleans, and despite Carmen's prayers to an Indian-faced Madonna statue holding "the brown Child with the Indian face" (*Ch* 76) they have never had another child. When Feliu finds a living girl among the corpses that are lying on the beach after the hurricane, he takes her home, which

---

134 In the following, for simplicity's sake, I will use *Ch* for *Chita: A Memory of Last Island* (1889).

brings back memories of their own lost child: "The child's hair was yellow—it was the flash of it that had saved her; yet her eyes and brows were beautifully black. She was comely, but with such a curious, delicate comeliness—totally unlike the robust beauty of Concha" (*Ch* 91). Adding to her appearance that is so different from that of the Vioscas, they are not able to communicate with the girl until a French Creole addresses her. The linguistic recognition of her mother tongue is framed in racial terms as an "embryonic feeling of race-affinity quickening in the little brain—some intuitive, inexplicable sense of kindred" (*Ch* 100). Although the girl is able to produce the names of her parents as Julien and Adèle, which are common names in the colonial quarter of New Orleans, she is never identified (*Ch* 106).

In part three the girl, who is now called Conchita by her foster parents, becomes acculturated and learns "another tongue," Spanish (*Ch* 144). Her renaming might be read as the reversal of the colonial practice of naming and of taking 'possession.' Yet, her inherited nature, including social prejudices, seems untouched by her forced adaptation:

> Occasional swarthy visitors,—men of the Manilla settlements,—she spoke of contemptuously as negues-marrons; and once she shocked Carmen inexpressibly by stopping in the middle of her evening prayer, declaring that she wanted to say her prayers to a white Virgin; Carmen's Senora de Guadalupe was only a negra! (*Ch* 134)

Feliu decides that Chita has to learn to swim in order to overcome her fears, the trauma of her near-drowning, that still haunt her in her dreams. She learns to swim and the sea almost magically transforms her into a woman and into the Other: "Her delicate constitution changed;—the soft, pale flesh became firm and brown, the meagre limbs rounded into robust symmetry, the thin cheeks grew peachy with richer life; for the strength of the sea had entered into her" (*Ch* 161). In the same summer of 1867 in which Chita learns to swim, a yellow fever epidemic ravages in New Orleans. Pointing to the "black heat," "the acrid air," the "venomous vapors, with morbific dews," and "the torpid moisture" (*Ch* 165) Hearn suggests an atmospheric manifestation of the disease in the city as opposed to the Gulf Islands to which many fled. Yet flight means an equal peril: "Men, who might have been saved by the craft of experienced nurses at home, hurriedly departed in apparent health, [...] died upon their way, by the road-side, by the river-banks, in woods, in deserted stations, on the cots of quarantine hospitals" (*Ch* 165–66). Doctor Julien La Brierre is called to attend to an old friend of his father, who has a heart condition and lies sick in Feliu Viosca's house. Despite the raging fever and plenty of work in the city, La Brierre boards a ship. When he arrives, his patient is dead and La Brierre comes down with yellow fever himself. What the reader already knows is never confirmed for the doctor: he continues to believe that the vision of his daughter, who has the smile and the whisper of his dead wife and even the brown speck between neck and cheek, is due to his high fever. Carmen is most afraid that Chita will catch the fever, but she is not infected, while Julien La Brierre dies. The reunion of father and daughter is thwarted by yellow fever.

What makes this novella so interesting is the transformation and de-culturation of its protagonist, of a fair blond French Creole girl into a dark-skinned girl of nature who is apparently immune to the city's and her own father's disease. Hearn plays with racial expectations and stereotypes and exemplifies the influence of heredity and environment. His obvious scientific interest in a Darwinian model of nature is thus extended toward gaining a more profound understanding of the inexplicable disease yellow fever.

5.4 Yellow Fever and the African American Experience

The last section in this larger chapter dealing with racial relations and the intersectionality of race, gender, ethnicity and class turns to the voices of African Americans, representing their versions of the yellow fever experience. They were politically blamed in narratives such as Mathew Carey's *Account* and culturally silenced in novels such as Charles Brockden Brown's *Arthur Mervyn*. The first and most influential African American text of yellow fever and efforts of community building as a means to control the disease remains the *Narrative* by Absalom Jones and Richard Allen (see ch. 2.3). Several authors followed their lead. In the following I will focus on the abolitionist writer William Wells Brown, and the activist and journalist Ida B. Wells, realizing that other African American writers of the nineteenth century, such as Alice Dunbar-Nelson and Frances Harper, have also—at least cursorily—treated the subject. In the latter's *Iola Leroy, or, Shadows Uplifted* (1892) the beautiful young mixed-race protagonist only finds out about her black ancestry after her father dies from yellow fever, and she is defrauded of her family's estate and sold into slavery in the Deep South. Iola Leroy is freed by Union soldiers during the war and forthwith refuses to 'pass' as white. Although based on the sentimental trope of the tragic mulatta, Harper suggests a gradual empowerment of African Americans through racial identification. The heroine, who continues to identify as black, moves to North Carolina with her mixed-race husband to work for 'racial uplift,' proving that racially hybrid forms of community existed before and after the end of slavery.

Alice Dunbar-Nelson's vignette "The Praline Woman" from *The Goodness of St. Rocque, and Other Stories* (1899) is constructed as a long monologue by a black Creole woman seated close to a chapel during the Carnival season, selling her pralines. Although her racial identity is never explicitly mentioned, readers may infer her dark complexion from the remark of the "I'ishman" (Dunbar-Nelson 178) who asks her "'Auntie, what fo' you talk so?'" (Dunbar-Nelson 180). African Americans were often disparagingly addressed with 'aunt' or 'uncle.' The praline woman refers to herself as "po' Tante Marie" who is "all alone" because of the yellow fever death of her daughter and the death of her son: "[m]y lil' gal, she's daid of de yellow fever; my lil' boy, he's daid" (Dunbar-Nelson 178). The loss defines her and she defines herself through it. Yet she also enjoys the autonomy she has as a vendor of goods, and from her vantage point at the marketplace the praline woman comments on the other ethnicities passing by.

William Wells Brown, who was born into slavery, became a renowned anti-slavery lecturer and writer after his escape via Ohio and after temporarily serving as a conductor of the Underground Railroad, being a steamboatsman on Lake Erie. His anti-slavery novel *Clotel, or, The President's Daughter: A Narrative of Slave Life in the United States* (1853) and his closet drama *The Escape, or A Leap for Freedom* (1858) reference yellow fever. Focusing on the sexual abuse of black enslaved women *The Escape* critically explores the intersectionality of race and gender within the slavery system. Yellow fever is briefly featured in the first scene of the play to characterize the scrupulous Dr. Gaines, who constantly sexually harasses and torments his mixed-race slave Melinda. The disease is paralleled to slavery, namely as something horrifying that Gaines and his wife benefit from. The physician wishes for yellow fever, which rages in New Orleans to the financial advantage of the doctors there, to be imported to his vicinity. In his hubris he believes that he "could invent a medicine that would cure it" and thus sustain his system of oppression (W. W. Brown, "The Escape" 44).

In *Clotel* Brown functionalizes yellow fever in a much more versatile way. The novel was first published in London as *Clotel, or, The President's Daughter: A Narrative of Slave Life in the United States* (1853)[135] before it appeared in the United States in serialized form with the title *Miralda, or The Beautiful Quadroon: A Romance of American Slavery Founded on Fact* (1860–61). The first American book version was substantially revised and appeared as *Clotelle: A Tale of the Southern States* (1864) and *Clotelle, or The Colored Heroine: A Tale of the Southern States* (1867). The novel is based on Lydia Maria Child's short story "The Quadroons" (1842) and uses the tragic mulatta trope as well as fictionalizes separation

135 In the following I will use C for *Clotel, or, The President's Daughter: A Narrative of Slave Life in the United States* (1853).

and the destruction of the family by force of slavery and of yellow fever. Brown could—like Child—be called a 'romantic racialist.' A second source for *Clotel* is the widely held belief that President Thomas Jefferson had fathered children with his slave Sally Hemings. What had circulated as a rumor in the early nineteenth century had—by the 1850s—become part of abolitionist discourse. Rather than presenting a unified narrative voice, the novel features a mixture of different texts and text forms, from slave life vignettes, newspaper reports, songs and poems to abolitionist oratory. The inclusion of historical facts also gives plausibility and lends authenticity to the presented story, a feature which is also reminiscent of the slave narrative.

At the beginning of the novel Currer—contemporary readers would recognize Sally Hemings—and her daughters Clotel and Althesa are sold as slaves in an auction. Clotel is bought by Horatio Green who takes her with him to his Virginia home and treats her like his wife, although—of course—the relationship is not legally binding. Currer is sold to Natchez, Mississippi and Althesa is bought by Dr. Henry Morton, a transplanted Northerner. Not realizing that Southern law does not sanction their marriage, they live as Mr. and Mrs. Morton in New Orleans. The experiences of yellow fever are all connected to the Deep Southern strand of the narrative. Firstly, Althesa learns from their servant Salome that she was not always a slave, but "was born in Germany, on the banks of the Rhine" (*C* 140) and immigrated to America. Salome's father worked at the wharf and—as a recent immigrant—was quite susceptible to yellow fever, of which he died. To escape poverty she finds work as a nurse but is brutally captured during an outing with her employers and sold as a slave. She first works on a farm and is later hired out in New Orleans. Secondly, Currer dies of yellow fever—having been a slave for all her life and shortly before her intended emancipation by her preacher owners, Mr. and Mrs. Carlton. Thirdly, yellow fever reaches New Orleans in the summer of 1831 and thus the home of the Mortons. With this Brown inserts a longer, more detailed and physically realistic description of yellow fever's symptoms and of its progression into his narrative:

> Soon the breath infected the air with a fetid odour, the lips were glazed, despair painted itself in the eyes, and sobs, with long intervals of silence, formed the only language. From each side of the mouth spread foam, tinged with black and burnt blood. Blue streaks mingled with the yellow all over the frame. All remedies were useless. This was the Yellow Fever. (*C* 204)

Brown also employs the trope of "the fear of contagion" which added to the devastating effect of the disease. "Nearly 2000 dead bodies lay uncovered in the burial-ground" as people were afraid of "becoming infected" (*C* 204). By informing his readers that [t]he Negro, whose home is in a hot climate, was not proof against the disease" (*C* 204), Brown makes an important point against the still commonly held but false assumption of black immunity.

Indeed, together with 13,000 inhabitants of the region, the white Mr. Morton and the mixed-race Mrs. Morton both die of yellow fever. Their daughters Ellen and Jane are shocked to discover their mixed-race identity. They are sold as slaves to satisfy their father's creditors. Ellen commits suicide rather than submit to the sexual advances of her master, and Jane dies of heartbreak after her lover, a young Frenchman and a former assistant in her father's office, tries to rescue her and is shot during the attempt.

In Virginia Clotel is sold by her 'husband' Horatio Green after he marries a white woman to advance his career. Their daughter Mary remains in the household as a servant to Green's new wife. Clotel escapes to Ohio but returns to Virginia—in the disguise of a white man—to rescue her daughter. Captured in Richmond, she is imprisoned in Washington, deceives her captors, but is eventually cornered on a bridge, from where she leaps into the Potomac river and dies. Brown makes very clear that "[t]hus died Clotel, the daughter of Thomas Jefferson, a president of the United States; a man distinguished as the author of the Declaration of American Independence, and one of the first statesmen of that country" (*C* 218). Clotel's daughter Mary is rescued by a Frenchman who takes her to Europe where he dies and thus leaves Mary free to marry her old love George Green, another fugitive and participant in Nat Turner's insurrection.

Particularly with the explicit reference to the Jefferson-Hemings relationship, Brown's novel critically exposes the hypocrisy between the aspirations and ideals expressed in the nation's foundational document and the cruel slave-owning practice of the same nation. Clotel's daughter is only able to enjoy the freedom and equality promised in the Declaration of Independence outside the jurisdiction of the United States in Europe. With Currer's death of yellow fever, the novel exposes the practice of slavery-condoning Christians who postpone emancipation long enough that another—but equally cruel—disease (yellow fever) takes her away. The intersectionality of class and ethnicity (i.e. poverty and exposure to disease) is foregrounded in the episode of the yellow fever death of Salome's father and her being sold into slavery. For Brown race meant "a dramatic role one can inhabit, imitate, and perform" (Crane 64). For example, Clotel's imitation of a white man during her flight challenges the fact that racial roles are fixed. Accordingly, appearance and designation can make a person either 'black' or 'white'—a practice the novel challenges. Finally, the horrifying description of yellow fever's course in New Orleans, which robs Jefferson's granddaughters of their parents, can be read as metaphor for the horrors of slavery. The threat and fear of disease was something white readers were familiar with, while they could only be made to 'feel' with fictional protagonists of slavery.

The last example of this study is taken from yellow fever life writing. The African American journalist, editor, activist, and cultural critic Ida B. Wells not only fought to end lynching in the United States and was active for women's rights, she also completed an autobiography as well as three diaries. Ida B. Wells was born a slave in Holly Springs, Mississippi, on July 16, 1862 as the oldest of eight children (Duster xiv). When yellow fever was raging in the Mississippi Valley in 1878, Holly Springs equally suffered under the epidemic. Two thirds of the town's population of 3,500 fled Holly Springs, and many of those who remained fell sick. Wells's parents and her nine-month old brother Stanley were among the 304 victims. To avoid her remaining siblings being separated and raised by different friends and neighbors, Wells became their primary caretaker, which also abruptly ended her education (Duster xv–xvi).

Wells's autobiography is an "historical memoir," in which she uses genuine newspaper articles to "authenticate" her narrative (Braxton 100). In the way she frames the yellow fever epidemic and also places it at the very beginning of her autobiography, it structurally serves as Wells's rite of passage or coming-of-age experience. Although Wells was sixteen years old in 1878, she refers to herself as has having been "only fourteen years old" (*Crusade for Justice* 16)—either an autobiographical oversight or the age she believes and perceives herself to have been when becoming an orphan. She describes herself as "being a happy, light-hearted schoolgirl" who "suddenly found [her]self at the head of a family" (Wells, *Crusade for Justice* 16).

When the epidemic broke out at Holly Springs, Wells was away visiting her paternal grandmother's mistress whom she refers to as "this grandmother" when she hears "that yellow fever was raging in Memphis, Tennessee, fifty miles away, as it had done before, and that the mayor of our town refused to quarantine against Memphis. Our little burg opened its doors to any who wanted to come in. That summer the fever took root in Holly Springs" (Wells, *Crusade for Justice* 10). The criticism directed against the mayor's policy not to quarantine Holly Springs becomes apparent in Wells's writing. Wells recalls trusting that her father would take the family out to the country. Even when she did not get any word from her family, she attributed this to the fact that the mail had been too irregular to expect letters. At her grandmother's place she is herself suffering from a bout of malarial fever when friends of the family personally deliver a letter from a doctor in Memphis:

> I read the first page of this letter through, telling the progress of the fever, and these words leaped out at me, "Jim and Lizzie Wells have both died of the fever. They died within twenty-four hours of each other. The children are all at home and the Howard Association has put a woman there to take care of them. Send word to Ida." That is as far as I read. The next thing I knew grandmother, aunt, and uncle were all in the house and ours indeed became a house of mourning. I wanted to go home at once, but not until three days later, on the receipt of a letter from the doctor in charge, who said I ought to come home, were they willing to let me go. (Wells, *Crusade for Justice* 11)

Although many people urge her not to go, she eventually boards a train to take her home, "[t]hey were sure that coming from the country I would fall victim at once, and that it was better for me to stay until the epidemic was over, so that I could take care of the children if any were left" (Wells, *Crusade for Justice* 11). On her way, she explains to the conductor why she is going home: she believes it her duty to look after her siblings. She describes the yellow fever scene as follows: "When I got home I found two of the children in bed with the fever—all had had slight attacks of it save Eugenia, my older sister, who was a paralytic and seemingly immune. The baby, Stanley, had died" (Wells, *Crusade for Justice* 12). Wells is scolded by the family physician and by her sister Eugenia for returning to the scene. Her sister tells her about her father who

> went about his work nursing the sick, making coffins for the dead; that he would come to the gate bringing food and finding out how all were getting along. She said our mother was taken first and a young Irish woman had been sent to nurse her. The first thing the nurse did was to take the nine-month-old baby from the breast, which increased our mother's fever. The milk clotted in her breast, and when she knew she was going to die asked what would become of her children. (Wells, *Crusade for Justice* 12).

Although seemingly described in a factual manner, the harmfulness of the nurse's therapy for Wells's mother cannot be denied. While critical of her mother's Irish nurse, Wells describes the white doctor, Dr. Gray, who took care of her family, with the highest praise. Since Eugenia, Ida's next younger, paralyzed sister, had seen her father's nurse go through his pockets, she had asked the doctor to take their father's money and lock it in a safe downtown—which he did in return for a receipt. When Wells also comes down with a fever, she describes it as malarial in kind. An old black nurse from New Orleans—a fact that characterizes her as a woman particularly experienced with yellow fever patients—puts her to bed and sweats her for four days until she recovers. The nurse was sent by Dr. Gray to take care of Wells's younger siblings after their parents' death. From Dr. Gray Wells also learns how much he had admired their father as "one of the best aids in helping to nurse, since he was cheerful and always inspired confidence. [...] Everyone liked him and missed him when he was gone" (Wells, *Crusade for Justice* 13).[136] From the old nurse Wells hears the rest of the story: "That Dr. Gray sure loved your pa." He had promised the nurse that she would be paid when sending her to the Wells's house "although no one was sick there" (Wells, *Crusade for Justice* 14). She closes her account by referencing Dr. Gray as "one good white man" (Wells, *Crusade for Justice* 14), and Wells does the same in her written words echoing the nurse's appraisal.

Compared to her autobiography, Wells's diary—which she began when she was twenty-five years old—represents a more intimate portrait of her life. It is particularly interesting with regard to how she refers—or does not refer—to the painful yellow fever experience. Throughout the diaries she hardly ever touches upon personal memories painful to her, such as the death of her brother Eddie or that of her paralyzed sister Eugenia. Yet in her first diary entry on December 29, 1885, she not only describes her trip to Rust University at Holly Springs to visit friends and former teachers, but she also visits the graves of her parents, who—with other yellow fever victims—were buried in Hillcrest Cemetery close to the Rust campus: "Visited the cemetery & found my father's and possibly my mother's grave, and was present at a burying. Came home very tired" (Wells, *Memphis Diary* 24). The reference is short and rather matter of fact. Yet Wells does not hide the fact that the experience at the cemetery strained her.

Wells's diary and her autobiography are unique documents that offer a rare personal glimpse into the realities and consequences of yellow fever in the late 1870s. In her autobiography, written from 1928 until her death in 1931, Wells primarily wanted to record her activities during the anti-lynching crusade with a focus on her public life from 1893 to 1927 (Duster xxx). Yet she begins her narrative by describing the yellow fever epidemic that changed the course of her life in early adulthood. The autobiography would not be Ida B. Wells's had she not taken the opportunity to also critically assess the events around the epidemic. The mayor of Holly Springs refuses to enforce a quarantine and thus—in Wells's opinion—invites yellow fever into the city. Wells also criticizes the white Irish nurse for prescribing the wrong treatment to her mother, and for trying to take advantage of them by searching for their father's money. The old black nurse serves Wells as a mother figure. Her experience is even valued by the white doctor, who

136 Jim Wells was a carpenter by trade who was politically active in the African American community as a Master mason and a trustee of Rust University. During the 1878 yellow fever epidemic he tended to victims and made coffins for those who died (DeCosta-Willis 7).

is an equal admirer of Jim Wells. Wells's critique is not framed in racial terms but in terms of community action: while she judges the behavior of the mayor and the nurse, she commends the old nurse and the doctor. That Wells is inspired by her father and aspires to emulate him becomes clear with the visit to the cemetery she describes in her diary. She not only visits her former teachers at Rust, but sets out from the University to look for the grave of her father's and possibly [her] mother's" (Wells, *Memphis Diary* 24)—the people and the experience that greatly affected the course of her life.

As diverse as the ethnic and racial relationships become in the course of the late eighteenth and throughout the nineteenth century, so diverse are the imagined and real places of yellow fever. Yellow fever and racism have been linked at least since the political debates of Mathew Carey, Absalom Jones and Richard Allen after the 1793 Philadelphia yellow fever epidemic. Beyond these texts, the many examples from sea stories, fictional renditions of New Orleans, and African American voices substantiate Samuel Otter's statement that "fever and race are yoked" (31) in much of U.S.-American fiction. That race is not limited to a simple black and white-binary is amply proven in the yellow fever texts that touch upon the themes of slavery, abolitionism, and immigration and feature African American as well as Irish American, German American, and Creole experiences with yellow fever.

A common trope used in the texts is the fever-stricken ship as "micro-political system in motion" (Gilroy 4) or "social microcosm" (McCarthy 409) that signifies the diseased American nation suffering under the ill practices of class distinction and slavery. We see this in Melville's *White Jacket* and *Redburn*, as well as in Sleeper's *Jack in the Forecastle*. A remedy is possible with an acceptance of the more heterogeneous makeup of U.S. society that is, in fact, a direct result of the slavery system. The same remedy of embracing hybridization is suggested in Edgar Allan Poe's *Narrative of Arthur Gordon Pym*, Melville's *Omoo*, and James Fenimore Cooper's *Jack Tier*.

Many of the narratives discussed use yellow fever and the fears surrounding the disease as an allegory for slavery and for racial fears, such as *The Narrative of Arthur Gordon Pym*, Melville's "Benito Cereno," James Fenimore Cooper's *Ned Myers*, George Washington Cable's *The Grandissimes*, and William Wells Brown's *Clotel*. A variation of this theme draws on the fact that the fear of diseases—and especially an unexplainable one like yellow fever—was something everybody understood, whereas particularly white Northerners were usually not threatened by slavery. Lydia Maria Child makes this point in her *Romance of the Republic*, in which she both demonstrates and compares the cruel separation of families by yellow fever and by slavery. While whites are most afraid of yellow fever in Cable's "Tite Poulette," blacks suffer under racial stigmatization.

Special aspects with regard to yellow fever and race were also brought up by several other writers discussed in this chapter: The French Souvestre presents an allegorical approach by linking yellow fever to existential fears in his novella "Mathieu Ropars." Yellow fever is horrifying because of its invisibility and location of origin in the West Indies and the Americas. While Cable returns to an older understanding of disease as divine retribution in "The Entomologist," his *Dr. Sevier* and Hearn's *Chita: A Memory of Last Island* turn away from a mere functionalization of the fever in metaphoric terms toward a naturalistic presentation which also weighs the influence of heredity and environment on it. Harper's *Iola Leroy* presents hybrid forms in African American community creation that actually go back to Allen and Jones. Dunbar-Nelson stresses the autonomy of a racialized subject who has suffered under yellow fever in "The Praline Woman." Ida B. Wells finally confronts her readers with the strength she gained from her experience with yellow fever framed in terms of community rather than race. With this, she also features as the most modern of the authors and points toward a post-racial society, yet not without disease.

6 Conclusion

I agree with Shirley Samuels who notes that "[t]o study the fiction of the nineteenth-century United States remains a practice full of discoveries" (*Reading the Novel* 151). The project of working with nineteenth-century fiction in the United States is open-ended. My wide and inclusive definition of yellow fever texts has pointed me to many previously critically disregarded texts, yet more texts in yet-to-be-digitized (and thus made more readily discoverable and searchable) magazines and newspapers will most certainly continue to appear. For these—yet to be recovered—texts *Yellow Fever Years* provides a matrix of how they may be grouped, analyzed and read together with other examples. My analysis of yellow fever texts under the lens of nation, gender, and race allowed for new assessments of epidemic threats and their fictional representations and new ways to read familiar novels as well as newly (re)discovered ones. Indeed, scrutinizing nineteenth-century fiction through the socio-political and biomedical lens of yellow fever discourse has enabled me to look at many of the canonized texts from a different angle and to make new discoveries. Fictional, non-fictional, and visual representations of yellow fever experiences and epidemic events are influential in the construction of medical and cultural knowledges of these phenomena. The metaphorical choices describing yellow fever epidemics in the texts additionally reveal anxieties of a more profound kind, such as social and political uncertainties, states of (perceived) crisis, and uncontrollable threats to the body politic. Between the Philadelphia yellow fever epidemic in 1793 and the devastating 1878 epidemic that gripped large portions of the South the United States had become a smaller place despite its continuous geographical expansion. The railroad and ships moved people and goods at ever faster speed, and the mosquitoes moved with the people. News reporting was revolutionized through wire cables. Illustrations could be produced more quickly with Frank Leslie's woodblock printing technique. Newspapers enabled people all over the nation to partake in the yellow fever experience from a safe distance. Advances in communication and transportation brought the epidemic that largely affected the Southern regions of the United States by the second half of the nineteenth century to the North and West.

Through my analyses I reach the following conclusions: First, a more stable nationhood and the formation of a national identity are achieved through the reporting and fictionalization of biomedical threats to the nation. The yellow fever discourse symbolically aligns the many suffering individual bodies with the disease-affected body politic. This can be seen in works such as those by

Charles Brockden Brown and in the writings that served him as blueprints for *Arthur Mervyn*, specifically Mathew Carey's *Short Account* and Absalom Jones and Richard Allen's *Narrative*. All three texts address questions of inclusion and exclusion from the national project by means of the representation of yellow fever. While also taken up by Charles Brockden Brown, Philip Freneau and Henry Wadsworth Longfellow critically approach the ideal of Agrarianism versus unhealthy city dwelling in their yellow fever poems. Catharine Maria Sedgwick implicitly references the nation's foundational documents by pointing out that the granting of freedom of religion that pertains to both sexes must lead to a more tolerant nation and society. Like *Arthur Mervyn*, S. Weir Mitchell's *The Red City* functionalizes yellow fever in Philadelphia as a metaphor for a nation in crisis, in his case the growing imperialist involvements of the United States at least since the events that led to the Spanish-American War (1898).

Second, medical and newspaper illustrations as well as photographic representations of yellow fever patients provide for a touristic or removed gaze upon the disease experience. The pictures convey other people's pain from a safe temporal or spatial distance. They generate a spectatorial self-consciousness of observing the Other, which may result in acts of benevolence or acts of self-protection, both of which are represented in specific examples. The yellow fever representations furthermore embody striking contradictions between an aestheticization of the abject and ethical questions that emerge from voyeuristic engagements with the suffering and dying. The frequent appropriation of the deathbed iconography uses women and children in particular and relies on the visual salience of bodies in agony. As witnesses to abjection and calamity, these pictures demand a political rather than an aesthetic response. What can be said about the visual representations is also applicable to popular nineteenth-century yellow fever texts. The graphic depictions of the painful yellow fever experience and reporting of sensationalist detail similarly satisfies voyeuristic enjoyment, but also—just like in the illustrations—stirs the capacity for empathy. This shows just how visualized fictional writing had become.

Third, *Yellow Fever Years* affirms the centrality of discourses of gender in the formation of nationhood in the nineteenth century in connection to crisis situations metaphorically represented as yellow fever threats. The disease functions as a metaphor for women's struggles for emancipation and equality. In Mary Floyd's novel *The Nereid* yellow fever enables the heroine to continue a professional occupation, even after her marriage. The two protagonists of Mollie E. M. Davis's novel *The Queen's Garden* are scarred from yellow fever; yet, their experience enables a marital relationship on equal terms. Wesley Bradshaw also puts forth a vision of female emancipation and of a medical profession that acknowledges the role of women. Elizabeth Stuart Phelps goes farthest in her yellow fever text by enabling a companionship across gender and social divisions and thus also symbolically healing the nation after the Civil War and Reconstruction. On many levels, discourses of gender intersect with those of race and are equally featured in the narratives.

Fourth and lastly, the intricate connection of yellow fever, racial relations, and racism as pivotal for defining the nation's future social makeup and cohesion has been moved into the center of cultural attention since the 1793 Philadelphia yellow fever epidemic. The yellow fever texts that are yoked to racial, ethnic and class issues and feature African American, Irish American, German American, and Creole characters employ allegorical strategies as well as positively focus on cross-racial and post-racial visions of community, society, and nation. The latter vision is particularly exemplified in such African American texts as Harper's *Iola Leroy* and Ida B. Wells's writings. More allegorical approaches introduce the fever-stricken ship as signifying the diseased American nation suffering from the aberration of the slave trade, or they use yellow fever and the fear of contagion as metaphor for slavery's aberrations.

Many yellow fever studies to date present historiographic analyses of very specific localities, such as Philadelphia in 1793, New Orleans in 1854, and Memphis in 1878. While these dates and places certainly play a major role in this book, I have tried to free myself from an approach relying merely on years and locales in order to look at the broader issues of the nineteenth century in connection with the medical crises yellow fever epidemics posed. With reference to the larger epidemiological connections and embeddedness of yellow fever into the Atlantic system in which it circulated, it needs to be noted that U.S. American, mainly Southern, ports "shared the microorganisms of Cuba, Vera Cruz, and Rio de Janeiro because their ships and people traveled frequently to and from these localities" (Humphreys, "Appendix II" 193). With regard to the fictional and visual productivity of the disease, *Yellow Fever Years* thus provides the typological groundwork for a broader hemispheric approach which connects perspectives and communities of the Caribbean, Central and South America, and the west coast of Africa. American studies practitioners, historians, and literary and cultural studies scholars will need to continue to engage in the field of empire studies in connection with epidemic diseases and to question medical imperialism with regard to issues of international public health. I agree with Margaret Humphreys, who declares: "yes, there is still much to be done on this fascinating and horrible disease" ("Appendix II" 195).

In face of the Zika virus circulating in about 30 countries since 2014 the United States National Institutes of Health investigate how virus infection affects reproduction, pregnancy and the developing fetus. The National Institutes of Health traces its roots to 1887 when it was part of the Marine Hospital Service. It was influential in facilitating Reed's discovery of the mosquito vector in the transmission of yellow fever in 1900. Historical fiction and the Hollywood film industry picked up on Reed's Cuba experiments and featured it as a success story of American medicine in the early 1930s (De Kruif; Howard and De Kruif). Yet Walter Reed's contribution was never acknowledged on the level of his medical excellence. He never received a Nobel Prize for his finding because he died in 1902, and Alfred Nobel had stipulated that the prize was not to be awarded posthumously. Efforts to have the prize awarded to Carlos Finlay in subsequent years were futile. Finlay first suggested the presence of a mosquito vector, tried unsuccessfully to prove it in several experimental studies and later worked with Walter Reed. For his work in proving yellow fever to be a viral disease and for subsequently producing a successful yellow fever vaccine in 1937, Max Theiler received the Nobel Prize in 1951. Theiler's and Hugh Smith's 17-D vaccine actually helped the United States win World War II because it immunized U.S. American soldiers against the disease; particularly those fighting in the North African war zones benefited (Frierson). Reed and his colleague William C. Gorgas, who was influential in abating the transmission of yellow fever in the Panama Canal region by controlling mosquitoes, were elected to the New York University Hall of Fame of Great Americans. The semicircular neo-classical arc that originated in 1900 includes 102 bronze portrait busts from Alexander Graham Bell to Eli Whitney. It stands as a U.S.-American version of the German Walhalla hall of fame, which was conceived in 1807 by Crown Prince Ludwig and was erected near Regensburg. The inclusion of Reed and Gorgas in the Hall of Great Americans testifies to the continued significance of an imperial power of interpretation over epidemic disease displayed in such public works of memorial architecture. That yellow fever was a continuous presence in the minds and the imagination of Americans is reflected in the many fictional and non-fictional texts that refer to it since its first major manifestation in the United States in 1793. They anchor it within an American storehouse of yellow fever memory that continues to be tapped to this day.

Fig. 30. Hall of Fame of Great Americans. Bronx Community College. Photo by H0n0r. Wikimedia Commons. Web.

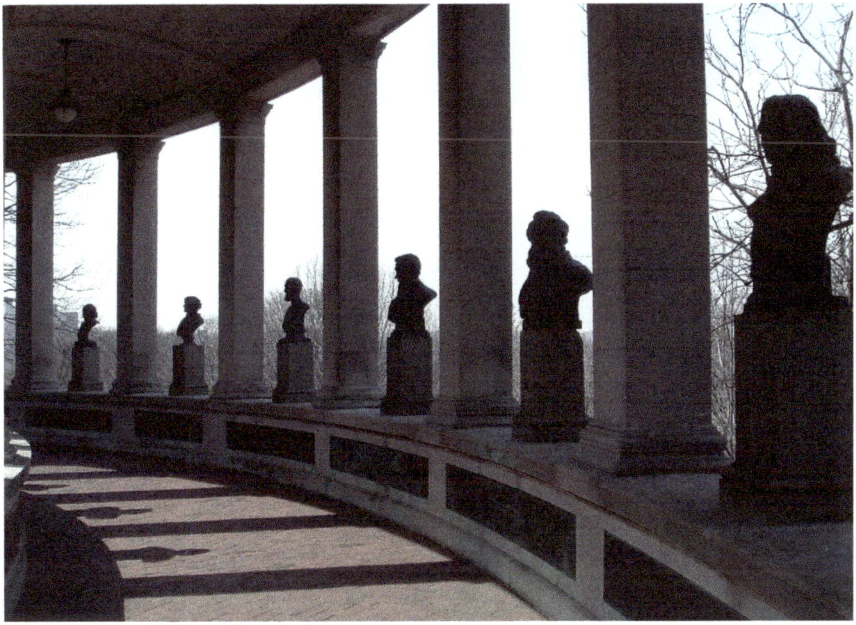

7 Bibliography

7.1 Yellow Fever Fiction, Poetry, and Drama 1793–1916

Abbot, Belle K., *Leah Mordecai* (1875)

Adams, F. Colburn, *An Outcast, or, Virtue and Faith* (1861)

Adams, F. Colburn, *Justice in the By-Ways* (1856)

Adams, F. Colburn, *Manuel Pereira, or, The Sovereign Rule of South Carolina* (1853)

Adams, Nehemiah, *The Sable Cloud* (1861)

Allen, Richard, and Absalom Jones, *A Narrative of the Proceedings of the Black People during the Late Awful Calamity in Philadelphia in the Year 1793* (1794)

Anon. (A Lady), *Alice Granger* (1852)

Anon., *Arrest, Confession and Suicide of Almira Cathcart …* (1869)

Anon., *Julia Tremaine* (1855)

Anon., *Nepenthe* (1864)

Anon., *Old Haun, the Pawnbroker, or, The Orphan's Legacy* (1857)

Anon., *Quest* (1864)

Anon., *Sea Stories* (1858)

Anon., *Swell Life at Sea, or, Fun, Frigates and Yachting* (1854)

Anon., *The Old Pine Farm, or, The Southern Side* (1859)

Anon., *The Recorded Will, or, Truth and Not Fiction* (1855)

Anon., *The Sisters of Orleans* (1871)

Armstrong, George D., *The Summer of the Pestilence: A History of the Ravages of the Yellow Fever in Norfolk, Virginia, A.D. 1855* (1856)

Arthur, T. S., *Cast Adrift* (1873)

Arthur, T. S., *Danger, or, Wounded in the House of a Friend* (1875)

Arthur, T. S., *The Mother's Rule, or, The Right Way and the Wrong Way* (1856)

Arthur, T. S., *The Way to Prosper, or, In Union There Is Strength* (1851)

Avery, Samuel Putnam, *Mrs. Partington's Carpet-bag of Fun* (1854)

Baker, William M., *Inside: a Chronicle of Secession* (1866)

Baldwin, Joseph G., *The Flush Times of Alabama and Mississippi* (1853)

Barclay, George Lippard, *"Little Cuba," or, Circumstantial Evidence* (1873)

Barker, Benjamin, *The Bandit of the Ocean, or, The Female Privateer* (1855)

Barnes, Euphemia, *Ellen Durand* (1855)

Bartlett, Napier, *Clarimonde* (1863)

Beckwith, J. R., *The Winthrops* (1864)

Bowen, Sue Petigru, *Busy Moments of an Idle Woman* (1854)

Brackenridge, Hugh Henry, *Modern Chivalry* (1804–1815)

Bradbury, Osgood, *Ellen Grant, or, Fashionable Life in New-York* (185?)

Bradshaw, Wesley, *Angel Agnes, or, The Heroine of the Yellow Fever Plague in Shreveport* (1873)

Bradshaw, Wesley, *Mattie Stephenson: The Sweet Young Martyr of Memphis* (1873)

Bristed, Charles Astor, *The Upper Ten Thousand* (1852)

Brown, Charles Brockden, *Arthur Mervyn, or, Memoirs of the Year 1793* (1799/1800)

Brown, Thurlow W., *Why I Am a Temperance Man* (1853)

Brown, William Wells, *Clotel, or, The President's Daughter: A Narrative of Slave Life in the United States* (1853)

Brown, William Wells, *Clotelle, or, The Colored Heroine* (1867)

Brown, William Wells, *Clotelle: A Tale of the Southern States* (1864)

Brown, William Wells, *The Escape; or, A Leap for Freedom* (1858)

Bruce, E. M., *The Sun-beam* (1863)

Buckingham, Emma May, *A Self-made Woman, or, Mary Idyl's Trials and Triumphs* (1873)

Bullard, A. T. J., *Love Affairs in Our Village Twenty Years* Ago (1852)

Bullard, A. T. J., *Matrimony, or, Love Affairs in Our Village Twenty Years Ago* (1853)

Bunkley, Josephine M., *The Testimony of an Escaped Novice From the Sisterhood of St. Joseph, Emmettsburg, Maryland* (1855)

Buntline, Ned, *Clarence Rhett, or, The Cruise of a Privateer* (1866)

Buntline, Ned, *Ella Adams, or, The Demon of Fire* (1862)

Buntline, Ned, *Magdalena, the Outcast, or, The Millionaire's Daughter* (1866)

Butt, Martha Haines, *The Leisure Moments of Miss Martha Haines Butt, A.M.* (1860)

Cable, George Washington, "The Entomologist" (1899)

Cable, George Washington, "Tite Poulette" ((1879, 1883))

Cable, George Washington, *The Creoles of Louisiana* (1884)

Cable, George Washington, *The Grandissimes: A Story of Creole Life* (1880)

Caldwell, John H., *The Mysterious Messenger* (1860)

Cannon, Charles James, *Bickerton, or, The Immigrant's Daughter* (1855)

Cannon, Charles James, *Ravellings from the Web of Life* (1855)

Carey, Matthew, *A Short Account of the Malignant Fever, Lately Prevalent in Philadelphia* (1793)

Catherwood, Mary Hartwell, *A Woman in Armor* (1875)

Challen, James, *Frank Elliott, or, Wells in the Desert* (1859)

Child, Lydia Maria Francis, *A Romance of the Republic* (1867)

Cleveland, Cecilia Pauline, *The Story of a Summer, or, Journal Leaves from Chappaqua* (1874)

Cooper, James Fenimore, *Elinor Wyllys; or, The Young Folk at Longbridge, A Tale* (1846)

Cooper, James Fenimore, *Jack Tier* (1848)

Cooper, James Fenimore, *Ned Myers; or, A Life before the Mast* (1843)

Cooper, James Fenimore, *The Two Admirals* (1842)

Cooper, James Fenimore, *The Wing-and-Wing; or, Le Feu-Follett* (1842)

Cooper, James Fenimore, *Wept of Wish Ton-Wish* (1829)

Cornwallis, Kinahan, *Pilgrims of Fashion* (1862)

Cowdin, V. G., *Ellen, or, The Fanatic's Daughter* (1860)

Crozier, R. H., *The Confederate Spy* (1866)

Davis, Andrew Jackson, *Tale of a Physician, or, The Seeds and Fruits of Crime* (1869)

Davis, Mollie E. M., *The Queen's Garden* (1900)

Davis, Rebecca Harding, *Margret Howth* (1862)

Davis, Richard Harding, *The Dictator* (1904; 1909)

De Forest, John William, *Miss Ravenel's Conversion from Secession to Loyalty* (1867)

Denison, Mary A., *Led to the Light* (1867)

Denison, Mary A., *Out of Prison* (1864)

Derby, George Horatio, *The Squibob Papers* (1865)

Dickens, Charles, *Life and Adventures of Martin Chuzzlewit* (1843)

Dixon, Edward H., *Scenes in the Practice of a New York Surgeon* (1855)

Doesticks, Q. K. Philander, *Doesticks, What He Says* (1855)

Dorsey, Sarah A., *Agnes Graham* (1869)

Dorsey, Sarah A., *Lucia Dare* (1867)

Dugan, James, *Doctor Dispachemquic: A Story of the Great Southern Plague of 1878* (1879)

Dupuy, Eliza A., *Emma Walton, or, Trials and Triumph* (1854)

Dupuy, Eliza A., *The Discarded Wife, or, Will She Succeed* (1875)
Eggleston, George Cary, *A Man of Honor* (1873)
Elliot, Samuel H., *New England's Chattels, or, Life in the Northern Poor-House* (1858)
Evans, Augusta J., *Beulah* (1859)
Fabens, Joseph Warren, *In the Tropics* (1863)
Falconbridge, *The Humors of Falconbridge* (1856)
Fern, Fanny, *Fresh Leaves* (1857)
Fern, Fanny, *Rose Clark* (1856)
Field, Margaret, *Bertha Percy, or, L'Espérance* (1860)
Fleming, May Agnes, *A Wonderful Woman* (1873)
Fleming, May Agnes, *Eulalie, or, The Wife's Tragedy* (1866)
Floyd, Mary Faith, *The Nereid* (1871)
Foxton, E., *Agnes Wentworth* (1869)
Foxton, E., *Herman, or, Young Knighthood* (1866)
Freeman, Theresa J., *Silver Lake, or, The Belle of Bayou Luie* (1867)
Freneau, Philip, "Pestilence: Written during the Prevalence of a Yellow Fever" (1793)
Furber, George C., *Ike McCandliss, and Other Stories, or, Incidents in the Life of a Soldier* (1852)
Gayarré, Charles, *Fernando de Lemos* (1872)
Giles, Daphne S., *Half-past Ten* (1860)
Goodwin, Hannah Bradbury, *Madge, or, Night and Morning* (1863)
Gordon, Clarence, *Christmas at Under-Tor* (1864)
Greene, Talbot, *American Nights' Entertainments* (1860)
Gringo, Harry, *Captain Brand of the "Centipede"* (1864)
Gringo, Harry, *Tales for the Marines* (1855)
Haco, Dion, *Dr. Blackburn: The Yellow Fever Fiend* (1866)
Hale, Edward Everett, *His Level Best, and Other Stories* (1873)
Hale, Sarah Josepha Buell, *Traits of American Life...* (1835)
Hall, Baynard Rush, *Something for Every Body: Gleaned in the Old Purchase, from Fields Often Reaped, by Robert Carlton* (1846)
Hall, Baynard Rush, *The New Purchase, or, Seven and a Half Years in the Far West, by Robert Carlton* (1843)
Hall, James, *Legends of the West...* (1832)

Hammett, Samuel Adams, *Piney Woods Tavern, or, Sam Slick in Texas* (1858)
Harland, Marion, *Miriam* (1862)
Harland, Marion, *The Hidden Path* (1855)
Hay, John, *Not Pretty, but Precious* (1872)
Hazel, Harry, *Marie, or, The Gambler of the Mississippi* (18--)
Hazel, Harry, *The Smuggler King! or, The Rovers of the Antilles* (1855)
Hazel, Harry, *Virginia Graham* (1867)
Hearn, Lafcadio, *Chita: A Memory of Last Island* (1889)
Hentz, Caroline Lee, *Rena, or, The Snow Bird* (1851)
Hentz, Caroline Lee, *The Victim of Excitement* (1853)
Hiatt, James M., *The Test of Loyalty* (1864)
Hicks, Rebecca, *The Milliner and the Millionaire* (1852)
Hildreth, Richard, *The White Slave, or, Memoirs of a Fugitive…* (1852)
Hill, L. C., *Laure: The History of a Blighted Life* (1869)
Holmes, Mary Jane, *Rose Mather* (1868)
Holmes, Mary Jane, *Tempest and Sunshine, or, Life in Kentucky* (1854)
Holmes, Mary Jane, *The Homestead on the Hillside* (1856)
Holt, John Saunders, *What I Know About Ben Eccles* (1869)
Hunt, Sara Keables, *The Brook, and The Tide Turning* (1875)
Huntington, J. V., *Alban* (1851)
Huntington, J. V., *The Forest* (1852)
Illinoian, *The Heart of the West: An American Story* (1871)
Ingersoll, Justine, "The Commodore" (1898)
Ingraham, Joseph Holt, *Blanche Talbot; or, The Maiden's Hand. A Romance of the War of 1812* (1847)
Ingraham, Joseph Holt, *The Odd Fellow; or, The Secret Association, and Foraging Peter* (1846)
Ingraham, Joseph Holt, *The South-West, by a Yankee* (1835)
Irving, Thomas J., *In the Rapids* (1871)
Irving, Washington, *A History of New York, from the Beginning of the World to the End of the Dutch Dynasty* (1809)
Irving, Washington, *The Beauties of Washington Irving…* (1835)
Jackson, Helen Hunt, *Saxe Holm's Stories* (1874)
Jay, W. M. L., *Holden with the Cords* (1874)

Johnson, Virginia W., *Joseph the Jew* (1874)

Johnston, Maria I., *The Siege of Vicksburg* (1869)

Keener, John C., *Post-oak Circuit* (1857)

Kelvin, Kit, *Kit Kelvin's Kernels* (1860)

Leslie, Eliza, *The Dennings and Their Beaux, and Alina Derlay…* (1851)

Leslie, Eliza, *The Maid of Canal Street, and the Bloxhams* (1851)

Lever, Charles, "A Day's Ride: A Life's Romance" (1860)

Lippard, George, *Memoirs of a Preacher: A Revelation of the Church and the Home* (1849)

Lippard, George, *Paul Ardenheim, the Monk of Wissahikon* (1848)

Locke, David Ross, *Eastern Fruit On Western Dishes; The Morals of Abou Ben Adhem* (1875)

Locke, David Ross, *Ekkoes from Kentucky* (1875)

Locke, David Ross, *The Struggles (Social, Financial and Political) of Petroleum V. Nasby* (1872)

Longfellow, Henry Wadsworth, "Evangeline: A Tale of Acadie" (1847)

Lunt, George, *Eastford, or, Household Sketches* (1855)

MacLeod, Xavier Donald, *The Bloodstone* (1853)

Maitland, James A., *The Cabin Boy's Story* (1854)

Maitland, James A., *The Wanderer* (1856)

Massett, Stephen C., *Drifting About, or, What "Jeems Pipes, of Pipesville" Saw-and-Did* (1863)

Mayfield, Millie, *Carrie Harrington, or, Scenes in New Orleans* (1857)

McAlpine, Emily Eliza Jours, *Doings in Maryland, or Matilda Douglas* (1871)

McConnel, John Ludlum, *The Glenns* (1851)

McElgun, John, *Annie Reilly, or, the Fortunes of an Irish Girl in New York* (1873)

Meeker, Nathan Cook, *Life and Adventures of Capt. Jacob D. Armstrong* (1852)

Meeker, Nathan Cook, *Life in the West, or, Stories of the Mississippi Valley* (1868)

Melville, Herman, "Benito Cereno" (1855, 1856)

Melville, Herman, *Omoo* (1847)

Melville, Herman, *Redburn* (1849)

Melville, Herman, *The Piazza Tales* (1856)

Melville, Herman, *White Jacket* (1850)

Mitchell, S. Weir, *The Red City* (1907)

Montgomery, Cora, *Eagle Pass, or, Life on the Border* (1852)
Morris, John, *Wanderings of a Vagabond* (1873)
Neal, John, *Authorship: A Tale* (1830)
Neal, John, *Errata; or, The Works of Will. Adams* (1823)
Neal, John, *Randolph: A Novel* (1823)
Neal, John, *The Down-Easters* (1833)
Newell, R. H., *The Cloven Foot* (1870)
Oliver, Optic, *Hatchie, the Guardian Slave, or, The Heiress of Bellevue* (1853)
Osborne, Elise, *Life and Its Aims* (1854)
Parker, Helen F., *Sunrise and Sunset* (1854)
Paulding, James Kirke, *John Bull in America; or, The New Munchausen* (1825)
Paulding, James Kirke, *Tales of the Good Woman. By a Doubtful Gentleman…* (1829)
Payson, George, *Golden Dreams and Leaden Realities* (1853)
Peacocke, James S., *The Creole Orphans, or, Lights and Shadows of Southern Life* (1856)
Peck, William H., *The Confederate Flag on the Ocean* (1868)
Peterson, Charles J., *The Old Stone Mansion* (1859)
Phelps, Elizabeth Stuart, "Zerviah Hope (1880)
Philadelphia Relief Committee, *Report of the Philadelphia Relief Committee, Appointed to Collect Funds for the Sufferers by Yellow Fever, at Norfolk & Portsmouth, Va., 1855* (1856)
Pinckard, M. E., *Bread of Heaven and Husks of Swine, or, The Curse of Jealousy* (1874)
Poe, Edgar Allan, "The Masque of the Red Death" (1842)
Poe, Edgar Allan, *The Narrative of Arthur Gordon Pym of Nantucket* (1838)
Potter, Eliza, *A Hairdresser's Experience in High Life* (1859)
Powell, Thomas, *Chit-chat of Humor, Wit and Anecdote* (1857)
Quad, M., *Quad's Odds: Anecdote, Humor and Pathos, and Other Things* (1875)
Quincy, Edmund, *Wensley* (1854)
Rees, James, *The Tinker Spy* (1855)
Reizenstein, Ludwig Baron von, *The Mysteries of New Orleans (Die Geheimnisse von New Orleans)* (1854–1855)
Remington, E. F., *The City of Sin and Its Capture by Immanuel's Army* (1857)
Richards, A. M., *Memories of a Grandmother* (1854)

Richards, A., *Zilla Fitz James, the Female Bandit of the South-West, or, The Horrible, Mysterious and Awful Disclosures in the Life of the Creole Murderess, Zilla Fitz James…* (1852)

Ritchie, Anna Cora Ogden Mowatt, *The Clergyman's Wife* (1867)

Roath, David L., *The Five Love Adventures of Solomon Slug* (1852)

Robinson, John Hovey, *Catholina, or, the Niche in the Wall* (1861)

Robinson, Solon, *Hot Corn* (1854)

Robinson, Solon, *Me-Won-I-Toc* (1867)

Robinson, William L., *The Diary of a Samaritan* (1860)

Roe, A. S., *Like and Unlike* (1862)

Roe, A. S., *The Cloud on the Heart* (1869)

Rush, Caroline E., *Way-marks in the Life of a Wanderer* (1855?)

Sargent, Epes, *Peculiar* (1864)

Schiller, Edward, *Cherry Blossom; or, "Love Thy Neighbor as Thyself"* (1860)

Schoolcraft, Henry R., *The Black Gauntlet* (1860)

Sealsfield, Charles, *Frontier Life, or, Scenes and Adventures in the South West* (1853)

Searson, John, "Mount Vernon, a poem…" (1800)

Sedgwick, Catharine Maria, *A New-England Tale, or, Sketches of New-England Character and Manners…* (1822)

Sedgwick, Catharine Maria, *Redwood: A Tale* (1824)

Sheppard, F. H., *Love Afloat* (1875)

Shillaber, B. P., *Life and Sayings of Mrs. Partington and Others of the Family* (1854)

Silvervale, Lumina, *An Orphan of the Old Dominion* (1873)

Simmons, J. F., *The Welded Link and Other Poems* (1881)

Simms, William Gilmore, "Paddy McGann; or, The Demon of the Stump" (1863)

Simms, William Gilmore, *Border Beagles: A Tale of Mississippi, Volume 1 and Volume 2* (1840)

Simms, William Gilmore, *Katharine Walton, or, The Rebel of Dorchester* (1851)

Simms, William Gilmore, *Southward Ho!* (1854)

Sleeper, John Sherburne, *Jack in the Forecastle, or, Incidents in the Early Life of Hawser Martingale* (1860)

Smith, Elizabeth Oakes Prince, *The Newsboy* (1854)

Smith, F. Irene Burge, *Nina, or, Life's Caprices* (1861)

Smith, Tom Washington, *The Bridle on the Heart, or, Pictures from Life* (1860)

Son of the Ocean, *A Home on the Deep, or, The Mariner's Trials on the Dark Blue Sea* (1857)

Soper, T. N., *Green Bluff: A Temperance Story* (1874)

Southworth, E.D.E.N., *The Haunted Homestead* (1860)

Southworth, E.D.E.N., *The Missing Bride, or, Miriam the Avenger* (1855)

Southworth, E.D.E.N., *The Spectre Lover* (1875)

Souvestre, Émile, "Mathieu Ropars" (1868)

Souvestre, Émile, *The Isle of the Dead, or, The Keeper of the Lazaretto: A Tale of the Yellow Fever* (1863)

Stephens, Ann Sophia, *Bertha's Engagement* (1875)

Stimson, A. L., *Waifwood* (1864)

Stowe, Harriet Beecher, *The Minister's Wooing* (1859)

Stowe, Harriet Beecher, *Uncle Tom's Cabin, or, Life Among the Lowly* (1852)

Summerton, Winter, *Will He Find Her? A Romance of New York and New Orleans* (1860)

Thomas, Frederick W., *John Randolph of Roanoke* (1853)

Thomes, William Henry, *A Slaver's Adventures on Land and Sea* (1872)

Thomes, William Henry, *The Gold Hunters' Adventures, or, Life in Australia* (1864)

Throop, George Higby, *Bertie, or, Life in the Old Field* (1851)

Towles, Catharine Webb Barber, *Stories for the American Freemason's Fireside* (1868)

Townsend, George Alfred, *Lost Abroad…* (1870)

Townsend, Virginia F., *The Battle-fields of Our Fathers* (1864)

Tracy, A., *Dear Little Marchioness: The Story of a Child's Faith and Love* (1895)

Trevor, Roland, *Roland Trevor, or, The Pilot of Human Life* (1853)

Trusta, H., *The Tell-tale, or, Home Secrets Told by Old Travellers* (1853)

Tuthill, Louisa C., *Reality, or, The Millionaire's Daughter* (1856)

von Kleist, Heinrich, *Die Verlobung in St. Domingo* (1811)

Wakeman, Joel, *The Mysterious Parchment; or, The Satanic License* (1853)

Walworth, Jeannette H., *Dead Men's Shoes* (1872)

Ward, Artemus, *Artemus Ward in London* (1867)

Ward, Artemus, *Sandwiches* (1870)

Warner, Susan, *Daisy* (1868–1869)

Warner, Susan, *The Hills of the Shatemuc* (1856)

Wells, Ida B., *The Autobiography of Ida B. Wells* (1928–31, 1970)
Whitaker, Mary Scrimzeour Furman, *Albert Hastings* (1868)
Whitney, Adeline Dutton Train, *The Gayworthys* (1865)
Williamson, Roland, "Uncle Phil" (1916)
Wilson, Harriet E., *Our Nig, or, Sketches from the Life of a Free Black in a Two-story White House, North* (1859)
Wise, H. A., "Captain Brand, of the Schooner 'Centipede': A Pirate of Eminence in the West Indies" (1860)
Wright, Julia McNair, *Secrets of the Convent and Confessional* (1872)

7.2 Yellow Fever Fiction of the Late Twentieth and Twenty-First Century

Anderson, Laurie Halse, *Fever, 1793* (2000)
Armstrong, Sally, *The Nine Lives of Charlotte Taylor* (2007)
Brown, Diana, *The Hand of a Woman* (1984)
Buckey, Sarah, *Marie-Grace and the Orphans* (2011)
Buckey, Sarah, *Marie-Grace Makes a Difference* (2011)
Dacus, Kaye, *Ransome's Crossing* (2010)
Fleischman, *Paul, Path of the Pale Horse* (1983)
Forney, Melissa, *The Astonishing Journey of Teddy Bodain* (2009)
Hicks, Robert, *A Separate Country* (2009)
Kohl, Susan, *The Ghost of Gracie Mansion* (1999)
Myers, Anna, *Graveyard Girl* (1995)
Patrick, Denise, *Cécile's Gift* (2011)
Patrick, Denise, *Troubles for Cécile* (2011)
Russell, Josh, *Yellow Jack* (1999)
Thoene, Bodie, *Winds of Promise* (1997)
Waring, William, *Yellow Fever: The Slave's Revenge* (1994)
Wideman, John Edgar, "Fever"
Wideman, John Edgar, *The Cattle Killing* (1996)

8 Works Cited

Allen, Richard, and Absalom Jones. *A Narrative of the Proceedings of the Black People, During the Late Awful Calamity in Philadelphia, in the Year 1793*. Philadelphia: William W. Woodward, 1794. Print.

American Anxieties. Spec. issue of *aspeers* 7 (2014). Web. 7 Mar. 2016.

Ammons, Elizabeth. "Gender and Fiction." *The Columbia History of the American Novel*. Ed. Emory Elliott and Cathy N. Davidson. New York: Columbia UP, 1991. 267–84. Print.

"Ancient and Modern Plagues." *Frank Leslie's Illustrated Newspaper* 13 Oct. 1888: 146. Print.

Anderson, Benedict R. *Imagined Communities: Reflections on the Origin and Spread of Nationalism*. Rev. and extended. London: Verso, 1983. Print.

Anderson, Laurie. *Fever, 1793*. New York: Simon & Schuster, 2000. Print.

Arejula, Juan Manuel de. *Breve descripcion de la fiebre amarilla padecida en Cadiz y pueblos comarcanos en 1800, en Medinasidonia en 1801, en Malaga en 1803 y en esta misma plaza y otras del Reyno en 1804*. Madrid: Imprenta Real, 1806. Print.

Armstrong, George D. *The Summer of the Pestilence: A History of the Ravages of the Yellow Fever in Norfolk, Virginia, A.D. 1855*. Philadelphia: J.B. Lippincott, 1856. Print.

Armstrong, Sally. *The Nine Lives of Charlotte Taylor*. Toronto: Vintage Canada, 2007. Print.

Arner, Katherine. "Making Yellow Fever American: The Early American Republic, the British Empire and the Geopolitics of Disease in the Atlantic World." *Atlantic Studies* 7.4 (2010): 447–71. Print.

Baker, T. Hart. "Yellowjack: The Yellow Fever Epidemic of 1878 in Memphis, Tennessee." *Bulletin of the History of Medicine* 42 (1968): 241–64. Print.

Bakhtin, Mikhail. *The Dialogic Imagination: Four Essays*. Austin: U of Texas P, 1992. Print.

Banerjee, Mita. "Civilizational Critique in Herman Melville's *Typee*, *Omoo*, and *Mardi*." *Amerikastudien / American Studies* 48.2 (2003): 207–25.

—. *Ethnic Ventriloquism: Literary Minstrelsy in Nineteenth-Century American Literature*. Vol. 159. Heidelberg: Winter, 2008. Print. American Studies—A Monograph Series.

Barnard, Philip, and Stephen Shapiro. "Related Texts." *Arthur Mervyn, or, Memoirs of the Year 1793, with Related Texts*. Ed. Philip Barnard and Stephen Shapiro. Indianapolis: Hackett, 2008. 331–426. Print.

Barnett, Elizabeth D. "Yellow Fever: Epidemiology and Prevention." *Clinical Infectious Diseases* 44.6 (2007): 850–56. *cid.oxfordjournals.org*. Web. 27 July 2013.

Barthes, Roland. *Image, Music, Text*. 1977. Trans. Stephen Heath. New York: Hill and Wang, 1996. Print.

Baym, Nina. *American Women Writers and the Work of History, 1790–1860*. New Brunswick, NJ: Rutgers UP, 1995. Print.

—. *Woman's Fiction: A Guide to Novels by and About Women in America, 1820–70*. 2nd ed., with new introd. and suppl. bibliography. Urbana: U of Illinois P, 1993. Print.

Beecher, Catherine E. "How to Redeem the Woman's Profession." *Harpers New Monthly Magazine* 31 (1865): 710–15. Print.

Bell, Andrew McIlwaine. *Mosquito Soldiers: Malaria, Yellow Fever, and the Course of the American Civil War*. Baton Rouge: Louisiana State UP, 2010. Print.

Bennett, Paula, ed. *Nineteenth-Century American Women Poets: An Anthology*. Malden, MA: Blackwell, 1998. Print. Blackwell Anthologies.

Bercovitch, Sacvan. *The Office of the Scarlet Letter*. Baltimore, MD: Johns Hopkins UP, 1991. Print. Parallax: Re-Visions of Culture and Society.

Berlant, Lauren Gail. *The Anatomy of National Fantasy: Hawthorne, Utopia, and Everyday Life*. U of Chicago P, 1991. Print.

Birkle, Carmen. "Infecting the City Upon a Hill: American Plague Narratives." European Association of American Studies: "E Pluribus Unum" or "E Pluribus Plura"? Oslo. 2008.

—. *Literature and Medicine*. 2011. Conference Proposal. Marburg.

—. "Saving the Circum-Atlantic World: Transnational (American) Memories in Julia Alvarez's Disease Narrative." *Media and Cultural Memory/Medien und Kulturelle Erinnerung*. Ed. Udo J. Hebel. Berlin: de Gruyter, 2009. 59–78.

—. "Traveling Nurses: Mary Seacole and the Nightingale Encounter: A Transatlantic Story." *"The Sea Is History": Exploring the Atlantic*. Ed. Carmen Birkle and Nicole Waller. Vol. 177. Heidelberg: Winter, 2009. 99–122. Print. American Studies—A Monograph Series.

Blair, Sara. "The Photograph's Last Word: Visual Culture Studies Now." *American Literary History* 22.3 (2010): 673–97. Print.

Blane, Gilbert. *Select Dissertations on Several Subjects of Medical Science*. London: Thomas and George Underwood, 1822. Print.

Bloom, Khaled J. *The Mississippi Valley's Great Yellow Fever Epidemic of 1878.* Baton Rouge: Louisiana State UP, 1993. Print.

Boelhower, William. "The Rise of the New Atlantic Studies Matrix." *American Literary History* 20.1–2 (2008): 83–101. Print.

Booss, John, and Marilyn J. August. *To Catch a Virus*. Washington, DC: ASM Press, 2013. Print.

Boudreau, Kristin. *Sympathy in American Literature: American Sentiments from Jefferson to the Jameses*. Gainesville: UP of Florida, 2002. Print.

Bradshaw, Wesley. *Angel Agnes, or, The Heroine of the Yellow Fever Plague in Shreveport*. Philadelphia: Old Franklin Publishing House, 1873. Print.

—. *Mattie Stephenson: The Sweet Young Martyr of Memphis*. Philadelphia: Old Franklin Publishing House, 1873. Print.

—. *The Volunteer Nurse! The Lovely Young Martyrs of Memphis, Grenada, New Orleans, Shreveport! The Yellow Fever Plague in the South! Being the Romantic, Heart-Touching History of Two Lovely Young Ladies*. Philadelphia: Old Franklin Publishing House, 1878. Print.

Brady, Patricia. "Mollie Moore Davis: A Literary Life." *Louisiana Women Writers: New Essays and a Comprehensive Bibliography*. Ed. Dorothy H. Brown and Barbara C. Ewell. Baton Rouge: Louisiana State UP, 1992. 99–118. Print.

Brandt, Allan M. "Behavior, Disease, and Health in the Twentieth-Century United States: The Moral Valence of Individual Risk." *Morality and Health*. Ed. Allan M. Brandt and Paul Rozin. New York: Routledge, 1997. 53–77. Print.

Brandt, Stefan L. "Exploring the 'Heart of the Wilderness': Cultural Self-Fashioning and the Aesthetics of the Body in Charles Brockden Brown's *Edgar Huntly*, or, *Memoirs of a Sleep-Walker*." *Making National Bodies: Cultural Identity and the Politics of the Body in (Post-)Revolutionary America*. Ed. Stefan L. Brandt and Astrid M. Fellner. Vol. 38. Trier: WVT, 2010. 133–52. Print. Mosaic.

Brandt, Stefan L., and Astrid M. Fellner. "Introduction: Making the Body, Making America." *Making National Bodies: Cultural Identity and the Politics of the Body in (Post-)Revolutionary America*. Vol. 38. Trier: WVT, 2010. 1–6. Print. Mosaic.

Braxton, Joanne M. "Crusader for Justice: Ida B. Wells." *African American Autobiography: A Collection of Critical Essays*. Ed. William L. Andrews. Englewood Cliffs: Prentice Hall, 1993. 90–112. Print. New Century Views.

Brooks, Joanna. *American Lazarus: Religion and the Rise of African American and Native American Literatures*. Oxford: Oxford UP, 2003. Print.

Brown, Charles Brockden. *An Address to the Government of the United States, on the Cession of Louisiana to the French and on the Late Breach of Treaty by the Spaniards Including the Translation of a Memorial, on the War of St. Domingo, and Cession of the Missisippi [i.e., Mississippi] to France, Drawn up by a French*

Counsellor of State. New ed., rev., corrected and improved. Philadelphia: John Conrad & Co., 1803. Early American Imprints 2nd Ser. No. 3880.

—. *Arthur Mervyn, oder, die Pest in Philadelphia: Denkwürdigkeiten aus dem Jahre 1793*. Leipzig: Christian Ernst Kollmann, 1859. Print.

—. *Arthur Mervyn, or, Memoirs of the Year 1793, with Related Texts*. Ed. Philip Barnard and Stephen Shapiro. Indianapolis: Hackett, 2008. Print.

Brown, Diana. *The Hand of a Woman*. New York: St. Martin's, 1984. Print.

Brown Elspeth H. "Affect, Empire and Photography." Roundtable Abstract. American Studies Association Annual Meeting, Puerto Rico, 17 Nov. 2012. Web. 3 Mar. 2013.

—. and Thy Phu, eds. *Feeling Photography*. Durham, NC: Duke UP, 2014. Print.

Brown, JoAnne. "Purity and Danger in Colour: Notes on Germ Theory and the Semantics of Segregation, 1895–1915." *Heredity and Infection: The History of Disease Transmission*. Ed. Jean-Paul Gaudillière and Ilana Löwy. London: Routledge, 2001. 101–32. Print.

Brown, William Wells. *Clotel; or, The President's Daughter: A Narrative of Slave Life in the United States*. London: Partridge & Oakey, 1853. Print.

—. *The Escape, or A Leap for Freedom. The Roots of African American Drama: An Anthology of Early Plays, 1858–1938*. Ed. Leo Hamalian. Detroit, MI: Wayne State UP, 1992. 42–95. Print.

Bryan, Violet Harrington. *The Myth of New Orleans in Literature: Dialogues of Race and Gender*. Knoxville: U of Tennessee P, 1993. Print.

Buckey, Sarah. *Marie-Grace and the Orphans*. Middleton, WI: American Girl, 2011. Print.

—. *Marie-Grace Makes a Difference*. Middleton, WI: American Girl, 2011. Print.

Burke, Edmund. *A Philosophical Enquiry into the Origin of Our Ideas of the Sublime and Beautiful*. London: Printed for R. and J. Dodsley, 1757. Print.

Burke, Kenneth. *The Philosophy of Literary Form: Studies in Symbolic Action*. 2nd ed. Baton Rouge: Louisiana State UP, 1967. Print.

Burns, Sarah. *Inventing the Modern Artist: Art and Culture in Gilded Age America*. New Haven, CT: Yale UP, 1996. Print.

Butler, Judith. *Frames of War: When Is Life Grievable?* Verso, 2009. Print.

—. *Krieg und Affekt*. Zürich: Diaphanes, 2009. Print.

—. "Photography, War, Outrage." *PMLA* 120.3 (2005): 822–27. Print.

Cable, George Washington. *Dr. Sevier*. Boston, MA: James Osgood and Co., 1885. Print.

—. *The Creoles of Louisiana*. New York: Charles Scribner's Sons, 1884. Print.

—. "The Entomologist." *Strong Hearts*. New York: Charles Scribner's Sons, 1899. 91–214.

—. *The Grandissimes: A Story of Creole Life*. New York: Charles Scribner's Sons, 1887. Print.

—. "Tite Poulette." *Old Creole Days*. New York: Charles Scribner's Sons, 1883. 213–43. Print.

Caldwell, Charles. *A Reply to Dr. Haygarth's Letter to Dr. Percival, on Infectious Fevers, and, His Address to the College of Physicians at Philadelphia, on the Preventing of the American Pestilence, Exposing the Medical, Philosophical, and Literary Errors of That Author, and Vindicating the Right Which Is the Faculty of the United States Have to Think and Decide for Themselves, Respecting the Diseases of Their Own Country, Uninfluenced by the Notions of the Physicians of Europe*. Philadelphia: Thomas and William Bradford, 1802. Early American Imprints 2nd Ser. No. 1981.

—. *A Semi-Annual Oration, on the Origin of Pestilential Diseases, Delivered before the Academy of Medicine of Philadelphia, on the 17th Day of December, 1798*. Philadelphia: Thomas and Samuel F. Bradford, 1799. Early American Imprints 1st Ser. No. 35263.

Cappel, Constance. *The Smallpox Genocide of the Odawa Tribe at L'Arbre Croche, 1763: The History of a Native American People*. Lewiston, NY: Edwin Mellen, 2007. Print.

Carey, Mathew. *A Short Account of the Malignant Fever, Lately Prevalent in Philadelphia: With a Statement of the Proceedings That Took Place on the Subject in Different Parts of the United States. To Which Are Added, Accounts of the Plague in London and Marseilles; and a List of the Dead, from August 1, to the Middle of December, 1793*. 4th ed., improved. Philadelphia: Printed by the Author, 1794. Early American Imprints 1st Ser. No. 26737.

—. *Address of M. Carey to the Public*. Philadelphia: Mathew Carey, 1794. Print.

Carrigan, Jo Ann. *The Saffron Scourge: A History of Yellow Fever in Louisiana, 1796–1905*. Lafayette: Center for Louisiana Studies, U of Southwestern Louisiana, 1994. Print.

—. "Yellow Fever: Scourge of the South." *Disease and Distinctiveness in the American South*. 1st ed. Ed. Todd Lee Savitt and James Harvey Young. Knoxville: U of Tennessee P, 1988. 55–78. Print.

Cartwright, Lisa, and Marita Sturken. *Practices of Looking: An Introduction to Visual Culture*. Oxford: Oxford UP, 2001. Print.

Castronovo, Russ. *Fathering the Nation: American Genealogies of Slavery and Freedom*. Berkeley: U of California P, 1995. Print.

—. ed. *The Oxford Handbook of Nineteenth-Century American Literature*. New York: Oxford UP, 2012. Print.

Child, Lydia Maria Francis. *A Romance of the Republic*. Boston: Ticknor and Fields, 1867. Print.

Chisholm, Colin. *A Manual of the Climate and Diseases of Tropical Countries; in Which a Practical View of the Statistical Pathology and of the History and Treatment of the Diseases of Those Countries Is Attempted to Be Given: Calculated Chiefly as a Guide to the Young Medical Practitioner on His First Resorting to Those Countries*. London: Burgess and Hill, 1822. Print.

—. *An Essay on the Malignant Pestilential Fever Introduced into the West Indian Islands from Boullam, on the Coast of Guinea, as It Appeared in 1793 and 1794*. London: C. Dilly, 1795. Print.

Christophersen, Bill. *The Apparition in the Glass: Charles Brockden Brown's American Gothic*. Athens: U of Georgia P, 1993. Print.

Cirillo, Vincent J. *Bullets and Bacilli: The Spanish-American War and Military Medicine*. New Brunswick, NJ: Rutgers UP, 2004. Print.

Clarkson, Thomas. *Memoirs of the Private and Public Life of William Penn*. London: R. Taylor for Longman, Hurst, Rees, Orme, and Brown, 1813. Print.

Colbert, Charles. *A Measure of Perfection: Phrenology and the Fine Arts in America*. Chapel Hill: U of North Carolina P, 1997. Print.

Coleman, William. *Yellow Fever in the North: The Methods of Early Epidemiology*. Madison: U of Wisconsin P, 1987. Print. Wisconsin Publications in the History of Science and Medicine 6.

Commager, Henry Steele. "The Search for a Usable Past." *The Search for a Usable Past, and Other Essays in Historiography*. New York: Knopf, 1967. 3–27. Print.

Cooper, James Fenimore. *Jack Tier, or, The Florida Reef*. New York: W.A. Townsend, 1860. Print.

—. *Ned Myers, or, A Life Before the Mast*. London: Richard Bentley, 1843. Print.

Coultrap-McQuin, Susan Margaret. *Doing Literary Business: American Women Writers in the Nineteenth Century*. Chapel Hill: U of North Carolina P, 1990. Print. Gender & American Culture.

Cowie, Alexander. *The Rise of the American Novel*. New York: American Book, 1951. Print.

Crane, Gregg David. *The Cambridge Introduction to the Nineteenth-Century American Novel*. Cambridge: Cambridge UP, 2007. Print. Cambridge Introductions to Literature.

Crosby, Molly Caldwell. *The American Plague: The Untold Story of Yellow Fever, the Epidemic That Shaped Our History*. New York: Berkley Books, 2006. Print.

Currie, William. *An Impartial Review of That Part of Dr. Rush's Late Publication, Entitled "An Account of the Bilious Remitting Yellow Fever, as It Appeared in the City of Philadelphia, in the Year 1793, Which Treats of the Origin of the Disease," in Which His Opinion Is Shewn to Be Erroneous; the Importation of the Disease Established; and the Wholesomeness of the City Vindicated.* Philadelphia: Thomas Dobson, 1794. Print.

Cutrer, Emily Fourmy. "Visualizing Nineteenth-Century American Culture." *American Quarterly* 51.4 (1999): 895–909. Print.

Dacus, Kaye. *Ransome's Crossing.* Eugene: Harvest House, 2010. Print.

Dallmann, Antje. "'Doctors Are Never Mistaken': Doctor Romances and Re-Negotiations of the Nature of Marriage in Late Nineteenth-Century America." *Communicating Disease: Cultural Representations of American Medicine.* Ed. Carmen Birkle and Johanna Heil. Vol. 236. Heidelberg: Winter, 2013. 119–44. Print. American Studies—A Monograph Series.

—. "To 'the General Reformation of American Manners': Popular Icons, Transnational Nursing Narratives, and the (Medical) Gaze Returned in *Wonderful Adventures of Mrs. Seacole in Many Lands* (1857)." *Transnational American Studies.* Ed. Udo J. Hebel. Vol. 222. Heidelberg: Winter, 2012. 423–44. Print. American Studies—A Monograph Series.

Davidson, Cathy N. *Revolution and the Word: The Rise of the Novel in America.* 1986. Expanded ed. New York: Oxford UP, 2004. Print.

Davidson, Cathy N., and Jessamyn Hatcher, eds. *No More Separate Spheres! A Next Wave American Studies Reader.* Durham, NC: Duke UP, 2002. Print. Next Wave: Women's Studies Beyond the Disciplines.

Davis, Cynthia J. *Bodily and Narrative Forms: The Influence of Medicine on American Literature, 1845–1915.* Stanford, CA: Stanford UP, 2000. Print.

Davis, Mollie E. M. *The Queen's Garden.* Boston: Houghton, Mifflin and Company, 1900. Print.

Davis, Richard Harding. *The Dictator: A Play in Three Acts.* New York: Charles Scribner's Sons, 1909. *Internet Archive.* Web. 9 Aug. 2013.

Däwes, Birgit. "Transgressive Television: Preliminary Thoughts." *Transgressive Television: Politics and Crime in 21st-century American TV Series.* Ed. Birgit Däwes, Alexandra Ganser, and Nicole Poppenhagen. Vol. 264. Heidelberg: Winter, 2015. 17–31. Print. American Studies—A Monograph Series.

Decker, Christof, "American Studies as Media and Visual Culture Studies: Observations on a Revitalized Research Tradition." *Amerikastudien / American Studies* 57.1 (2012): 115–28. Print.

De Kruif, Paul. *Microbe Hunters.* New York: Harcourt, Brace, 1926. Print.

DeCosta-Willis, Miriam. "Introduction." *The Memphis Diary of Ida B. Wells*. Ed. Miriam DeCosta-Willis. Boston: Beacon, 1995. 1–16. Print.

DeSalle, Robert, ed. *Epidemic! The World of Infectious Diseases*. New York: New Press, 1999. Print.

DeSalle, Robert, and Marla Jo Brickman. "Outbreaks." *Epidemic! The World of Infectious Diseases*. Ed. Robert DeSalle. New York: New Press, 1999. 113–16. Print.

Desowitz, Robert S. *Who Gave Pinta to Santa Maria? Torrid Diseases in a Temperate World*. Harcourt Brace, 1997. Print.

Dickerson, James L. *Yellow Fever: A Deadly Disease Poised to Kill Again*. Amherst: Prometheus, 2006. Print.

Dine, Sarah Blank. "Diaries and Doctors: Elizabeth Drinker and Philadelphia Medical Practice, 1760–1810." *Pennsylvania History* 68.4 (2001): 413–34. Print.

Donaldson, Susan V. "Elizabeth Stuart Phelps, Realism, and Literary Debates on Changing Gender Roles." *Realism and Its Discontents*. Ed. Danuta Zadworna-Fjellestad and Elizabeth Kella. Karlskrona: Blekinge Inst. of Technology, 2003. 87–111. Print.

Douglas, Ann. *The Feminization of American Culture*. 1977. 2nd ed, with a new preface by the author. New York: Noonday Press and Farrar, Straus and Giroux, 1998. Print.

Douglas, Mary. *Purity and Danger: An Analysis of Concepts of Pollution and Taboo*. London: Routledge & Kegan Paul, 1978. Print.

Downs, Jim. *Sick from Freedom: African-American Illness and Suffering during the Civil War and Reconstruction*. New York: Oxford UP, 2012. Print.

Duffy, John. *Sword of Pestilence: The New Orleans Yellow Fever Epidemic of 1853*. Baton Rouge: Louisiana State UP, 1966. Print.

—. *The Sanitarians: A History of American Public Health*. Urbana: U of Illinois P, 1990. Print.

Dugan, James. *Doctor Dispachemquic: A Story of the Great Southern Plague of 1878*. New Orleans: Clark & Hofeline, 1879. Print.

Dunbar-Nelson, Alice Moore. "The Praline Woman." *The Goodness of St. Rocque, and Other Stories*. New York: Dodd, Mead and Co., 1899. 175–80. Print.

Duster, Alfreda M. "Introduction." *Crusade for Justice: The Autobiography of Ida B. Wells*. Ed. Alfreda M. Duster. Chicago: U of Chicago P, 1970. xiii–xxxii. Print.

Eagleton, Terry. *Criticism and Ideology: A Study in Marxist Literary Theory*. Verso, 2006. Print.

Early American Visual Culture. Ed. Karsten Fitz and Klaus-Dieter Gross. Spec. issue of *Amerikastudien / American Studies* 50.3 (2005). Print.

Elias, Norbert. *The Civilizing Process: Sociogenetic and Psychogenetic Investigations*. Malden, MA: Blackwell, 2009. Print.

Elliott, Emory. "Diversity in the United States and Abroad: What Does It Mean When American Studies Is Transnational?" *American Quarterly* 59.1 (2007): 1–22. Print.

—. *Revolutionary Writers: Literature and Authority in the New Republic, 1725–1810*. New York: Oxford UP, 1982. Print.

Ellis, John Hubert. *Yellow Fever & Public Health in the New South*. Lexington: UP of Kentucky, 1992. Print.

Eschborn, Ulrich. *Stories of Survival: John Edgar Wideman's Representations of History*. Vol. 42. Trier: WVT, 2011. Print. Mosaic.

Espinosa, Mariola. *Epidemic Invasions: Yellow Fever and the Limits of Cuban Independence, 1878–1930*. Chicago: U of Chicago P, 2009. Print.

Esty, Joshua. "Oceanic, Traumatic, Post-Paradigmatic: A Response to William Boelhower." *American Literary History* 20.1–2 (2008): 102–07. Print.

Fahs, Alice. *The Imagined Civil War: Popular Literature of the North and South, 1861–1865*. Chapel Hill: U of North Carolina P, 2003. Print.

Fetterley, Judith, ed. *Provisions: A Reader from 19th-Century American Women*. Bloomington: Indiana UP, 1985. Print. Everywoman.

"Finale of Swill Milk." *American Medical Times* (1862): 278–80. Print.

Finger, Simon. *The Contagious City: The Politics of Public Health in Early Philadelphia*. Ithaca, NY: Cornell UP, 2012. Print.

Fish, Cheryl J. *Black and White Women's Travel Narratives: Antebellum Explorations*. Gainesville: UP of Florida, 2004. Print.

Fisher, Philip. *Hard Facts: Setting and Form in the American Novel*. New York: Oxford UP, 1985. Print.

Fishkin, Shelley Fisher. "Crossroads of Cultures: The Transnational Turn in American Studies—Presidential Address to the American Studies Association, November 12, 2004." *American Quarterly* 57.1 (2005): 17–57. Print.

Flavin, Francis. "A Pox on Amherst: Smallpox, Sir Jeffrey, and a Town Named Amherst." *Historical Journal of Massachusetts* 30.1 (2002): n. pag. Print.

Fleischman, Paul. *Path of the Pale Horse*. New York: Harper & Row, 1983. Print.

Floyd, Charles Rinaldo et al. "Floyd-McAdoo Families Papers." n. pag. Print.

"Floyd-McAdoo Families Papers: A Finding Aid to the Collection in the Library of Congress." 2009. Web. 19 Sept. 2012.

Fluck, Winfried. *Das kulturelle Imaginäre: Eine Funktionsgeschichte des amerikanischen Romans, 1790–1900*. Frankfurt/M.: Suhrkamp, 1997. Print.

—. "Literature as Symbolic Action." *Amerikastudien / American Studies* 28.3 (1983): 361–71. Print.

Forney, Melissa. *The Astonishing Journey of Teddy Bodain*. Orange City, FL: Buttery Moon Multimedia, 2009. Print.

Forrest, Tuomi J. "Writing the Fever." *Clean, Green, Machine: Philadelphia's Fairmount Water Works, 1800–1860*. Web. 16 Sept. 2013.

Foucault, Michel. *The Birth of the Clinic: An Archaeology of Medical Perception*. New York: Vintage, 1975. Print.

Fox, John P., Carrie E. Hall, and Lila R. Elveback. *Epidemiology: Man and Disease*. New York: Macmillan, 1970. Print.

Francis, William A. "Yellow Fever in Mollie Davis's Novel *The Queen's Garden*." *Louisiana Literature: A Review of Literature and Humanities* 8 (1991): 61–68.

Freneau, Philip Morin. *Poems Written and Published During the American Revolutionary War, and Now Republished from the Original Manuscripts: Interspersed with Translations from the Ancients, and Other Pieces Not Heretofore in Print*. Lydia R. Bailey, 1809. Print.

Frierson, J. Gordon. "The Yellow Fever Vaccine: A History." *Yale Journal of Biology and Medicine* 83.2 (2010): 77–85. Print.

Furneaux, Holly. *Queer Dickens: Erotics, Families, Masculinities*. Oxford: Oxford UP, 2009. Print.

Garrett, Laurie. *The Coming Plague: Newly Emerging Diseases in a World Out of Balance*. New York: Farrar, Straus and Giroux, 1994. Print.

Gasché, Rodolphe. "… And the Beautiful? Revisiting Edmund Burke's 'Double Aesthetics.'" *The Sublime: From Antiquity to the Present*. Ed. Timothy M. Costelloe. Cambridge: Cambridge UP, 2012. 24–36. Print.

Gayarré, Charles. *History of Louisiana*. 4th ed. New Orleans: F.F. Hansell & Bro., Ltd., 1903. Print.

Gessner, Ingrid. "'A country life and estate I like best for my children': Spatial Dialectics and the Contagiousness of Fear." *Rural America*. Ed. Antje Kley and Heike Paul. Heidelberg: Winter, 2015. 227–46. Print.

—. "Contagion, Crisis, and Control: Tracing Yellow Fever in Nineteenth-Century American Literature and Culture." *Communicating Disease: Cultural Representations of American Medicine*. Ed. Carmen Birkle and Johanna Heil. Heidelberg: Winter, 2013. 219–42. Print.

—. "Epidemic Iconographies: Towards a Disease Aesthetics of the Destructive Sublime." Spec. issue of *Amerikastudien / American Studies* 58.4 (2013). Ed. Ingrid Gessner and Susanne Leikam. 559–82. Print.

—. "Heroines of Health: Examining the Other Side of the 'Splendid Little War.'" *European Journal of American Studies* 10.1 (2015). Web. 8 Mar. 2016.

—. "Of He-Nurses and She-Doctors: Gendered Accounts of Yellow Fever in Postbellum American Literature." *Gender and Disease in Literary and Medical Cultures*. Ed. Anne-Julia Zwierlein, and Iris M. Heid. Heidelberg: Winter, 2014: 137–55. Print.

—. and Susanne Leikam, "Introduction: Iconographies of the Calamitous in American Visual Culture." Spec. issue of *Amerikastudien / American Studies* 58.4 (2013). Ed. Ingrid Gessner and Susanne Leikam. 533–42. Print.

Gilbert, Sandra M., and Susan Gubar. *The Madwoman in the Attic: The Woman Writer and the Nineteenth-Century Literary Imagination*. New Haven, CT: Yale UP, 1979. Print.

Gillman, Susan. "The Mulatto, Tragic or Triumphant? The Nineteenth-Century American Race Melodrama." *The Culture of Sentiment: Race, Gender, and Sentimentality in Nineteenth-Century America*. Ed. Shirley Samuels. New York: Oxford UP, 1992. 221–43. Print.

Gilman, Charlotte Perkins. "*The Yellow Wall-paper*." Ed. Shawn St. Jean. Athens: Ohio UP, 2006. Print.

Gilman, Sander L. *Disease and Representation: Images of Illness from Madness to AIDS*. Ithaca, NY: Cornell UP, 1988. Print.

Gilroy, Paul. *The Black Atlantic: Modernity and Double Consciousness*. Cambridge, MA: Harvard UP, 1993. Print.

Glassner, Barry. *The Culture of Fear: Why Americans Are Afraid of the Wrong Things: Crime, Drugs, Minorities, Teen Moms, Killer Kids, Mutant Microbes, Plane Crashes, Road Rage, & So Much More*. New York: Basic Books, 2010. Print.

Godwin, William. *Enquiry Concerning Political Justice and Its Influence on Modern Morals and Happiness*. Harmondsworth: Penguin, 1985. Print. Penguin Classics.

Goffman, Erving. *Stigma: Notes on the Management of Spoiled Identity*. 1963. New York: Simon & Schuster, 1986. Print.

Gould, Philip. "Race, Commerce, and the Literature of Yellow Fever in Early National Philadelphia." *Early American Literature* 35.2 (2000): 157–86. Print.

Grabo, Norman S. *The Coincidental Art of Charles Brockden Brown*. Chapel Hill: U of North Carolina P, 1981. Print.

Grant, Michael, and John Hazel. *Lexikon der antiken Mythen und Gestalten*. 11th ed. München: Deutscher Taschenbuch Verlag, 1995. Print.

Greenberg, Stephen. RE: Context and Usage of Two Images (IHM). 23 Oct. 2012. E-mail.

Greenblatt, Stephen. "Culture." *Critical Terms for Literary Study*. 2nd ed. Ed. Frank Lentricchia and Thomas McLaughlin. Chicago: U of Chicago P, 1995. 225–32. Print.

—. *Shakespearean Negotiations: The Circulation of Social Energy in Renaissance England*. Berkeley: U of California P, 1988. Print. New Historicism 4.

Gysin, Fritz. "John Edgar Wideman's 'Fever.'" *Callaloo* 22.3 (1999): 715–26. Print.

Haakonssen, Lisbeth. *Medicine and Morals in the Enlightenment: John Gregory, Thomas Percival and Benjamin Rush*. Amsterdam: Rodopi, 1997. Print.

Haas, Astrid. *Stages of Agency: The Contributions of American Drama to the AIDS Discourse*. Vol. 204. Heidelberg: Winter, 2011. Print. American Studies—A Monograph Series.

Haco, Dion. *Dr. Blackburn: The Yellow Fever Fiend*. New York: Hurst, 1866. Vol. 24. Print. Popular Series of Fiction, Fancy and Fact.

Hall, Gwendolyn Midlo. "The Formation of Afro-Creole Culture." *Creole New Orleans: Race and Americanization*. Ed. Arnold R. Hirsch and Joseph Logsdon. Baton Rouge: Louisiana State UP, 1992. 58–90. Print.

Harrison, Mark. *Contagion: How Commerce Has Spread Disease*. New Haven, CT: Yale UP, 2012. Print.

—. "Disease, Diplomacy and International Commerce: The Origins of International Sanitary Regulation in the Nineteenth Century." *Journal of Global History* 1 (2006): 197–217. Print.

—. *Medicine in an Age of Commerce and Empire: Britain and Its Tropical Colonies, 1660–1830*. New York: Oxford UP, 2010. Print.

Hauptman, Laurence M. *Tribes and Tribulations: Misconceptions About American Indians and Their Histories*. Albuquerque: U of New Mexico P, 1995. Print.

Hayne, Barrie. "S[ilas]. Weir Mitchell (1892–1914)." *American Literary Realism, 1870–1910* 2.2 (1969): 149–55. Print.

Hearn, Lafcadio. *Chita: A Memory of Last Island*. New York: Harper & Brothers, 1889. Print.

Hebel, Udo J. "'American' Pictures and (Trans-)National Iconographies: Mapping Interpictorial Clusters in American Studies." *American Studies Today: New Research Agendas*. Ed. Winfried Fluck, Erik Redling, Sabine Sielke, and Hubert Zapf. Vol. 230. Heidelberg: Winter, 2014. 401–32. Print. American Studies—A Monograph Series.

—. "Der amerikanische New Historicism der achtziger Jahre: Bestandsaufnahme einer neuen Orthodoxie kulturwissenschaftlicher Literaturinterpretation." *Amerikastudien / American Studies* 37.2 (1992): 325–47. Print.

—. and Christine Moreth-Hebel. "The Pictorial Turn and the Teaching of American Cultural Studies: Repositioning the Visual Narrative of Norman Rockwell's 'Freedom from Want' (1943)." *Text, Kontext und Fremdsprachenunterricht: Festschrift für Gerhard Bach zum 60. Geburtstag*. Ed. Dagmar Abendroth-Timmer, Britta Viebrock, and Michael Wendt. Frankfurt/M.: Lang, 2003. 187–201. Print. Kolloquium Fremdsprachenunterricht 16.

Herget, Winfried. "Villains for Pleasure: The Paradox of Nineteenth-Century (American) Melodrama." *Melodrama! The Mode of Excess from Early America to Hollywood*. Ed. Frank Kelleter, Barbara Krah, and Ruth Mayer. Vol. 145. Heidelberg: Winter, 2007. 19–34. Print. American Studies—A Monograph Series.

Herringshaw, Thomas William. *Herringshaw's National Library of American Biography*. Chicago: American Publishers' Association, 1909. Print. Harvard Medicine Preservation Microfilm Project. Part 4. Biographies.

Herzlich, Claudine, and Janine Pierret. *Illness and Self in Society*. Baltimore, MD: Johns Hopkins UP, 1987. Print.

Hicks, Robert. *A Separate Country*. New York: Grand Central, 2009. Print.

Hirsch, Arnold R., and Joseph Logsdon. "Preface." *Creole New Orleans: Race and Americanization*. Ed. Arnold R. Hirsch and Joseph Logsdon. Baton Rouge: Louisiana State UP, 1992. ix–xiii. Print.

Hornung, Alfred. "Transnationalism and American Studies: The View from Abroad." *Encyclopedia of American Studies*. Ed. Simon J. Bronner. Baltimore, MD: John Hopkins UP, 2014. Web. 10 Mar. 2016.

Howard, Jean Elizabeth, and Marion F. O'Connor, eds. *Shakespeare Reproduced: The Text in History and Ideology*. New York: Methuen, 1987. Print.

Howard, Sidney Coe, and Paul De Kruif. *Yellow Jack: A History*. New York: Harcourt, Brace, 1934. Print.

Humphreys, Margaret. "Appendix II: Yellow Fever Since 1793: History and Historiography." *A Melancholy Scene of Devastation: The Public Response to the 1793 Philadelphia Yellow Fever Epidemic*. Ed. J. Worth Estes and Billy G. Smith. Canton, MA: College of Physicians of Philadelphia and the Library Company of Philadelphia, Science History Publications, 1997. 183–98. Print.

—. *Intensely Human: The Health of the Black Soldier in the American Civil War*. Baltimore, MD: Johns Hopkins UP, 2008. Print.

—. *Yellow Fever and the South*. Baltimore, MD: Johns Hopkins UP, 1999. Print.

Iconographies of the Calamitous in American Visual Culture. Ed. Ingrid Gessner and Susanne Leikam. Spec. issue of *Amerikastudien / American Studies* 58.4 (2013). Print.

Iser, Wolfgang. *The Act of Reading: A Theory of Aesthetic Response*. Baltimore, MD: Johns Hopkins UP, 1978. Print.

Jackson, Robert. *A Treatise on the Fevers of Jamaica, with Some Observations on the Intermitting Fever of America, and an Appendix, Containing Some Hints on the Means of Preserving the Health of Soldiers in Hot Climates.* London: J. Murray, 1791. Print.

—. *An Outline of the History and Cure of Fever, Endemic and Contagious; More Expressly the Contagious Fever of Jails, Ships, and Hospitals, the Concentrated Endemic, Vulgarly the Yellow Fever of the West Indies.* Edinburgh: Mundell & Son, 1798. Print.

Jagow, Bettina von, and Florian Steger, eds. *Jahrbuch Literatur und Medizin.* Heidelberg: Winter, 2007ff. Print.

—. *Was treibt die Literatur zur Medizin? Ein kulturwissenschaftlicher Dialog.* Göttingen: Vandenhoeck & Ruprecht, 2009. Print.

Jameson, Frederic. "Ideology and Symbolic Action." *Critical Inquiry* 5.2 (1978): 417–22. Print.

—. *The Political Unconscious: Narrative as a Socially Symbolic Act.* Ithaca, NY: Cornell UP, 1981. Print.

—. "The Symbolic Inference; or, Kenneth Burke and Ideological Analysis." *Critical Inquiry* 4.3 (1978): 507–23. Print.

—. *Valences of the Dialectic.* London: Verso, 2009. Print.

Jehle, Oliver. "'The Conqueror of Canada'—Benjamin West and the Heroes of Sentimentalism." *Pictorial Cultures and Political Iconographies.* Ed. Udo J. Hebel and Christoph Wagner. Berlin: de Gruyter, 2011. 85–104. Print.

Johnson, Edward. *A History of New-England [Wonder-Working Providence of Sions Saviour].* London: Nath Brooke at the Angel in Cornhill, 1654. Print.

Johnson, Samuel. *Samuel Johnson's Dictionary of the English Language.* London: Studio Editions, 1994. Print.

Jones, Marian Moser. *The American Red Cross: From Clara Barton to the New Deal.* Baltimore, MD: Johns Hopkins UP, 2013. Print.

Kaplan, Amy. "Manifest Domesticity." *American Literature* 70.3 (1998): 581–606. Print.

Keith, Jeanette. *Fever Season: The Story of a Terrifying Epidemic and the People who Saved a City.* New York: Bloomsbury, 2012. Print.

Kelley, Mary. "Introduction." *The Power of Her Sympathy: The Autobiography and Journal of Catharine Maria Sedgwick.* Ed. Mary Kelley. Boston: Massachusetts Historical Society, Northeastern UP, 1993. 1–41. Print.

Kelly, Maura. "Trickle-Down Distress: How America's Broken Meritocracy Drives Our National Anxiety Epidemic." *The Atlantic.* 3 July 2012. Web. 31 July 2013.

Kerber, Linda K. *Women of the Republic: Intellect and Ideology in Revolutionary America*. Chapel Hill: U of North Carolina P, 1980. Print.

Kessler, Carol Farley. *Elizabeth Stuart Phelps*. Boston: Twayne, 1982. Vol. 434. Print. Twayne's United States Authors Series (TUSAS).

Kilcup, Karen L., ed. *Nineteenth-Century American Women Writers: A Critical Reader*. Malden, MA: Blackwell, 1998. Print.

Kiple, Kenneth F. "Response to Sheldon Watts, 'Yellow Fever Immunities in West Africa and the Americas in the Age of Slavery and Beyond: A Reappraisal.'" *Journal of Social History* 34.4 (2001): 969–74. Print.

—. and Virginia H. Kiple. "Black Yellow Fever Immunities, Innate and Acquired, as Revealed in the American South." *Social Science History* 1.4 (1977): 419–36. Print.

Klepp, Susan E. "Appendix I: 'How Many Precious Souls Are Fled'?: The Magnitude of the 1793 Yellow Fever Epidemic." *A Melancholy Scene of Devastation: The Public Response to the 1793 Philadelphia Yellow Fever Epidemic*. Ed. J. Worth Estes and Billy G. Smith. Canton, MA: College of Physicians of Philadelphia and the Library Company of Philadelphia, Science History Publications, 1997. 163–76. Print.

Kley, Antje. *Ethik medialer Repräsentation im britischen und US-amerikanischen Roman, 1741–2000*. Vol. 166. Heidelberg: Winter, 2009. Print. American Studies—A Monograph Series.

Knight, Lucian Lamar. *Biographical Dictionary of Authors*. 1909. Print.

Koch, Tom. *Disease Maps: Epidemics on the Ground*. Chicago: U of Chicago P, 2011. Print.

Kohl, Susan. *The Ghost of Gracie Mansion*. New York: Silver Moon, 1999. Print.

Kolodny, Annette. *The Land Before Her: Fantasy and Experience of the American Frontiers, 1630–1860*. Chapel Hill: U of North Carolina P, 1984. Print.

Kornfeld, Eve. "Crisis in the Capital: The Cultural Significance of Philadelphia's Great Yellow Fever Epidemic." *Pennsylvania History* 51.3 (1984): 189–205. Print.

Kress, Gunther R., and Theo Van Leeuwen. *Reading Images: The Grammar of Visual Design*. 2nd ed. London: Routledge, 2006. Print.

Krieg, Joann P. *Epidemics in the Modern World*. New York: Twayne, 1992. Print.

Kunow, Rüdiger. "In Sickness and in Health: Transnationalism Reconsidered." *Virtually American?* Ed. Mita Banerjee. Heidelberg: Winter, 2009. 23–36. Print.

—. "The Rhetoric of Crisis: Cultural Reformulations and Social Change in the United States in the 1980s." *Amerikastudien / American Studies* 32.4 (1987): 467–80. Print.

Laffrado, Laura. *Uncommon Women: Gender and Representation in Nineteenth-Century U.S. Women's Writing*. Columbus: Ohio State UP, 2009. Print.

Lapsansky, Philip. "'Abigail, a Negress': The Role and the Legacy of African Americans in the Yellow Fever Epidemic." *A Melancholy Scene of Devastation: The Public Response to the 1793 Philadelphia Yellow Fever Epidemic*. Ed. J. Worth Estes and Billy G. Smith. Canton, MA: College of Physicians of Philadelphia and the Library Company of Philadelphia, Science History Publications, 1997. 61–78. Print.

Lawlor, Clark. *Consumption and Literature: The Making of the Romantic Disease*. Basingstoke: Palgrave Macmillan, 2006. Print.

Leikam, Susanne. *Framing Spaces in Motion: Tracing Visualizations of Earthquakes into Twentieth-Century San Francisco*. Vol. 255. Heidelberg: Winter, 2015. Print. American Studies—A Monograph Series.

Le Moyne de Morgues, Jacques, and Theodor de Bry. *Brevis Narratio Eorum Quae in Florida Americae Provi[n]cia Gallis Acciderunt Secunda in Illam Nauigatione, Duce Renato de Laudo[n]niere Classis Praefecto, Anno M D Lxiiii: Quae Est Secunda Para Americae : Additae Figurae & Incolarum Eicones Ibiden Ad Vivu[um] Expressae, Brevis Item Declaratio Religionis, Rituum, Vivendiq́ue Ratione Ipsorum*. Frankfurt/M.: Johannes Wecheli, 1591. Print.

Lempriere, William. *Practical Observations on the Diseases of the Army in Jamaica, as They Occurred Between the Years 1792 and 1797; on the Situation, Climate, and Diseases of That Island; and on the Most Probable Means of Lessening Mortality Among the Troops, and Among Europeans in Tropical Climates*. London: T. N. Longman and O. Rees, 1799. Print.

Leverenz, David. *Manhood and the American Renaissance*. Ithaca, NY: Cornell UP, 1989. Print.

Levine, Robert S. *Conspiracy and Romance: Studies in Brockden Brown, Cooper, Hawthorne, and Melville*. Cambridge: Cambridge UP, 1989. Print.

—. *Dislocating Race & Nation: Episodes in Nineteenth-Century American Literary Nationalism*. Chapel Hill: U of North Carolina P, 2008. Print.

Lewis, Penelope Barlow, and Donald W. Lewis. "Deathstorm: The Yellow Fever Epidemic of 1855." *Virginia Medical Quarerly* 122 (1995): 38–42. Print.

Lining, John. *A Description of the American Yellow Fever, Which Prevailed at Charleston, in South Carolina, in the Year 1748*. Philadelphia: Thomas Dobson, 1799. Print.

Link, Bruce G., and Jo C. Phelan. "Conceptualizing Stigma." *Annual Review of Sociology* 2001: 363–85. Print.

Liptak, Adam. "Reaction to Supreme Court's Health Decision a Rarity, Study Finds." *The New York Times* 1 Oct. 2012. *NYTimes.com*. Web. 1 Aug. 2013.

Long, Gretchen. *Doctoring Freedom: The Politics of African American Medical Care in Slavery and Emancipation*. Chapel Hill: U of North Carolina P, 2012. Print.

Long, Lisa A. "The Post-Bellum Reform Writings of Rebecca Harding Davis and Elizabeth Stuart Phelps." *The Cambridge Companion to Nineteenth-Century American Women's Writing*. Ed. Dale M. Bauer and Philip Gould. Cambridge: Cambridge UP, 2001. 262–83. Print. Cambridge Companions to Literature.

Longfellow, Henry Wadsworth. *Evangeline: A Tale of Acadie*. Champaign, IL: Project Gutenberg. *EBSCOhost*. Web.

Lowe, Lisa. *The Intimacies of Four Continents*. Durham, NC: Duke UP, 2015. Print.

Lupton, Deborah. *Medicine as Culture: Illness, Disease and the Body in Western Societies*. London: Sage, 1994. Print.

Lynch, Lisa. "The Fever Next Time: The Race of Disease and the Disease of Racism in John Edgar Wideman." *American Literary History* 14.4 (2002): 776–804. Print.

M'Cabe, James. *Military-Medical Reports: Containing Pathological and Practical Observations Illustrating the Diseases of Warm Climates*. Cheltenham: G.A. Williams, 1825. Print.

Mackenthun, Gesa. *Fictions of the Black Atlantic in American Foundational Literature*. London: Routledge, 2004. Print. Routledge Transatlantic Perspectives on American Literature 4.

Maddox, Lucy. *Removals: Nineteenth-Century American Literature and the Politics of Indian Affairs*. New York: Oxford UP, 1991. Print.

"Major U.S. Epidemics." *Information Please Database, Pearson Education*. 2007. Web. 29 Sept. 2011.

Makittrick, Jacob Barter. *Dissertatio Medica Inauguralis de Febre Indiae Occidentalis Maligna Flava*. Edinburgh: A. Donaldson, 1764. Print.

Manganelli, Kimberly Snyder. *Transatlantic Spectacles of Race: The Tragic Mulatta and the Tragic Muse*. New Brunswick, NJ: Rutgers UP, 2012. Print.

Masteller, Jean Carwile. "The Women Doctors of Howells, Phelps, and Jewett: The Conflict of Marriage and Career." *Critical Essays on Sarah Orne Jewett*. Ed. Gwen L. Nagel. Boston: Hall, 1984. 135–47. Print. Critical Essays on American Literature.

Mayor, Adrienne. "The Nessus Shirt in the New World: Smallpox Blankets in History and Legend." *Journal of American Folklore* 108.427 (1995): 54–77. Print.

Mazet, André, and Etienne Pariset. *Observations Sur La Fièvre Jaune, Faites a Cadiz, En 1819*. Paris: Audot, Libraire, 1820. Print.

McAuley, Louis Kirk. "'Periodical Visitations': Yellow Fever as Yellow Journalism in Charles Brockden Brown's *Arthur Mervyn*." *Eighteenth-Century Fiction* 19.3 (2007): 307–40.

McCarthy, Harold T. "Meville's *Redburn* and the City." *The Midwest Quarterly* 12 (1971): 395–410. Print.

Melville, Herman. *Omoo: A Narrative of Adventures in the South Seas.* London: John Murray, 1847. Print.

—. *Redburn: His First Voyage Being the Sailor-Boy Confessions and Reminiscences of the Son of a Gentleman in the Merchant Service.* Vol. 5. New York: Russel & Russell, 1963. Print. The Works of Herman Melville.

—. *White Jacket, or, The World in a Man-of-War. The Writings of Herman Melville: The Northwestern-Newberry Edition.* Ed. Harrison Hayford. Evanston, IL: Northwestern UP, 1983. 341–770. Print.

"Memphis Under Quarantine Rule." *Frank Leslie's Illustrated Newspaper* 20 Sept. 1879: 43. Print.

Meyer, Anne-Rose. "Zwischen Zeugenschaft und Voyeurismus: Visuelle Medien und die Berichterstattung über Krieg und Terrorismus als ästhetisches Problem und literarisches Thema." *Kriegsdiskurse in Literatur und Medien nach 1989.* Ed. Carsten Gansel and Heinrich Kaulen. Göttingen: V&R unipress, 2011. 357–78. Print.

Meyers, Jeffrey. *Disease and the Novel, 1880–1960.* London: Macmillan, 1985. Print.

Mills, Theodora. "Charles Wesley Alexander." *Dictionary of Literary Biography.* Vol. 49. *American Literary Publishing Houses, 1638–1899.* Ed. Peter Dzwonkoski. Detroit, MI: Thomson Gale, 1986. 7. Print.

Mirzoeff, Nicholas. *An Introduction to Visual Culture.* London: Routledge, 1999. Print.

Mitchell, W. J. Thomas. *Picture Theory: Essays on Verbal and Visual Representation.* Chicago: U of Chicago P, 1994. Print.

—. "Showing Seeing: A Critique of Visual Culture." *Journal of Visual Culture* 1.2 (2002): 165–81. Print.

Moore, Jennifer E. "'Ours Has Been No Pleasing Task': Sensationalism in Frank Leslie's Campaign Against Swill Milk." *Sensationalism: Murder, Mayhem, Mudslinging, Scandals, and Disasters in 19th-Century Reporting.* Ed. David B. Sachsman and David W. Bulla. New Brunswick, NJ: Transaction. 127–40. Print.

Moran, John J. "Memoirs of a Human Guinea Pig." 1949. Web. 11 Aug. 2013.

Morantz-Sanchez, Regina. *Sympathy and Science: Women Physicians in American Medicine.* New York: Oxford UP, 1985. Print.

Moreau de Jonnès, Alexandre. *Monographie historique et médicale de la fièvre jaune des Antilles.* Paris: Migneret, 1820. Print.

Morris, Timothy. "Professional Ethics and Professional Erotics in Elizabeth Stuart Phelps' *Doctor Zay*." *Studies in American Fiction* 21.2 (1993): 141–52. Print.

"Moscamed Launches Urban Scale Project Using Oxitec GM Mosquitoes in Battle Against Dengue." *PR Newswire* 20 June 2013. Web. 7 Mar. 2016.

Mott, Frank Luther. *A History of American Magazines 1741–1850*. 4th ed. Cambridge, MA: Belknap Press of Harvard UP, 1966. Print.

—. *A History of American Magazines 1850–1865*. 2nd ed. Cambridge, MA: Belknap Press of Harvard UP, 1957. Print.

—. *A History of American Magazines 1865–1885*. 2nd ed. Cambridge, MA: Belknap Press of Harvard UP, 1957. Print.

—. *A History of American Magazines 1885–1905*. Cambridge, MA: Belknap Press of Harvard UP, 1957. Print.

Myers, Anna. *Graveyard Girl*. New York: Walker, 1995. Print.

Nelson, Dana D. *National Manhood: Capitalist Citizenship and the Imagined Fraternity of White Men*. Durham, NC: Duke UP, 1998. Print. New Americanists.

Nemerov, Alexander. *Frederic Remington & Turn-of-the-century America*. New Haven, CT: Yale UP, 1995.

Newsom, Elizabeth Young. "South Carolina's Last Yellow Fever Epidemic: Manning Simons at Port Royal, 1877." *Journal of the South Carolina Medical Association* 7 (1995): 311–13. Print.

Nuwer, Deanne Stephens. *Plague Among the Magnolias: The 1878 Yellow Fever Epidemic in Mississippi*. Tuscaloosa: U of Alabama P, 2009. Print.

Orishima, Masahi. "Immersed in Palpable Darkness: Republican Virtue and the Spatial Topography of Charles Brockden Brown's *Arthur Mervyn*." *The Japanese Journal of American Studies* 13 (2002): 7–23. Print.

Orvell, Miles. "After 9/11: Photography, the Destructive Sublime, and the Postmodern Archive." *Michigan Quarterly Review* (2006): 239–56. Print.

—. *American Photography*. Oxford: Oxford UP, 2003. Print.

—. "Cultural Studies, Visual Studies, Historical Studies: Connecting the Dots." *American Studies / Amerikastudien* 47.2 (2006): 87–103. Print.

Ossoli Circle. *History of Ossoli Circle, Knoxville, Tenn. Founded November Twentieth, Eighteen Hundred Eighty-Five*. Knoxville, 1890. Print.

Otter, Samuel. *Philadelphia Stories: America's Literature of Race and Freedom*. New York: Oxford UP, 2010. Print.

Painter, Nell Irvin. *Exodusters: Black Migration to Kansas after Reconstruction*. Lawrence: UP of Kansas, 1986. Print.

Panofsky, Erwin. *Ikonographie und Ikonologie: Bildinterpretation nach dem Dreistufenmodell.* 1932/1955. Köln: DuMont, 2006. Print.

Pareene. "Study: Indians Gave You Syphilis." *Gawker.* 15 Jan. 2008. Web. 31 July 2013.

Patrick, Denise. *Cecile's Gift.* Middleton, WI: American Girl, 2011. Print.

—. *Troubles for Cecile.* Middleton, WI: American Girl, 2011. Print.

Patterson, K. David. "Yellow Fever Epidemics and Mortality in the United States, 1693–1905." *Social Science & Medicine* 34.8 (1992): 855–65. Print.

Patton, Cindy. *Globalizing AIDS.* Vol. 22. Minneapolis: U of Minnesota P, 2002. Print. Theory Out of Bounds.

Pernick, Martin S. "Contagion and Culture." *American Literary History* 14.4 (2002): 858–65. Print.

—. "Politics, Parties, and Pestilence: Epidemic Yellow Fever in Philadelphia and the Rise of the First Party System." *The William and Mary Quarterly* 29.4 (1972): 559–86. Print.

Phelps, Elizabeth Stuart. "The Experiment Tried." *Independent* 5 Mar. 1874: 1–2. Print.

—. "What Shall They Do?" *Harper's New Monthly Magazine* Sept. 1867: 519–23. Print.

—. "What They Are Doing." *Independent* 17 Aug. 1871: 1. Print.

—. "Zerviah Hope." *Scribner's Monthly* Nov. 1880: 78–88. Print.

Pierce, John R., and Jim Writer. *Yellow Jack: How Yellow Fever Ravaged America and Walter Reed Discovered Its Deadly Secrets.* Hoboken: J. Wiley, 2005. Print.

Pinckard, George. *Notes on the West Indies: Written During the Expedition Under the Command of the Late General Sir Ralph Abercromby: Including Observations on the Island of Barbadoes, and the Settlements Captured by the British Troops, Upon the Coast of Guiana; Likewise Remarks Relating to the Creoles and Slaves of the Western Colonies, and the Indians of South America: With Occasional Hints, Regarding the Seasoning, or Yellow Fever of Hot Climates.* 3 vols. London: Longman, Hurst, Rees, and Orme, 1806. Print.

Poe, Edgar Allan. *The Narrative of Arthur Gordon Pym of Nantucket. The Essential Tales and Poems of Edgar Allan Poe.* Ed. Benjamin F. Fisher. New York: Barnes & Noble Classics, 2004. 443–606. Print.

Powell, Charles. *A Treatise on the Nature, Causes, & Cure, of the Endemic, or Yellow Fever of Tropical Climates, as It Occurs in the West Indies: To Which Europeans Are More Particularly Subject on Their First Arrival. Founded on Principle, and Illustrated by the Writings of, and Cases from, Various Authors of Different Periods.* London: Printed for John Callow, 1814. Print.

Powell, John Harvey. *Bring Out Your Dead: The Great Plague of Yellow Fever in Philadelphia in 1793*. 1949. Philadelphia: U of Pennsylvania P, 1993. Print. Studies in Health, Illness, and Caregiving.

Preston, Richard. *The Hot Zone*. New York: Random House, 1994. Print.

Prettyman, Gib. "Harper's 'Weekly' and the Spectacle of Industrialization." *American Periodicals* 11 (2001): 24–48. Print.

Priewe, Marc. *Textualizing Illness: Medicine and Culture in New England, 1620–1730*. Vol. 249. Heidelberg: Winter, 2014. Print. American Studies—A Monograph Series.

Prosser, Jay. Introduction. *Picturing Atrocity: Photography in Crisis*. Ed. Geoffrey Batchen, Mick Gidley, Nancy K. Miller, and Jay Prosser. London: Reaktion Books, 2012. 7–13. Print.

Pryse, Marjorie, and Judith Fetterley. *Writing Out of Place: Regionalism, Women, and American Literary Culture*. Urbana: U of Illinois P, 2003. Print.

Pym, William. *Observations Upon the Bulam Fever, Which Has of Late Years Prevailed in the West Indies, on the Coast of America, at Gibraltar, Cadiz, and Other Parts of Spain: With a Collection of Facts Proving It to Be a Highly Contagious Disease*. London: J. Callow, 1815. Print.

Pyne, Kathleen. *Art and the Higher Life: Painting and Evolutionary Thought in Late Nineteenth-Century America*. Austin: U of Texas P, 1996. Print.

Rainey, Sue. *Creating Picturesque America: Monument to the Natural and Cultural Landscape*. Nashville, TN: Vanderbilt UP, 1994. Print.

Ramenofsky, Ann F., Alicia K. Wilbur, and Anne C. Stone. "Native American Disease History: Past, Present and Future Directions." *World Archeology* 35.2 (2003): 241–57. Print.

Rancière, Jacques. *The Future of the Image*. London: Verso, 2007. Print.

Reilly, Elizabeth Carroll. *A Dictionary of Colonial American Printers' Ornaments and Illustrations*. Worcester: American Antiquarian Society, 1975. Print.

Reizenstein, Ludwig Baron von. *The Mysteries of New Orleans*. Ed. Steven W. Rowan. Baltimore, MD: Johns Hopkins UP, 2002. Print. The Longfellow Series of American Languages and Literatures.

Reynolds, Larry J. "Introduction: American Cultural Iconography." *National Imaginaries, American Identities: The Cultural Work of American Iconography*. Ed. Larry J. Reynolds and Gordon Hutner. Princeton, NJ: Princeton UP, 2000. 3–28. Print.

Roach, Mary. "Contagion." *The New York Times* 5 Nov. 2006. *NYTimes.com*. Web. 29 Sept. 2011.

Robinson, William L. *The Diary of a Samaritan*. New York: Harper, 1860. Print.

Ross, Cheri Louise. "Catharine Maria Sedgwick: Critical Perspectives." *Legacy* 21.2 (2004): 246–47. Print.

Rothfield, Lawrence. *Vital Signs: Medical Realism in Nineteenth-Century Fiction.* Princeton, NJ: Princeton UP, 1992. Print. Literature in History.

Rowan, Steven W. "Baron von Reizenstein's *Die Geheimnisse von New Orleans* (*The Mysteries of New Orleans*)." Recent Research in American Studies. Regensburg. 2004.

—. "Introduction: Searching for a Key to *The Mysteries*." *The Mysteries of New Orleans.* Ed. Steven W. Rowan. Baltimore, MD: Johns Hopkins UP, 2002. xiii–xxxiii. Print. The Longfellow Series of American Languages and Literatures.

Rowe, John Carlos. *At Emerson's Tomb: The Politics of Classic American Literature.* New York: Columbia UP, 1997. Print.

Rubery, Matthew. "A Transatlantic Sensation: Stanley's Search for Livingstone and the Anglo-American Press." *US Popular Print Culture 1860–1920.* Ed. Christine Bold. Vol. 6. Oxford: Oxford UP, 2012. 501–18. Print.

Rupp, Leila J. "Women's History in the New Millennium: A Retrospective Analysis of Barbara Welter's 'The Cult of True Womanhood, 1820–1860.'" *Journal of Women's History* 14.1 (2002): 149. Print.

Rush, Benjamin. *An Account of the Bilious Remitting Yellow Fever, as It Appeared in the City of Philadelphia, in the Year 1793.* Philadelphia: Thomas Dobson, 1794. Print.

—. "Facts Intended to Prove the Yellow Fever Not to Be Contagious, and Instances of Its Supposed Contagion Explained Upon Other Principles." *Medical Repository* 6.2 (1803): 155–71. Print.

Russell, Josh. *Yellow Jack.* New York: Norton, 1999. Print.

Ryan, Mary P. *Civic Wars: Democracy and Public Life in the American City During the Nineteenth Century.* Berkeley: U of California P, 1997. Print.

Sahagún, Fray Bernardino de. *We People Here: Nahuatl Accounts of the Conquest of Mexico.* Ed. James Lockhart. Berkeley: U of California P, 1993. Print. Repertorium Columbianum.

Said, Edward W. "Molestation and Authority in Narrative Fiction." *Aspects of Narrative: Selected Papers from the English Institute.* Ed. J. Hillis Miller. New York: Columbia UP, 1971. 38–60. Print.

Samuels, Shirley. *Reading the American Novel, 1780–1865.* Chichester: Wiley-Blackwell, 2012. Print. Reading the Novel.

—. *Romances of the Republic: Women, the Family, and Violence in the Literature of the Early American Nation.* New York: Oxford UP, 1996. Print.

—. ed. *The Culture of Sentiment: Race, Gender, and Sentimentality in Nineteenth-Century America*. New York: Oxford UP, 1992. Print.

—. "The Identity of Slavery." *The Culture of Sentiment: Race, Gender, and Sentimentality in Nineteenth-Century America*. Ed. Shirley Samuels. New York: Oxford UP, 1992. 157–90. Print.

Sánchez-Eppler, Karen. "The Intersecting Rhetorics of Feminism and Abolition." *The Culture of Sentiment: Race, Gender, and Sentimentality in Nineteenth-Century America*. Ed. Shirley Samuels. New York: Oxford UP, 1992. 92–114. Print.

Saulsbury, Rebecca. "Cult of True Womanhood." *The Literary Encyclopedia* 30 June 2002. Web. 23 Oct. 2011.

Schell, Heather. "The Sexist Gene: Science Fiction and the Germ Theory of History." *American Literary History* 14.4 (2002): 805–27.

Schultz, Jane E. "The Inhospitable Hospital: Gender and Professionalism in Civil War Medicine." *Signs* 17.2 (1992): 363–92. Print.

—. *Women at the Front: Hospital Workers in Civil War America*. Chapel Hill: U of North Carolina P, 2004. Print. Civil War America.

Schulz, Martin. *Ordnungen der Bilder*. München: Fink, 2005. Print.

Searson, John. *Mount Vernon: A Poem, Being the Seat of His Excellency George Washington, in the State of Virginia; Lieutenant-General and Commander in Chief of the Land Forces of the United States of America: This Rural, Romantic and Descriptive Poem of the Seat of so Great a Character, It Is Hoped May Please, with a Copper-Plate Likeness of the General. It Was Taken from an Actual View on the Spot by the Author, 15th May, 1799: Also a Cursory View of Georgetown, City of Washington, and the Capital*. Philadelphia: Printed for the author by Folwell, 1800. Print.

Sedgwick, Catharine Maria. *A New England Tale, and Miscellanies*. New York: G. P. Putnam & Co., 1852. Print.

—. *Redwood: A Tale*. Rev. ed. New York: George P. Putnam, 1850. Print.

Seitz, George B. *Yellow Jack*. 1938. Film.

Shah, Nayan. *Contagious Divides: Epidemics and Race in San Francisco's Chinatown*. Vol. 7. Berkeley: U of California P, 2001. Print. American Crossroads.

Sheehan, Tanya. *Doctored: The Medicine of Photography in Nineteenth-Century America*. University Park: Pennsylvania State UP, 2011. Print.

Silber, Nina. *The Romance of Reunion: Northerners and the South, 1865–1900*. Chapel Hill: U of North Carolina P, 1993. Print. Civil War America.

Silva, Cristobal. *Miraculous Plagues: An Epidemiology of Early New England Narrative*. Oxford: Oxford UP, 2011. Print.

Silverman, Kenneth. *The Life and Times of Cotton Mather*. 1st ed. New York: Harper & Row, 1984. Print.

Simmons, John Franklin. *The Welded Link, and Other Poems*. Philadelphia: J.B. Lippincott, 1881. Print.

Skaggs, Merrill. "The Louisianas of Katherine Anne Porter's Mind." *Louisiana Women Writers: New Essays and a Comprehensive Bibliography*. Ed. Dorothy H. Brown and Barbara C. Ewell. Baton Rouge: Louisiana State UP, 1992. 155–68.

Skårdal, Dorothy Burton. "Scandinavian-American Literature: A Frontier for Research." *Swedish Pioneer Historical Quarterly* 28.4 (1977): 237–51. Print.

Sleeper, John Sherburne. *Jack in the Forecastle, or, Incidents in the Early Life of Hawser Martingale*. Boston: Crosby, Nichols, Lee, 1860. Print.

Smith, Mark A. "Andrew Brown's 'Earnest Endeavor': The Federal Gazette's Role in Philadelphia's Yellow Fever Epidemic of 1793." *Pennsylvania Magazine of History & Biography* 120.4 (1996): 321–42. Print.

Smith-Rosenberg, Carroll. *Disorderly Conduct: Visions of Gender in Victorian America*. New York: Oxford UP, 1985. Print.

—. *This Violent Empire: The Birth of an American National Identity*. Chapel Hill: Published for the Omohundro Institute of Early American History and Culture by the U of North Carolina P, 2010. Print.

Snell, A. B. et al. *Report of the Committee on the Yellow Fever Epidemic of 1873 at Shreveport, Louisiana*. Shreveport, LA: Howard Association, 1874. Print.

Sontag, Susan. *Illness as Metaphor and AIDS and Its Metaphors*. London: Penguin, 2002. Print. Penguin Classics.

—. *On Photography*. New York: Farrar, 1977. Print.

—. *Regarding the Pain of Others*. New York: Farrar, 2003. Print.

Souvestre, Émile. "Mathieu Ropars." *Mathieu Ropars et Cetera*. Ed. William Young. New York: Putnam, 1868. 7–75. Print.

—. *The Isle of the Dead, or, The Keeper of the Lazaretto*. London: Burns & Lambert, 1863. Print.

Starr, Paul. *The Social Transformation of American Medicine*. New York: Basic Books, 1982. Print.

Statistics of Population, Tables I–VIII Inclusive. Washington: GPO, 1872. Print.

Steel, Galterus (Walter). *Dissertatio Medica Inauguralis de Febre Insularum Indae Occidentalis*. Edinburgh: Stevenson & Co., 1818. Print.

Stern, Julia A. *The Plight of Feeling: Sympathy and Dissent in the Early American Novel*. Chicago: U of Chicago P, 1997. Print.

Stowe, Harriet Beecher. *Uncle Tom's Cabin*. Ed. Mary R Reichardt and Joseph Pearce. San Francisco: Ignatius, 2009. Print. Ignatius Critical Editions.

Swagerty, William R., and Henry F. Dobyns. *Their Number Become Thinned: Native American Population Dynamics in Eastern North America*. Knoxville, TN: U of Tennessee P and Newberry Library Center for the History of the American Indian, 1983. Print. Native American Historic Demography Series.

Sweet, Nancy F. "Dissent and the Daughter in *A New England Tale* and *Hobomok*." *Legacy* 22.2 (2005): 107–25.

"Swine Flu Lessons from SARS, Mad Cow & Bird Flu of Past (GILD, BCRX, NVAX, GNBT, VICL, AVII, CRXL, RHHBY, GSK, SFD, EWW, MXF)." *24/7 Wall St.* Web. 7 Nov. 2011.

Tanrisal, Meldan, and Tanfer Emin Tunç, eds. *The Health of the Nation*. Vol. 6. Heidelberg: Winter, 2014. Print. European Views of the United States.

Tardy, Mary T. *The Living Female Writers of the South*. Philadelphia: Claxton, Remsen & Haffelfinger, 1872.

"The Open Corner." *Philadelphia Photographer* 23.265 (1886): 20. Print.

"The Plague-Stricken South." *Frank Leslie's Illustrated Newspaper* 29 Sept. 1888: 103. Print.

"The Yellow Fever Visitation: Terrible Scenes in New Orleans and Memphis." *Frank Leslie's Illustrated Newspaper* 28 Sept. 1878: 56–59. Print.

"The Yellow Fever: No Cases in Little Rock—Subscriptions for the Aid of Shreveport and Memphis—The Quarantine on the Railroads." *Daily Arkansas Gazette* 7 Oct. 1873: col. D. Print.

"The Yellow-Fever Ravages." *Frank Leslie's Illustrated Newspaper* 22 Sept. 1888: 82. Print.

Theriot, Nancy M. "Women's Voices in Nineteenth-Century Medical Discourse: A Step Toward Deconstructing Science." *Signs* 19 (1993): 1–31.

Thoene, Bodie. *Winds of Promise*. Nashville: Thomas Nelson, 1997. Print.

Thompson, Gary R. *Reading the American Novel 1865–1914*. Malden, MA: Wiley-Blackwell, 2012. Print.

Thompson, Shirley Elizabeth. *Exiles at Home: The Struggle to Become American in Creole New Orleans*. Cambridge, MA: Harvard UP, 2009. Print.

Thucydides. *The Peloponnesian War*. Trans. Steven Lattimore. Indianapolis: Hackett, 1998. Print.

"To George Washington from John Searson, 2 August 1797." *National Archives: Founders Online*. Web. 16 Sept. 2013.

Tocqueville, Alexis de. *Democracy in America*. Ed. Phillips Bradley. Trans. Henry Reeve. Vol. 1. 2 vols. New York: A.A. Knopf, 1945. Print.

Tompkins, Jane P. *Sensational Designs: The Cultural Work of American Fiction, 1790–1860*. New York: Oxford UP, 1985. Print.

Toth, Emily. *Kate Chopin*. New York: Morrow, 1990. Print.

Tregle, Jr., Joseph G. "Creoles and Americans." *Creole New Orleans: Race and Americanization*. Ed. Arnold R. Hirsch and Joseph Logsdon. Baton Rouge: Louisiana State UP, 1992. 131–86. Print.

Trotter, Thomas. *Medicina Nautica: An Essay on the Diseases of Seamen: Comprehending the History of Health in His Majesty's Fleet, Under the Command of Richard Earl Howe, Admiral*. London: T. Cadell and W. Davies, 1797. Print.

"Under the Shadow of the Plague." *Frank Leslie's Illustrated Newspaper* 6 Oct. 1888: 123. Print.

Van Hook, Bailey. *Angels of Art: Women and Art in American Society, 1876–1914*. University Park: Pennsylvania State UP, 1996. Print.

Vicinus, Martha. *Independent Women: Work and Community for Single Women, 1850–1920*. Chicago: U of Chicago P, 1985. Print. Women in Culture and Society.

"Visual Culture and Public Health Posters: Exhibit Introduction." *U.S. National Library of Medicine*. Exhibitions. 8 Sept. 2011. Web. 10 Apr. 2013.

Vogel, Virgil J. *American Indian Medicine*. Vol. 95. Norman: U of Oklahoma P, 1990. Print. The Civilization of the American Indian Series.

Wald, Priscilla. *Contagious: Cultures, Carriers, and the Outbreak Narrative*. Durham, NC: Duke UP, 2008. Print.

—. "Imagined Immunities." *Cultural Studies & Political Theory*. Ed. Jodi Dean. Ithaca, NY: Cornell UP, 2000. 189–208. Print.

—, Nancy Tomes, and Lisa Lynch. "Contagion and Culture." *American Literary History* 14.4 (2002): 617–24. Print.

Warburg, Aby. *Der Bilderatlas Mnemosyne. 1924–1929*. Ed. Martin Warnke. Berlin: Akademie Verlag, 2001. Print.

Waring, William. *Yellow Fever: The Slave's Revenge*. Chapel Hill, NC: Professional Press, 1994. Print.

Waterman, Bryan. "Arthur Mervyn's Medical Repository and the Early Republic's Knowledge Industries." *American Literary History* 15.2 (2003): 213–47. Print.

—. *Republic of Intellect: The Friendly Club of New York City and the Making of American Literature*. Baltimore, MD: Johns Hopkins UP, 2007. Print. New Studies in American Intellectual and Cultural History.

Watts, Sheldon. "Yellow Fever Immunities in West Africa and the Americas in the Age of Slavery and Beyond: A Reappraisal." *Journal of Social History* 34.4 (2001): 955–67. Print.

Webster, Noah. *A Brief History of Epidemic and Pestilential Diseases with the Principal Phenomena of the Physical World, Which Precede and Accompany Them, and Observations Deduced from the Facts Stated in Two Volumes.* Hartford, CT: Hudson & Goodwin, 1799. Early American Imprints. 1st Ser. No. 36687.

—. *A Collection of Papers on the Subject of Bilious Fevers, Prevalent in the United-States for a Few Years Past.* New York: Hopkins, Webb, 1796. Print.

Wegener, Frederick. "'Few Things More Womanly Or More Noble': Elizabeth Stuart Phelps and the Advent of the Woman Doctor in America." *Legacy* 22.1 (2005): 1–17. Print.

Wells, Ida B. *Crusade for Justice: The Autobiography of Ida B. Wells.* Ed. Alfreda M. Duster. Chicago: U of Chicago P, 1970. Print.

—. *The Memphis Diary of Ida B. Wells.* Ed. Miriam DeCosta-Willis. Boston: Beacon, 1995. Print.

"Western Migration and Homesteading." *The African-American Mosaic (Library of Congress Exhibition).* 23 July 2010. Web. 20 Sept. 2013.

White, Barbara Anne, and Lucy M. Freibert, eds. *Hidden Hands: An Anthology of American Women Writers, 1790–1870.* New Brunswick, NJ: Rutgers UP, 1985. Print. Douglass Series on Women's Lives and the Meaning of Gender.

White, Morton Gabriel, and Lucia White. *The Intellectual versus the City, from Thomas Jefferson to Frank Lloyd Wright.* Cambridge, MA: Harvard UP, 1962. Print. Publications of the Joint Center for Urban Studies.

"WHO: Summary of Probable SARS Cases with Onset of Illness from 1 November 2002 to 31 July 2003." *WHO.* Web. 1 Aug. 2013.

Wideman, John Edgar. "Fever." *The Stories of John Edgar Wideman.* New York: Pantheon, 1992. 239–66. Print.

—. *The Cattle Killing.* Boston: Houghton Mifflin, 1996. Print.

Wilford, John Noble. "Genetic Study Bolsters Columbus Link to Syphilis." *The New York Times* 15 Jan. 2008. *NYTimes.com.* Web. 31 July 2013.

Wills, Christopher. *Yellow Fever, Black Goddess: The Coevolution of People and Plagues.* Reading, MA: Addison-Wesley, 1996. Print.

Winslow, Edward, *Good Newes from New-England: Or, A True Telation of Things Very Remarkable at the Plantation of Plimouth in New England. Shewing the Wondrous Providence and Goodnes of God, in their Preservation and Continuance, being Delivered from many Apparant Deaths and Dangers. Together with a Relation of such Religious, and Civill Lawes and Customes, as Are in Practise amongst the Indians, Adjoyning to Them at this Day. As also What Commodities Are There to Be Raysed for the Maintenance of That and Other Plantations in the Said Country.* London: W. Bladen and J. Bellamie, 1624. Print.

Winthrop, John. "Generall Considerations for the Plantation in New England, with an Answer to Severall Objections (1629)." *The Winthrop Papers*. Ed. Stewart Mitchell. Vol. 2. Boston: Massachusetts Historical Society, 1931. Print.

Wisecup, Kelly. *Medical Encounters: Knowledge and Identity in Early American Literatures*. Amherst: U of Massachusetts P, 2013. Print.

Woodworth, John Maynard. *Proceedings of the Board of Experts Authorized by Congress, to Investigate the Yellow Fever Epidemic of 1878: Meeting Held in Memphis, Tenn., December 26th, 27th, 28th, 1878*. New Orleans: L. Graham, 1878. Print.

Workman, M. "Medical Practice in Philadelphia at the Time of the Yellow Fever Epidemic, 1793." *Pennsylvania Folklife* 27.4 (1978): 33–39. Print.

Wright, F. M. "Annie Cook: The Mary Magdalene of Memphis." *West Tennessee Historical Society Papers* 43 (1989): 44–54. Print.

—. "The 1878 Yellow Fever Epidemic in Memphis." *Journal of the Mississippi State Medical Association* 42.1 (2001): 9–13. Print.

"Yellow Fever at Shreveport." *Daily Evening Bulletin* 30 Sept. 1873: col. D. Print.

"Yellow Fever in Florida." *Frank Leslie's Illustrated Newspaper* 25 Aug. 1888: 27. Print.

"Yellow Fever Kills Two-Thirds of the Wampanoag." *U.S. National Library of Medicine: Native Voices—Native Voices Native Peoples' Concepts of Health and Illness*. 31 July 2013. Web. 31 July 2013.

"Yellow Fever: The Plague at Memphis and Shreveport—Relief Contributions." *Milwaukee Daily Sentinel* 25 Oct. 1873: col. D. Print.

Young, Elizabeth. *Disarming the Nation: Women's Writing and the American Civil War*. Chicago: U of Chicago P, 1999. Print. Women in Culture and Society.

Zelizer, Barbie. *About to Die: how News Images Move the Public*. New York: Oxford UP, 2010. Print.

Zwierlein, Anne-Julia, and Iris M. Heid, eds. *Gender and Disease in Literary and Medical Cultures*. Heidelberg: Winter, 2014. Print.

9 Index

Regensburger Arbeiten zur Anglistik und Amerikanistik
Regensburg Studies in British and American Languages and Cultures

Band 1 Karl Heinz Göller: Romance und Novel. Die Anfänge des englischen Romans. Unter Mitarbeit von Manfred Markus und Rainer Schöwerling. 1972.

Band 2 Eberhard Griem: Form und Funktion der Englischen Geburtstagsdichtung im Klassizismus. 1971.

Band 3 Manfred Markus: Moderne Erzählperspektive in den Werken des Gawain-Autors. 1971.

Band 4 Thomas Ross: A Book of Elizabethan Magic. Thomas Hill's Natural and Artificial Conclusions. 1974.

Band 5 Alfred Becker: Franks Casket. Zu den Bildern und Inschriften des Runenkästchens von Auzon. 1973.

Band 6 Kurt-Michael Pätzold: Historischer Roman und Realismus. Das Erzählwerk Thomas Deloneys. 1972.

Band 7 Evelyn B. Jolles: G. A. Bürgers Ballade Lenore in England. 1974.

Band 8 Anton Bauer: Das melanesische und chinesische Pidginenglisch. Linguistische Kriterien und Probleme. 1974.

Band 9 Philip A. Luelsdorff (Ed.): Linguistic Perspectives on Black English. 1975.

Band 10 Ludwig Rothmayer: Der Mensch und das Schicksal in den Romanen Herman Melvilles. 1977.

Band 11 Hans-Martin Braun: Prototypen der amerikanischen Kriminalerzählung: Die Romane und Kurzgeschichten Carroll John Dalys und Dashiell Hammetts. 1977.

Band 12 Günter Tschöpl: Zur Identitätsthematik bei Robert Penn Warren: Die Ermittlung des Ich in *All the King's Men*. 1978.

Band 13 Henning Thies: Namen im Kontext von Dramen. Studien zur Funktion von Personennamen im englischen, amerikanischen und deutschen Drama. 1978.

Band 14 Wolfgang Riedel: Die Arbeit der Dichter. Vergleichende Studien zur dichterischen Subjektivität in der englischen Romantik und Moderne. 1979.

Band 15 Jochen Achilles: Drama als problematische Form. Der Wandel zu nichtrealistischer Gestaltungsweise im Werk Sean O'Caseys. 1979.

Band 16 Renate Haas: Die mittelenglische Totenklage, Realitätsbezug, abendländische Tradition und individuelle Gestaltung. 1980.

Band 17 Jean Ritzke-Rutherford: Light and Darkness in Anglo-Saxon Thought and Writing. 1979.

Band 18 Rainer Schöwerling: Chapbooks. Zur Literaturgeschichte des einfachen Lesers. Englische Konsumliteratur 1680-1840. 1980.

Band 19 Anke Janssen: Francis Godwins *The Man in the Moone*. Die Entdeckung des Romans als Medium der Auseinandersetzung mit Zeitproblemen. 1981.

Band 20 Michael Thomas: Studien zur Short Story als fiktional-narrative Textform und die Möglichkeiten einer Typenbildung. 1982.

Band 21 Werner Huber: James Stephen's frühe Romane. Rezeption - Text - Intention. 1982.

Band 22 Claus Gadau: How to write a Short Story. Zum historischen Wandel der Kurzgeschichtentheorie in amerikanischen Leitfäden zum Verfassen kurzer Prosaerzählungen. 1984.

Band 23 Reinhard Gleißner: Die 'zweideutigen' altenglischen Rätsel des *Exeter Book* in ihrem zeitgenössischen Kontext. 1984.

Band 24 Peter Lenz: Klerus, Gesellschaft, Literatur. Die moderne irische Erzählprosa zwischen innerem und äußerem Exil. 1985.

Band 25 Johann Aßbeck: Why are my Country-Men such Foes to Verse? Untersuchungen zur schottischen Dichtung des frühen 18. Jahrhunderts in ihrem Verhältnis zum englischen Klassizismus. 1986.

Band 26 Michael Baumann: Milton's Arianism. 1987.

Band 27 Thekla Zachrau: Mythos und Phantastik: Funktion und Struktur der Cthulhu-Mythologie in den phantastischen Erzählungen H.P. Lovecrafts. 1986.

Band 28 Manfred Pütz: Ralph Waldo Emerson: A Bibliography of Twenthieth-Century Criticism. With the assistance of J.K. Adams and J. Böck. 1986.

Band 29 Marion Soceanu: Das Federal Theatre Project und seine Dramen über amerikanische Geschichte. 1987.

Band 30 Wilhelm Bomke: Die Teufelsfiguren der mittelenglischen Dramen. 1990.

Band 31 Richard J. Utz: Literarischer Nominalismus im Spätmittelalter. Eine Untersuchung zu Sprache, Charakterzeichnung und Struktur in Geoffrey Chaucers *Troilus and Criseyde*. 1990.

Band 32 Markus Preußner: Poe und Baudelaire: Ein Vergleich. 1991.

Band 33 Ulrike Dirscherl: Ritterliche Ideale in Chrétiens *Yvain* und im mittelenglischen *Ywain and Gawain*. Von "amour courtois" zu "trew luf", vom "frans chevaliers deboneire" zum "man of mekyl myght". 1991.

Band 34 Paul Neubauer: Die Rezeption der US-amerikanischen Literatur der Postmoderne im deutschsprachigen Raum. 1991.

Band 35 Franz Meier: Die frühe Ding-Lyrik William Carlos Williams'. Genese und Poetologie. 1991.

Band 36 Christoph Houswitschka: Politik und Liebe in der Literatur des englischen Spätmittelalters am Beispiel von Thomas Malorys *Morte Darthur*. 1991.

Band 37 Klaus-Dieter Groß: Zwischen Romantik, Naturalismus und Moderne. Strömungen des Realismus in amerikanischen Romanen und Gemälden der Zeit zwischen 1920 und 1940. 1992.

Band 38 Paul Neubauer: Die Diskussion der US-amerikanischen Erzählliteratur der Postmoderne in der deutschsprachigen Amerikanistik. 1994.

Band 39 Helge Nowak: "Completeness is all". Fortsetzungen und andere Weiterführungen britischer Romane als Beispiel zeitübergreifender und interkultureller Rezeption. 1994.

Band 40 Vera Hölzl: His Motto is Service. Die Herr-Diener-Problematik in der englischen Literatur seit dem 18. Jahrhundert. 1999.

Band 41 Rainer A. Wirth: Welt / Spiegel / Buch: Theorie der Fiktionalität und James Joyces Prosa. 2000.

Band 42 Eva Hofmann: Decadence Revisited: F. Scott Fitzgerald und das europäische Fin de siècle. 2000.

Band 43 Karsten Fitz: Negotiating History and Culture. Transculturation in Contemporary Native American Fiction. 2001.

Band 44 Elmar Singer: Moving Beyond Nativism. Eine Betrachtung des irischen Gegenwartsromans aus dem Blickwinkel postkolonialer Theorien. 2002.

Band 45 Christin Galster: Hybrides Erzählen und hybride Identität im britischen Roman der Gegenwart. 2002.

Band 46 Lucia Krämer: Oscar Wilde in Roman, Drama und Film. Eine medienkomparatistische Analyse fiktionaler Biographien. 2003.

Band 47 Ulrich Miethaner: *I can look through muddy water*. Analyzing Earlier African American English in Blues Lyrics (BLUR). 2005.

Band 48 Susanne Auflitsch: Staging Separate Spheres. Theatrical Spaces as Sites of Antagonism in One-Act Plays by American Women, 1910–1930. Including Bibliographies on One-Act Plays in the United States, 1900–1940. 2006.

Band 49 Ursula Baumann: Sklavenhalter wider Willen und ein Krieg zwischen *Cause* und Chaos. Amerikanische Bürgerkriegsromane am Ende des 20. Jahrhunderts. 2009.

Band 50 Susanne Ehrenreich-Blažeković: Intermedial Representations of 9/11 in U.S. American and German Newspapers. 2010.

Band 51 Zeno Ackermann: Messing with Romance. American Poetics and Antebellum Southern Fiction. 2012.

Band 52 Ingrid Gessner: Yellow Fever Years. An Epidemiology of Nineteenth-Century American Literature and Culture. 2016.

www.peterlang.com

www.ingramcontent.com/pod-product-compliance
Ingram Content Group UK Ltd.
Pitfield, Milton Keynes, MK11 3LW, UK
UKHW020032121026
15625UKWH00043B/325

9 783631 674123